TROUBLESOME
DISGUISES

Troublesome Disguises

UNDERDIAGNOSED PSYCHIATRIC SYNDROMES

EDITED BY

DINESH BHUGRA

MA, MSc, MPhil, MB BS, FRCPsych
Senior Lecturer in Psychiatry
Institute of Psychiatry
London

AND

ALISTAIR MUNRO

MD, FRCPE, FRCPsych, FRCPC
Professor of Psychiatry
Dalhousie University
Canada

b

**Blackwell
Science**

© 1997 by
Blackwell Science Ltd
Editorial Offices:
Osney Mead, Oxford OX2 OEL
25 John Street, London WC1N 2BL
23 Ainslie Place, Edinburgh EH3 6AJ
350 Main Street, Malden
  MA 02148 5018, USA
54 University Street, Carlton
  Victoria 3053, Australia

Other Editorial Offices:
Blackwell Wissenschafts-Verlag GmbH
Kurfürstendamm 57
10707 Berlin, Germany

Blackwell Science KK
MG Kodenmacho Building
7–10 Kodenmacho Nihombashi
Chuo-ku, Tokyo 104, Japan

First published 1997

Set by Excel Typesetter Co., Hong Kong
Printed and bound in Great Britain
by Hartnolls Ltd, Bodmin, Cornwall

The Blackwell Science logo is a
trade mark of Blackwell Science Ltd,
registered at the United Kingdom
Trade Marks Registry

DISTRIBUTORS

Marston Book Services Ltd
PO Box 269
Abingdon, Oxon OX14 4YN
(*Orders*: Tel: 01235 465500
            Fax: 01235 465555)

USA
Blackwell Science, Inc.
Commerce Place, 350 Main Street
Malden, MA 02148 5018
(*Orders*: Tel: 800 759 6102
                 617 388 8250
           Fax: 617 388 8255)

Canada
Copp Clark Professional
200 Adelaide St West, 3rd Floor
Toronto, Ontario M5H 1W7
(*Orders*: Tel: 416 597-1616
                 800 815-9417
           Fax: 416 597-1617)

Australia
Blackwell Science Pty Ltd
54 University Street
Carlton, Victoria 3053
(*Orders*: Tel: 3 9347 0300
           Fax: 3 9347 5001)

A catalogue record for this title
is available from the British Library

ISBN 0-86542-674-0

Library of Congress
Cataloging-in-publication Data

Troublesome disguises/edited by
  Dinesh Bhugra and Alistair Munro.
      p.   cm.
    Includes bibliographical references
  and index.
    ISBN 0-86542-674-0
    1. Mental illness—Diagnosis.
  2. Diagnosis, Differential.
  I. Bhugra, Dinesh.   II. Munro, Alistair.
    [DNLM: 1. Mental Disorders—
  diagnosis.
  WM 141 T859 1997]
  RC469.T77   1997
  616.89'075–dc21
  DNLM/DLC
  for Library of Congress   97-4247
                                                 CIP

Contents

vi | *Contents*

List of Contributors

David S. Baldwin MRCPsych, Senior Lecturer in Psychiatry, Faculty of Medicine, Health and Biological Sciences, University of Southampton, Southampton SO14 OYG, UK

Dinesh Bhugra MA, MSc, MPhil, MB BS, FRCPsych, Senior Lecturer in Psychiatry, Institute of Psychiatry, De Crespigny Park, Denmark Hill, London SE5 8AF, UK

Ian W. Coffey MRCPsych, MB, BCh, BAO, DCh, NUI, St John's Hospital, Howden Road West, Livingston, West Lothian EH54 6PP, UK

Michael J. Crowe DM, FRCP, FRCPsych, Consultant Psychiatrist, Maudsley Hospital, Denmark Hill, London SE5 8AZ, UK

Padmal de Silva CPsychol, FBPsS, Senior Lecturer in Psychology, Institute of Psychiatry, De Crespigny Park, Denmark Hill, London SE5 8AF, UK

Hadyn D. Ellis PhD, DSc, FBPsS, Professor of Psychology and Pro Vice-Chancellor, School of Psychology, University of Wales, PO Box 901, Cardiff CF1 3YG, UK

Thomas A. Hughes MRCPsych, Lecturer in Psychiatry, Division of Psychiatry and Behavioural Sciences in Relation to Medicine, University of Leeds, Clinical Sciences Building, St James's University Hospital, Leeds LS9 7TF, UK

K.S. Jacob MD, Wellcome Overseas Fellow, Institute of Psychiatry, De Crespigny Park, Denmark Hill, London SE5 8AF, UK

Eve C. Johnstone MD, FRCP, FRCPsych, Professor of Psychiatry, Department of Psychiatry, The University of Edinburgh, Kennedy Tower, Royal Edinburgh Hospital, Morningside Park, Edinburgh EH10 5HF, UK

Paul E. Mullen MB BS, DSc, MPhil (PsychMed), FRANZCP, FRCPsych, Professor of Forensic Psychiatry, Monash University, and Director of Victorian Forensic Psychiatry Services, PO Box 266, Rosanna, Victoria 3084, Australia

Alistair Munro MD, FRCPE, FRCPsych, FRCPC, Professor of Psychiatry, Dalhousie University, Halifax, Nova Scotia, Canada

Brice Pitt MD, MB BS, FRCPsych, Director of the Memory Clinic, Royal Postgraduate Medical School, London w12, UK

Andrew C.P. Sims MA, MD, FRCPsych, FRCPEd, Professor of Psychiatry, Division of Psychiatry and Behavioural Sciences in Relation to Medicine, University of Leeds, Clinical Sciences Building, St James's University Hospital, Leeds ls9 7tf, UK

Julia M.A. Sinclair BSc, MB BS, Clinical Research Fellow, Mental Health Group, Faculty of Medicine, Health and Biological Sciences, University of Southampton, Southampton so14 0yg, UK

Michael R. Trimble MD, FRCP, FRCPsych, Professor in Behavioural Neurology and Consultant Physician in Psychological Medicine, Institute of Neurology, The National Hospital for Neurology and Neurosurgery, Queen Square, London wc1n 3bg, UK

Gabor S. Ungvari MD, PhD, FRANZCP, FHKCPsych, Associate Professor, Department of Psychiatry, Faculty of Medicine, The Chinese University of Hong Kong, Prince of Wales Hospital, Shatin, NT, Hong Kong

Preface

Several psychiatric disorders remain underdiagnosed in clinical practice. The first reason is that their presentations remain atypical and are often difficult to diagnose. Secondly, they are genuinely rare and their rarity makes the diagnosis and clinical management a problem. This volume aims to bridge this gap and make clinicians aware of the rare and not-so-rare conditions in psychiatry. Both the theoretical and the practical aspects of conditions that clinicians are likely to encounter are brought together. The diagnosis of the distress and symptoms and their management remain a joint endeavour between the patients and their clinicians. With increasing availability of powerful pharmaceutical agents which are becoming more sophisticated and more specifically targeted it is essential that diagnosis is accurate.

The collection of disorders described by the eminent authors in this volume are not rare curiosities: they are relatively common conditions which, with familiarity, can and should be recognized by any competent psychiatrist. We urge our readers to regard this book as an exercise in consciousness-raising as well as a warning to beware of diagnostic systems which, despite their many virtues, may become too influential and may perpetuate errors which are to the detriment of our patients. At present, these errors are as much of omission as of commission. It is our earnest hope that our efforts may go some way to highlighting and counteracting these omissions.

We have been fortunate indeed in getting our contributors together who have brought their expertise, skill and good humour to this volume. Our thanks to them.

Our deep appreciation is due to the staff at Blackwell Science, especially Stuart Taylor for keeping the faith, Katrina McCallum for putting in hard work beyond the call of duty, and Victoria Oddie for her support.

Dinesh Bhugra
Alistair Munro

CHAPTER I

Introduction

DINESH BHUGRA AND
ALISTAIR MUNRO

When a patient feels unwell and visits a doctor, he or she makes a complaint whose expression may be influenced by a variety of factors including verbal fluency, intelligence, knowledge of illness, confidence in the physician, and many others. It is one's task as a doctor to formulate the complaint in medical terms, make a diagnosis when an illness is present, institute the clinical management of the case, and estimate a prognosis. If possible, the underlying pathology of the illness should also be sought out. This process should involve informing and, if necessary, educating the patient and his or her relatives about the illness, and the formulation of the case should make communication of the facts to other physicians relatively straightforward. At a systems level, the process should also encourage the development of efficient treatment services.

Different branches of medicine have reached varying degrees of sophistication in making diagnoses and recognizing the accompanying pathology. Although important strides are beginning to be made in psychiatry, it has to be admitted that psychiatric diagnosis remains a disputatious topic.

Problems in reaching a diagnosis

We do not have to remind the reader about the difficulties in defining mental ill-health or in reaching a psychiatric diagnosis which has both validity and reliability. The many conceptualizations of mental illness present a bewildering array of theories but very few facts. In order to begin to understand the complexity of the subject, we try to construct paradigms which will give some cohesion to the subject. Unfortunately, when it is all theory and no fact, a given paradigm cannot be proved or disproved, but paradigms have a well-known tendency to multiply. As a result we have countless models of mental illness.

Then, we have to communicate with patients and colleagues and so we utilize metaphors which we hope represent state-of-the-art information: but remember, these are metaphors which are, at best, approximations to the truth. Unhappily, we often forget how lacking in substance our paradigms and metaphors are, and employ them as though they were scientifically proven data.

Quot homines, tot sententiae, so we have an enormous variety of interpretations of mental illness and its causative factors. As Clare (1980) noted, this bewildering array often leads the clinician and the layman in completely different directions. This can lead to acrimonious debate about whether psychiatric diagnosis has any inherent legitimacy and to attempts to replace the concept of mental illness with terms such as social disturbance, maladaptation, problems of living or community disorder. In the same vein, patients become users, consumers, clients or punters, and their problems are handled as variously as their designations.

In the field of cross-cultural psychiatry, Eisenberg (1977) and Kleinman (1980) made a distinction between disease and illness. Disease (or dis-ease) is a physiopathological change which may or may not be symptomatic, and it turns into illness when others around the individual are involved. Society or culture tends to define the norm in health matters so we find that the illness process and abnormal behaviours related to illness are very much dictated by society. However, the diagnosis of illness and its subsequent management have retained their value despite so much controversy and remain very much the province of the medical profession. We as physicians are committed to discovering the illness, identifying its pathology and returning the patient to good health: patients may be at the receiving end but obviously they have a profound interest in the process and are increasingly demanding in a participatory role. The diagnostic process is a highly interactive one and involves both participants negotiating towards a mutually acceptable understanding and course of action.

Nowadays in psychiatry we have increasingly precise guidelines for clinical diagnosis as well as operational criteria for research diagnoses, yet as already noted, we still have far to go. In 1980, Clare was concerned that the perception of disease as physiological phenomena under altered physiological conditions (essentially a 19th-century concept) had been over-influential in psychiatric diagnosis, tempting many psychiatrists to relate mental phenomena to an almost entirely physical basis. Just over a decade-and-a-half ago his concern was well founded because the study of cerebral anatomy, physiology, biochemistry and pathology had produced meagre results in psychiatry, but since then there has been an explosion of knowledge produced by modern investigative techniques and the conclusion seems inescapable: mind is, indeed, a product of brain.

In our field, the false dichotomy between somatic and psychic phenomena is coming to be seen as increasingly untenable. Real physical phenomena can result from psychological disturbances but when patients with psychiatric disorders have made predominantly physical complaints there has been a tendency to disparage the patients and their symptoms as being psychologically unsophisticated. There have been many speculations in this area and, for example, Leff (1988) argued that hysteria was the somatizing equivalent of schizophrenia. We would propose that psyche and soma are indivisible, that psychiatric illness can give rise to both physical symptoms and physical complaints in highly intelligent patients and, even if the brain be but the mediator of mental disorder, it too is both psyche and soma in itself.

When a patient becomes unwell or his or her relatives notice he or she is unwell, the first steps to deal with this are usually in the personal and folk realms and it is only when the problem comes to be seen as one of illness (often when simple remedies have not afforded cure) that professional, i.e. medical, help is sought. The actual route into health-care is very largely determined by patients and their families and this means that our patients come to us at varying stages of their disorders.

Clinical diagnosis can depend a great deal on the particular stage at which the disease is seen. In acute illnesses with well-defined pathologies and objectively determinable abnormalities, a cross-sectional diagnosis may be appropriate, based on observations made at one point in time. In psychiatric illnesses, the time-line and the course of the disorder over a prolonged period may be very important elements in diagnosis—for example, in distinguishing the deteriorative course of schizophrenia from the relapsing course of major mood disorder.

In psychiatry we have few 'hard' physical signs to aid us but we can readily observe phenomena such as alteration of movement, depressive appearance, tics and grimaces, mannerisms and so on. Other highly important phenomena such as delusions or hallucinations can only be inferred by the patient's description of them and the skilled observer's interpretation of these descriptions. We must also be aware of the influence on clinical appearances of factors such as premorbid personality, past experiences, biological influences and a variety of social influences such as employment status, poverty, the presence or lack of social support and others.

In the 19th and early 20th centuries there were virtually no psychiatric treatments and psychiatrists had all the time in the world to observe their patients and make their diagnoses at leisure. Nowadays we have treatments and cannot ethically withhold them, so we have to make our diagnoses much more rapidly, often on cases presenting at an earlier stage of the illness than used to be the case. We hope that our assessments are more accurate and more scientific than they used to be, but there are many barriers in our way, as we have noted.

Models of mental illness

The clinician's diagnostic perspective relies heavily on his or her preferred model of mental disorder and Tyrer and Steinberg (1993) have described four broad categories of approach—the disease model, the psychodynamic, the behavioural, and the social.

The disease model is regaining favour in psychiatry but often remains overmechanistic if applied too rigidly. The psychodynamic model is useful in conceptualizing illness as a consequence of maladaptive developments in psychic structure throughout life, but is high in theory and very low in demonstrable proof. The behavioural approach focuses on symptoms and the appropriate treatment for them without enquiring closely into their aetiology. The social model proposes that mental disorders can only be understood within the context of society at large and its processes and maladies.

Of course, each theory has its counterpart approach to treatment. Medicine seeks a specific, usually physical, treatment for each disorder whereas the psychodynamic school proposes a psychotherapeutic approach to encourage personal development and more effective adaptations. Behavioural and cognitive treatments aim to change symptoms in the here-and-now and to maintain improvement in the future with little concern to alter the effects of the past. The sociotherapeutic aim is to change the impact of perceived adverse societal factors. In fact, the most sophisticated diagnostic and treatment processes will tend to incorporate elements from all of these theoretical sectors, in varying proportions according to the individual case.

In recent years we have become used to the so-called multiaxial approach to psychiatric diagnosis in which we differentiate between discrete illnesses, background personality factors, medical illness, social circumstances and overall health performance. (Some critics decry the lack of a psychodynamic axis in our official classifications which would, as we have said, focus on developmental/aetiological influences.) The use of these axes emphasizes the need to define a specific Axis I illness in a particular individual in order to apply the most effective immediate treatment, but recognizes that there is a simultaneous requirement to deal with significant factors on the other axes. Failure to take these additional elements into account may well lead to a less-than-accurate diagnosis and poorly effective treatment.

In 1980, DSM-III appeared (the third edition of the *Diagnostic and Statistical Manual of Mental Disorders*, produced by the American Psychiatric Association) and this was very quickly seen to be a highly significant step forward in the area of psychiatric diagnosis. First, it introduced the multi-axial diagnostic system and, secondly, it eschewed speculation on aetiology, insisting on a straightforward description of the illness and its course. Also, it provided definitions of terms and it returned, in many ways, to the traditional medical model of psychiatric illness. DSM-III and its successors, DSM-III-R and DSM-IV, have been enormously influential and the other great diagnostic system, the *International Classification of Disease* (ICD), issued by the World Health Organization, has largely fallen in line. The language of psychiatry, the conceptualization of psychiatric illness and the diagnostic approach have all rapidly become much more international and more uniform. In addition, there has been an increasing demand for knowledge based on experiment rather than on tradition, which has meant quite radical changes in some diagnostic areas.

We pay a price for this massive overhaul in our diagnostic habits. DSM is an instrument with a decidedly American outlook and this sometimes means that valid viewpoints from other parts of the world are ignored. Also, there is a tendency to see a diagnostic manual as an infallible guide and to reduce diagnosis to a series of steps determined by numbers of items contained within defined categories in that manual. Patients often fail to oblige and so the manual has to have increasingly large 'residual' categories for the atypical cases which do not fit the official criteria.

In medicine in general and in psychiatry in particular, it is a not uncommon experience to discover that cases which are 'atypical' of some illness category are, in fact, typical of some other illness category. At present many psychiatric illnesses are probably heterogeneous in their basic pathology even if their clinical appearances suggest an affinity: for example, we increasingly suspect that schizophrenia is actually a complicated group of disorders whose symptoms pass through a final common pathway.

This book has taken the rather iconoclastic approach that ICD-10 and DSM-IV are not the founts of all wisdom in psychiatry and that they overlook certain groups of illnesses which have a valid existence and which are in danger of becoming obscure because they are not officially recognized. We also believe that certain other diagnoses which are more widely accepted are nevertheless underused because the cases are not sought out vigorously enough.

References

Clare, A. (1980) *Psychiatry in Dissent*. Tavistock, London.

Eisenberg, L. (1977) Disease and illness: distinctions between professional and popular ideas of sickness. *Culture, Medicine and Psychiatry* 1, 9–23.

Kleinman, A. (1980) *Patients and their Healers in the Context of Culture*. University of California, Berkeley, Calif.

Leff, J. (1988) *Psychiatry across the Globe*. Gaskell, London.

Tyrer, P. & Steinberg, D. (1993) *Models for Mental Disorders*. John Wiley, Chichester.

CHAPTER 2

Misidentification Syndromes

HADYN D. ELLIS

Humans have a quite amazing ability rapidly to discriminate one face from another to classify them in various ways (e.g. race, gender), to recognize whether it is familiar or not and, if known, to identify exactly whose it is: skills that no computer system has yet matched. Not only can we process faces to extract information about people's age, gender, race and familiarity, but we also possess a quite remarkable capacity accurately to infer from faces details of health, mood, and intention; in addition, we can make a host of other readings solely from others' faces, some but not all of which may be accurate (Ellis 1981).

Given also that we evince a measurable interest in faces from the moment of birth (Goren *et al.* 1975; Johnson *et al.* 1992), it seems reasonable to conclude that faces are extremely important sociobiological objects and that there are strong reasons for our facility in face processing. Presumably, the capacity to make rapid judgements about others, largely based upon physiognomic information concerning their identity and intentions towards us, has evolved as a result of the usual evolutionary pressures. As a species we have survived partly because of our ability to know friend from foe, kin from stranger, high status individual from low status person and the healthy from the diseased.

Although most of us share these skills, for some people they are not so evident; and for a small group the abilities become corrupted in interestingly systematic ways.

Delusional misidentification syndromes: cases

Before turning to a generic theoretical model that aims both to describe and to explain the mental processes underlying the way we look at faces, I shall illustrate a selection of face-processing disorders that are often, but not exclusively, associated with psychiatric illness. These are collectively known as the delusional misidentification syndromes (DMIs). In each case the cardinal symptoms include distortion errors in the perception of others. The DMIs have been extensively reviewed elsewhere (see Christodoulou 1988; Ellis *et al.* 1994a). Before adumbrating the historical background and nosological implications of the individual DMIs, I shall illustrate them with case histories of patients that my colleagues and I have examined over the last 10 years. Each reveals symptoms that are bizarre, that sometimes comprise their sole psychiatric problems; but above all the beliefs expressed are paradigmatic and classic. It is the attempt to provide a theoretical explanation for them that primarily motivates me and my colleagues.

Case No. 2.1

When first examined by me, KP was a 43-year-old man with a 25-year history of alcohol abuse and schizophrenia. During his ill periods, he spends much of his time looking into mirrors, where, after a while, one of two things can happen to his own image: his face may seem to disappear, leaving no gap in the reflection of the room, or his face may become progressively more distorted until it looks quite terrifying. Sometimes when KP looks at others their faces, too, may seem to change into grotesque masks. He is able to describe these experiences in a calm and articulate fashion, showing some insight but no ability to control these disturbing episodes.

Case No. 2.2

YD was a 37-year-old man, with a long history of paranoid schizophrenia. Among his many symptoms was his occasional violence towards his family, provoked by perceived changes in their faces. He attacked his mother once, for example, because, as she was putting on her spectacles, she suddenly seemed to be a neighbour whom YD disliked. A similar incident caused him to attack his father. YD's behaviour occurred within more general schizophrenic symptoms that, at times, included delusions both about his own identity and concerning his artistic abilities.

(Similar cases observed include DL who attacked a shopkeeper when his face took on the appearance of a famous snooker player; and NT who developed the delusion that all women looked either exactly like his girlfriend or her mother.)

Case No. 2.3

BC, a 66-year-old woman with a history of psychiatric illness, experienced transient ischaemic attacks, followed by a right-sided temporoparietal infarct. She developed the delusion that the father of her now adult illegitimate daughter was disguising himself in order to persecute her. The former lover and his current partner appeared in the guise of all sorts of people, but BC was always able to discern their presence and confront them or call the police. She never revealed any insight into her delusion: drugs therapy enabled her to cope but did not appear to diminish her belief in the veracity of her experiences.

Case No. 2.4

AP was a 43-year-old woman with a 6-year history of paranoid and somatic delusions. She asserted that her son, as well as other members of her family and neighbours, had been replaced by doubles. She also thought that her psychiatrist had been substituted by another doctor, who resembled him closely. These symptoms eventually disappeared but it was not clear whether AP was ever disabused of her beliefs.

Delusions

The systematic study of delusional belief systems, such as those just described, provides us, perhaps, with a unique opportunity to discover the genesis of personal ideas. By scientific examination of patients with specific delusions we may discover the ways in which not only bizarre notions develop and are sustained but also how everyday beliefs arise and are maintained or abandoned. Delusions, whether arising in a functional or an organic setting, are disorders in high-level cognition that, by definition, are specific to humans. Psychologists have long researched most aspects of thinking and problem solving; but, by comparison, they have neglected to address the very nature of belief.

Cognitive neuropsychiatry

I should like to propose that the only realistic way we can hope to understand how delusions occur is by the detailed and principled analysis of patients' cognitive integrity. Formerly it was customary for theorists to speculate wildly on what caused delusions without the discipline of testing their ideas in any empirical fashion. Indeed, many of the ideas on delusions in common currency can be traced to speculations made by Freud (1911) relating them to latent homosexuality. Other kinds of psychodynamic speculations have long flourished without check (de Pauw 1994). However plausible these ideas may be, they are *post hoc* and are usually incapable of generating testable predictions. The most persuasive exponents (Berson 1983; Enoch & Trethowan 1991) do remind us, though, of the need to consider the psychological background of individual cases, which, as Fleminger (1994a) points out is not necessarily incompatible with other explanatory approaches.

An approach to understanding specific cognitive deficit following brain injury, however, that is beginning to have some impact on scientific thinking is cognitive neuropsychology (Caramazza 1986; Coltheart 1986). This methodology uses models of particular cognitive processes, such as reading or face recognition, to understand specific types of cognitive difficulty following brain damage. In turn, it uses the results obtained from neurological patients to refine the cognitive models. A few years ago both Anthony David and I suggested that, *mutatis mutandis*, cognitive neuropsychiatry could be the label for the study of positive psychiatric symptoms similarly analysed by the systematic application of models of normal cognitive processes to help explain these symptoms (Ellis 1991; David 1993). *Cognitive Neuropsychiatry*, the title of a new journal first published in 1996 by Psychology Press, is concerned with the analysis of certain psychiatric and neurological symptoms within models of normal cognitive processing. The ways in which cognition can break down, malfunction or be perverted can then be interpreted within this framework. Moreover, where the models are inadequate to explain the specific condition, they should be modified to do so. This iterative process has proved successful when applied to patients with specific brain damage and could be an equally effective technique for understanding many psychotic behaviours.

It should be admitted, however, that the precepts of the cognitive neuropsychiatry approach are neither original nor yet particularly well articulated. None the less, for some years now researchers have been attempting to throw light on many psychiatric conditions by examining them from the perspective of normal information-processing mechanisms. What we have today, then, is the beginnings of a concerted effort to examine normal and abnormal cognitions together and to acknowledge the mutual benefits that can arise from incorporating them both within the same theoretical framework. As I shall show shortly, it is not too difficult to apply the principles of cognitive neuropsychiatry to DMIs and, I hope, one may quickly appreciate the benefits from doing so.

Delusional misidentification syndromes: history

In this section I shall outline the historical backgrounds to the principal DMIs. More definitive sources can be found in the collection of papers edited by Christodoulou (1986) and the proceedings of his first international conference on DMIs held in Paris (Ellis *et al.* 1994a). Translations into English from French of some of the original papers were published by Ellis *et al.* (1994b).

PARAPROSOPIA

Paraprosopia is the apparent transformation of a face, usually into a frightening appearance. Patients have described faces as monstrous, vampire-like or seeming to become that of a werewolf (Krauss 1852). According to Grüsser and Landis (1991), paraprosopia is most often associated with schizophrenia in childhood, but it is observed in adults too. Daniel Paul Schreber, for example, who was President of the Court of Appeal in Dresden, in describing his own schizophrenic illness once saw some men 'as devils with particularly red faces . . .' — a frightening apparition (Schreber 1903).

KP, whom I mentioned earlier, not only showed paraprosopia but also revealed it for his own face. This, I suggest, should be termed 'autoparaprosopia'. His other face symptom, the disappearance of his face in a mirror, is known as negative heautoscopy. This is also interesting but lies outside the scope of this chapter.

INTERMETAMORPHOSIS

The first description of the kinds of symptoms shown by YD, DL and NT was made by Courbon and Tusques (1932). They described a 49-year-old woman, whom they called Sylvie G, whose experiences included seeing animals and objects alter appearance. Her most striking symptoms, however, involved people. Many individuals looked almost exactly like her aunt or her son—indeed, when the latter's friends called at her house sometimes Sylvie G could only distinguish him from them by their feet: her son's being large and invariably shod in dirty shoes.

Intermetamorphosis is characterized by the often sudden switch in appearance of one person to someone else's face. Its occurrence as a psychiatric symptom was thought to be quite rare but Young *et al.* (1990b) tested the three cases mentioned earlier in a single hospital over a relatively short period of time. This suggests that the delusion may not be so uncommon, after all: instead it may be masked by the presence of other, more prominent symptoms.

FRÉGOLI DELUSION

Courbon and Fail (1927) were the first to report a case that they labelled the 'illusion de Frégoli' in honour of a famous Italian mimic, Léopoldo Frégoli. They described a 27-year-old woman who developed the delusion that the actresses Sarah Bernhardt and Robine were persecuting her while disguised as others. The patient sometimes attacked individuals in the belief that they were one of her tormentors and as a result would land in trouble with the police.

The essential feature of the Frégoli delusion is that the patients with the symptoms feel able to see through someone's outward appearance to discern, within, the person who usually is thought to be persecuting them. Like intermetamorphosis, the Frégoli delusion has not often been reported in the literature. When cases have been published they are usually found within a paranoid setting but a recent, unpublished, case in Cardiff suggests that this may not always be so. Here, a 23-year-old woman developed the delusion that members of a family, friendly with her own, were disguising themselves as others to look after her. Thus it would seem that the delusion can occur within a benign context (S. Sadler and A. Quayle, personal communication).

CAPGRAS DELUSION

Easily the most common DMI is the Capgras delusion in which patients insist that others usually, but not necessarily, close to them have been replaced by doubles, robots, etc. This delusion may provide the key to philosophical as well as psychological issues regarding identity (Dennett 1996).

Although this delusion was noted earlier (e.g. Kahlbaum 1866; Jaspers 1923/1963) it was not until the publication of two papers by Capgras and his

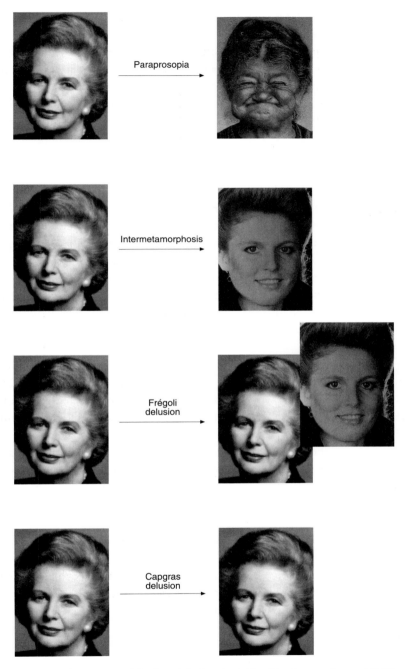

Fig. 2.1 Pictorial summary of the four delusional misidentification syndrome (DMI) symptoms described in the text.

colleagues that the delusion was properly documented (Capgras & Reboul-Lachaux 1923; Capgras *et al.* 1924). The original label '*l'illusion de sosies*' was quickly replaced by the term Capgras delusion and was subsequently reported in a wide range of psychiatric and neurological patients, of all ages, across most cultures (Ellis & de Pauw 1994). Estimates of the incidence vary between 1 and 5% of the psychiatric population (Ellis & de Pauw 1994; Joseph 1994; Kirov *et al.* 1994).

Whatever the true figure for its incidence, the Capgras delusion is clearly a significant symptom — but one that, curiously, has yet to receive singular identification in any psychiatric classification system (Ellis *et al.* 1994a). Parallel symptoms for inanimate objects have also been reported. Anderson (1988) described the case of an elderly man, with a large pituitary tumour, who believed his wife and her nephew had replaced more than 300 of his possessions with similar, but inferior doubles. Ellis *et al.* (1996) described two similar cases of Capgras delusion for objects but not people. These were found also to have difficulties in remembering non-facial objects, in contrast to the usual Capgras delusion cases who display a variety of face-processing difficulties (Bidault *et al.* 1986).

Figure 2.1 provides a visual summary of the four DMIs discussed here.

A model of face recognition

Over the last 20 years great efforts have been made by psychologists to try to understand how we recognize others (Ellis 1975, 1981, 1986; Bruce 1979; Bruce & Young 1986; Burton *et al.* 1990).

Although models of the process have become increasingly sophisticated, most are still predicated upon the following three, interconnected core elements:

1   initial structural encoding (early visual analysis leading to the construction of a facial precept);

2   face-recognition units (store of every known face, each unit signalling a sense of familiarity);

3   person identity nodes (either a repository or a gateway to episodic and biographical information about known individuals).

Ellis and Young (1990) offered an analysis of some of the DMIs within the framework of the simplified model outlines above. Although we can now extend their arguments a little, it still remains to be seen whether predictions arising from them will be borne out.

Figure 2.2 is an illustration of the simplified, generic face-recognition

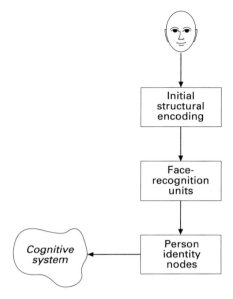

Fig. 2.2 Generic, simplified information-processing model of the stages involved in face recognition.

model used by Ellis and Young (1990) using that framework within which it is possible to identify three of the DMIs with different stages. It must be acknowledged at the outset that this particular application of cognitive neuropsychiatric principles is speculative, incomplete and not yet fully vindicated by results. But the attempt to understand abnormalities in the way some psychiatric and neurological patients perceived others within the framework of a model of normal face processing does provide a paradigm for future cognitive neuropsychiatric research in so far as the face-recognition model can accommodate most of the DMIs mentioned earlier but is incapable of easily explaining at least one of them. In theory of course, this aberrant example should lead to a modification of the model. I shall return to this point later.

First, how does the model shown in Fig. 2.2 cope with each of the DMIs described? As Fig. 2.3 indicates, three of them (paraprosopia, intermetamorphosis and the Frégoli delusion) can each be associated with faults presumed to occur at one or other of the three stages of the model.

Paraprosopia is a distortion in the appearance of facial features that may arise at the level at which faces are initially encoded and at which a structural description is derived. At this moment it is not possible to be precise as to the

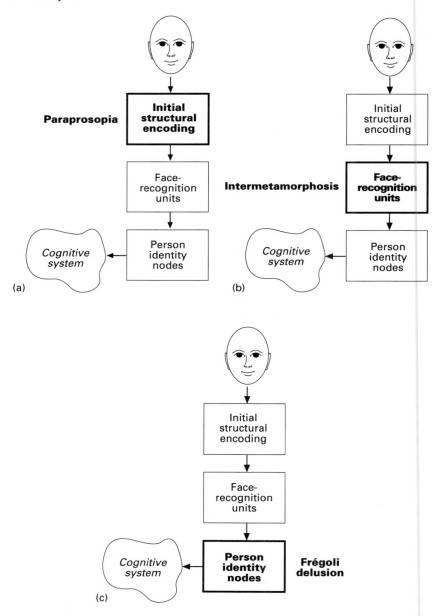

Fig. 2.3 Proposed sites of malfunction for: (a) paraprosopia; (b) intermetamorphosis; and (c) the Frégoli delusion.

nature of the problem: given the fact that these distortions are usually ugly or frightening, however, one could assume some non-random factor, culturally determined and implying the influence of some top down constraints. It is worth noting that in some forms of prosopagnosia, the acquired inability to recognize faces, chronic distortions occur in the appearance of others (Bodamer 1947; Ellis 1975). Also, there have been some reports of neurological cases for whom parts of people's faces seem altered in some way (Young *et al.* 1990a). In paraprosopia and autoparaprosopia, these delusions are transient and so it is reasonable to ask not only *how* they occur at, say, a neurophysiological level, but *why* they occur.

Intermetamorphosis may be associated with faults occurring at the face-recognition unit stage. This comprises a store of all known faces, a sort of physiognomic lexicon (Ellis 1981; Hay & Young 1982). Input from the structural encoding stage usually triggers the appropriate unit which in turn fires to signal that it is familiar and excites the appropriate semantic node at the next stage. Ellis and Young (1990) conjectured that if a face-recognition unit, for any reason, is hyperexcitable, it may be triggered by input that is similar but not identical to that which normally causes it to fire and thus gives rise to a false identification. It is noteworthy that when deluded, Courbon and Tusques' (1932) patient could distinguish her son from others by looking at the feet, which one must assume were recognized by some other mechanism than that involved in face processing.

At first sight the Frégoli delusion does not appear easily to fit an explanation couched in terms of face recognition because it does not involve a distortion or misidentification, as such. Patients assert that people are not what they seem to be, and that they can see beyond their outward appearance. In their attempts to understand the Frégoli delusion within the face-recognition model, Ellis and Young (1990) argued that it could arise from hyperexcitable nodes at the final stage of recognition. These could fire, be triggered, or whatever, quite inappropriately simply because the usual level of evidence was unnecessary. For the patient described by Courbon and Tusques, the nodes corresponding to Sarah Bernhardt and Robine were excited by many percepts so that, although there was enough evidence for her to see people veridically, one or other of these two nodes could be simultaneously fired giving her the sense that one of the actresses was before her, in disguise.

But what about the Capgras delusion? How may this be explained within the model? The answer is that, in its present form, the model does not easily seem capable of doing so. In episodes of Capgras delusion, patients have no difficulty identifying someone, even if they claim to discern small physical changes in the face: what they say, however, is that the person is an impostor.

One way of approaching this is to suggest that, while the face recognition mechanism is working in all its principal functions — the encoding is accurate, the correct face-recognition unit fires and the appropriate person identity mode is triggered—something, none the less, is missing. What?

We have to make a logical leap here. First we have to make the not unreasonable assumption that every face one encounters engenders a feeling of familiarity or of strangeness. It is a well-known experience that seeing people out of their usual context can sometimes induce a feeling of familiarity, with absolutely no further information about them (Young *et al.* 1985).

If the mechanism that gives rise to the sense of familiarity is not functioning properly, it could form the genesis of the Capgras delusion. Patients would recognize an individual they know but, lacking any concurrent feeling of familiarity, would confabulate by believing him or her to be an impostor. It is not surprising, I think, that patients do not describe their feelings and belief processes in this way: the underlying processes would be largely unconscious and therefore difficult to articulate. The explanation is speculative but it does have the merit of accounting for the fact that patients with the Capgras delusion do not assert that all people have been replaced, but usually do so for those, such as family, who have a long-term emotional significance; or others, such as medical staff, who have a more immediate and transient significance.

One characteristic of all four DMIs is their specificity for faces. Where the Capgras-type delusion for inanimate objects occurs, it does so independently, not alongside a problem with faces. The idea that the mind, in some respects, is organized in a modular fashion, of course, is neither new nor original. Fodor (1983) first expounded this idea and both cognitive neuropsychology and cognitive neuropsychiatry are predicated upon it. The DMIs reinforce the idea of a face-recognition module, itself comprising subcomponents, that may be damaged or malfunction while all other systems may operate normally.

For the cognitive neuropsychiatric approach to DMIs to have any real plausibility, however, it must, unlike earlier psychodynamic explanations, in principle be capable of generating predictions that are falsifiable. Ellis and Young (1990) addressed this issue by predicting that intermetamorphosis would be most likely to occur when the real and delusional person shared some physical resemblance; and, further, that because allegedly it occurs at the face-recognition unit stage, which is entirely face specific, it should not occur for voices: the patient ought not to be deluded by the voice, only the face. The Frégoli delusion, on the other hand, arising from problems at a multimodel site, where information from face, voice, gait, etc. can all access data on people's biographies, could occur from any of these inputs.

To illustrate the difference in predictions for intermetamorphosis and the Frégoli delusion, consider how patients with either of these symptoms would react upon encountering someone on the telephone. The one with intermeta-morphosis should never 'hear' someone other than the speaker; but the one with Frégoli delusion could well believe that the person he or she is speaking to is someone else disguising his or her voice.

The Capgras delusion was also defined by Ellis and Young (1990) as a face-specific problem. Moreover, they predicted that patients with the Capgras delusion would not reveal at least one response to familiar faces that is normally evoked. When skin conductance responses are measured while faces are shown, familiar faces elicit a larger autonomic response than do the faces of strangers (Tranel *et al.* 1985). This occurs even when the faces are presented at a speed too fast for conscious registration (Ellis *et al.* 1993). Ellis and Young's (1990) prediction is that patients with Capgras delusion will not display these differential skin conductance responses. That is to say, whatever causes the differential skin conductance responses for faces that are known, compared with faces that are unknown, is not likely to operate for them. The mechanism signalling emotional significance or, simply, famili-arity just is not functioning normally. Although Dennett (1996) recently described this as 'an ingenious and plausible hypothesis' (p. 112), it remains to be tested and the precise underlying neural mechanisms have yet to be determined.

Having outlined at least one advantage of the cognitive neuropsychiatric approach to DMIs, namely its ability to generate predictable data, it would be remiss of me if I did not reiterate that, as yet, data either to confirm or dis-confirm any of the predictions have yet to be published; and that some theo-rists argue that apparently identical DMIs may occur for different reasons; that, for example, patients may show quite different onset patterns and respond differently to drug treatments. Therefore, it could be argued, that more than one explanation for the same symptoms may be required (Malloy *et al.* 1992; Fleminger & Burns 1993).

Another factor which must not be overlooked has been put forward, in different ways, by Fleminger (1994b) and by Ellis and Young (1996). Fleminger (1994a, 1994b) argues cogently that delusions need to be inter-preted within a wider context: that a patient's psychological history has a direct bearing on his or her symptoms, and, therefore, that one should look at both organic aetiologies as well as psychological ones that are specific to the patient.

Ellis and Young (1996) were exercised by the fact that DMI patients, while perhaps suffering from some deficit within the cognitive system dealing with faces, should form such bizarre beliefs. Maher (1974) had addressed this in relation to delusions in general and decided that when perceptual experiences are so anomalous, there is no need to posit any further problem: odd experiences are sufficient to produce delusions, a view first tentatively expressed by Southend (1912). Ellis and Young (1996), however, suggest a two-stage model in which unusual experiences, resulting from cognitive deficits, are a necessary precursor but that for a full-blown DMI to occur patients must also have a malfunction in those cognitive processes that underly belief, judgement or attribution. In other words, they claim that one can have problems at either stage without developing a delusion. To sustain the belief, however, that a face has been radically changed and that someone is in disguise or even an impostor, it is necessary for this higher-order monitoring system also to have failed in some way as well as there to be a fault within the face-recognition system.

Overview

In this chapter I have attempted to give an outline of some of the issues concerning the DMIs that are of current interest. My primary aim was to demonstrate the potential of the cognitive neuropsychiatric approach in helping us to understand these bizarre person-centred delusions. In doing so, I have not given much prominence either to more psychologically oriented approaches or to identifying likely neural substrates. These important considerations, as well as others, can be further explored, for example, by consulting the latest collection of papers on DMIs published as a special issue of *Psychopathology* (Ellis *et al.* 1994a).

The DMIs, it is argued, provide not only a paradigm case for the cognitive neuropsychiatric approach but, as do other delusions, they also prompt questions about the nature of belief within the normal as well as pathological populations. It is the study of the system when it is malfunctioning that may provide a window on an important aspect of human cognition.

Acknowledgements

The author's work on DMIs and delusions in general has been funded by grants from the EJLB Foundation and the Wellcome Trust (to Ellis, de Pauw and Young). The assistance of Angela Quayle and Ikbal Bahia is also gratefully acknowledged.

References

Anderson, D.N. (1988) The delusion of inanimate doubles: Implications for understanding the Capgras phenomenon. *British Journal of Psychiatry* **153**, 694–699.

Berson, R.J. (1983) Capgras' syndrome. *American Journal of Psychiatry* **140**, 969–978.

Bidault, E., Luauté, J.-P. & Tzavaras, A. (1986) Prosopagnosia and the delusional misidentification syndromes. *Bibliotheca Psychiatrica* **164**, 80–91.

Bodamer, J. (1947) Die prosop-agnosie. *Archiv für Psychiatrie und Nerven Krank-Leiten* **179**, 6–54.

Bruce, V. (1979) Searching for politicians: An information-processing approach to face recognition. *Quarterly Journal of Experimental Psychology* **31**, 373–395.

Bruce, V. (1988) *Recognising Faces*. Lawrence Erlbaum, Hove.

Bruce, V. & Young, A. (1986) Understanding face recognition. *British Journal of Psychology* **77**, 305–327.

Burton, A.M., Bruce, V. & Johnston, R.A. (1990) Understanding face recognition with an interactive activation model. *British Journal of Psychology* **81**, 361–380.

Capgras, J. & Reboul-Lachaux, J. (1923) L'illusion des 'sosies' dans un délire systématisé chronique. *Bulletin de la Societé Clinique de Médecine Mentale* **11**, 6–16.

Capgras, J., Lucchini, P. & Schiff, P. (1924) Du sentiment d'étrangeté à l'illusion des sosies. *Bulletin de la Societé de Médecine Mentale* **12**, 210–217.

Caramazza, A. (1986) On drawing inferences about the structure of normal cognitive systems from the analysis of patterns of impaired performance: The case for single-patient studies. *Brain and Cognition* **5**, 41–66.

Christodoulou, G.A. (1986) *The Delusional Misidentification Syndromes*. Karger, Basel.

Coltheart, M. (1986) Cognitive neuropsychology. In: *Attention and Performance, XI* (eds M. Pasner & V.S.M Marin). Lawrence Erlbaum, Hillsdale, N.J.

Courbon, P. & Fail, G. (1927) Syndrome d'illusion de Frégoli et schizophrenie. *Bulletin de la Societé de Médicine Mentale* **15**, 121–124.

Courbon, P. & Tusques, J. (1932) Illusion d'intermétamorphose et de charme. *Annales Médico-Psychologiques* **90**, 401–405.

David, A.S. (1993) Cognitive neuropsychiatry? *Psychological Medicine* **25**, 1–5.

Dennett, D.C. (1996) *Kinds of Minds: Towards an Understanding of Consciousness*. Weidenfeld & Nicholson, London.

de Pauw, K.W. (1994) Psychodynamic approaches to the Capgras delusion: A critical historical review. *Psychopathology* **27**, 154–160.

Ellis, H.D. (1975) Recognising faces. *British Journal of Psychology* **66**, 409–426.

Ellis, H.D. (1981) Theoretical aspects of face recognition. In: *Perceiving and Remembering Faces* (eds G. Davies, H. Ellis & J. Shepherd). Academic Press, London.

Ellis, H.D. (1986) Processes underlying face recognition. In: *The Neuropsychology of Face Perception and Facial Expressions* (ed. R. Bruyer). Lawrence Erlbaum, Hillsdale, N.J.

Ellis, H.D. (1991) Delusional misidentification syndromes: a cognitive neuropsychiatric approach. Paper presented at the *International Symposium on the Neuropsychology of Schizophrenia*, 1991. London.

Ellis, H.D. & de Pauw, K.W. (1994) The cognitive neuropsychiatric origins of the Capgras delusion. In: *The Neuropsychology of Schizophrenia* (eds A. David & J. Cutting). Lawrence Erlbaum, Hove.

Ellis, H.D. & Young, A.W. (1990) Accounting for delusional misidentification. *British Journal of Psychiatry* 160, 293–303.

Ellis, H.D. & Young, A.W. (1996) Problems of person perception in schizophrenia. In: *Neuropsychology of Schizophrenia* (eds C. Pantelis, H. Nelson & T. Barnes). Wiley, Chichester.

Ellis, H.D., Luauté, J.-P. & Retterstol, N. (1994a) The delusional misidentification syndromes. Proceedings of the Conference on delusional misidentification syndromes, Paris 1993. *Psychopathology* 27, whole issue.

Ellis, H.D., Luauté, J.-P. & Whitley, J. (1994b) Delusional misidentification: The three original papers on the Capgras, Frégoli and intermetamorphosis delusions. *History of Psychiatry* 5, 117–146.

Ellis, H.D., Quayle, A.H. & de Pauw, K.W. (1996) Delusional misidentification of inanimate objects: A literature review and neuropsychological analysis of cognitive deficits in two cases. *Cognitive Neuropsychiatry* 1, 27–40.

Ellis, H.D., Young, A.W. & Köhnken, G. (1993) Covert face recognition without prosopagnosia. *Behavioural Neurology* 6, 27–32.

Enoch, D. & Trethowan, W. (1991) *Uncommon Psychiatric Syndromes*, 3rd edn. Butterworth-Heinemann, Oxford.

Fleminger, S. (1994a) Top-down preconscious perceptual processing and delusional misidentification in neuropsychiatric disorder. In: *The Neuropsychology of Schizophrenia* (eds A. David & J. Cutting). Lawrence Erlbaum, Hove.

Fleminger, S. (1994b) Delusional misidentification: An exemplary symptom illustrating an interaction between organic brain disease and psychological processes. *Psychopathology* 27, 161–167.

Fleminger, S. & Burns, A. (1993) The delusional misidentification syndromes in patients with and without evidence of organic cerebral disorder: A structured review of case reports. *Biological Psychiatry* 33, 22–32.

Fodor, G. (1983) *The Modularity of the Mind*. MIT Press, Cambridge, Mass.

Freud, S. (1911) Psychoanalytic notes on an autobiographical account of a case of paranoia (dementia paranoides). In: *Standard Edition of the Complete Works of Sigmund Freud*, Vol. 12. Hogarth, London.

Goren, C.C., Sarty, M. & Wu, P.Y.K. (1975) Visual following and pattern discrimination of face-like stimuli by new-born infants. *Pediatrics* 56, 544–549.

Grüsser, O.J. & Landis, T. (1991) *Vision and Visual Dysfunction*, Vol. 12. *Visual Agnosias and Other Disturbances of Visual Perception and Cognition*. Macmillan Press, London.

Hay, D.C. & Young, A.W. (1982) The human face. In: *Normality and Pathology in Cognitive Functions* (ed. A. Ellis). Academic Press, London.

Jaspers, K. (1923/1963) *General Psychopathology*. Springer-Verlag, Berlin. (Trans. J. Hoenig & M. Hamilton.) Manchester University Press, Manchester.

Johnson, M.H., Dziurawiec, S., Ellis, H.D. & Morton, J. (1992) Newborns' preferential tracking of face-like stimuli and its subsequent decline. *Cognition* 40, 1–21.

Joseph, A.B. (1994) Observations on the epidemiology of the delusional misidentification syndromes in the Boston Metropolitan area: April 1983–June 1984. *Psychopathology* 27, 150–153.

Kahlbaum, K.L. (1866) Die Sinnesdelirien c. die Illusion. *Allgemeine Zeitschrift für Psychiatrie* 23, 56–78.

Kirov, G., Jones, P. & Lewis, S. (1994) Prevalence of delusional misidentification syndromes. *Psychopathology* 27, 148–149.

Krauss, F. (1852) *Nothschreieines*. Magnetisch-Vergifteten Selbstverlag, Stuttgart.

Maher, B.A. (1974) Delusional thinking and perceptual disorder. *Journal of Individual Psychology* 30, 98–113.

Malloy, P., Cimino, C. & Westlake, R. (1992) Differential diagnosis of primary and secondary Capgras delusions. *Neuropsychiatry, Neuropsychology and Behavioral Science* 5, 83–96.

Schreber, D.P. (1903) *Denkwürdigkeiten einer Nervenkranken*. Reprinted in: *Bürgerliche Wahnweltum 1900* (eds P. Heiligenthal & R. Volk). Focus, Wiesbaden.

Southend, E.E. (1912) On the somatic sources of somatic delusions. *Journal of Abnormal Psychology* 7, 326–339.

Tranel, D., Fowles, D.C. & Damasio, A.R. (1985) Electro-dermal discrimination of familiar and unfamiliar faces: A methodology. *Psychophysiology* 22, 403–408.

Young, A.W., De Haan, E.H.F., Newcombe, F. & Hay, D.C. (1990a) Facial neglect. *Neuropsychologia* 28, 391–415.

Young, A.W., Ellis, H.D., Szulecka, T.K. & de Pauw, K.W. (1990b) Face processing impairments and delusional misidentification. *Behavioural Neurology* 3, 153–168.

Young, A.W., Hay, D.C. & Ellis, A.W. (1985) The faces that launched a thousand ships: Everyday difficulties and errors in recognizing people. *British Journal of Psychology* 76, 495–523.

CHAPTER 3

Paranoia or Delusional Disorder

ALISTAIR MUNRO

A fanatic is one who can't change his mind and won't change the subject.
[Winston Churchill]

Introduction

By the end of the 19th century, paranoia was a well-established diagnosis and a not-infrequently recognized illness. Yet, by 1977, Gregory and Smeltzer expressed the view of many authorities when they commented that the concept of paranoia was largely theoretical (Gregory & Smeltzer 1977). And, in 1980, the *British Medical Journal* stated in an editorial that 'Paranoia is no longer a fashionable term' (Editorial 1980).

Despite this, in 1987, paranoia was firmly reinstated in DSM-III-R (American Psychiatric Association (APA) 1987), albeit renamed 'delusional disorder', and is now an important diagnostic entity in DSM-IV (APA 1994) and in ICD-10 (World Health Organization (WHO) 1992–1993) under this new rubric. How can an illness gain prominence, apparently disappear, and now flourish again like this? In the course of this chapter, as well as describing the illness itself, a brief attempt will be made to explain the vagaries of its existence during this past century. Needless to say, it is unlikely to be the illness itself which varies all that much, but rather the beliefs of those who do or do not diagnose it.

What do we mean by paranoia?

This chapter will describe an illness characterized by a stable and persistent delusional system to which the patient usually clings with fanatical intensity but which is relatively encapsulated and which leaves personality and psychosocial functioning intact to a considerable extent. Hallucinations may

occur but are usually not prominent and typically are related to the delusional belief. The illness is chronic and often lifelong, but does not have the
principal characteristics of schizophrenia (Criterion A in APA 1994).

Unfortunately, the nomenclature associated with this disorder is, to put it
mildly, confusing. Terms like 'paranoia', 'paranoid', 'paraphrenia', etc., are
used indiscriminately in the professional and lay literatures, and many psychiatrists would have difficulty in defining them. We often find that a technical word like 'paranoia', denoting a specific psychiatric syndrome, is
confused with the term 'paranoid' which, depending on the user, can mean a
group of psychotic illnesses, a personality type or, more likely nowadays, a
layman's vague concept of certain personality traits or attitudes, usually
involving a negative connotation. Such looseness of meaning often makes it
impossible to know what a particular author is describing.

Fish (1962) noted that English-speaking psychiatrists habitually used
'paranoid' to mean 'persecutory' and Case No. 3.1 is typical of what many
people conceptualize as paranoia. It is indeed a case of paranoia and the
main delusion is a persecutory one, but, as will be shown later, this is only
one subtype among several. Fish maintained that 'paranoid' should have the
general meaning of 'delusional', but common usage has decreed that 'paranoia' and 'paranoid' usually mean 'angrily suspicious' without any necessary
implication of delusional thinking. To compound the confusion, 'paranoid
personality disorder' is an officially accepted diagnosis in which delusions
play no part. So, to make matters more straightforward, DSM-III-R, and
now ICD-10, have dropped the term 'paranoia' and refer to the illness as
'delusional disorder'. In this chapter, paranoia and delusional disorder are
used interchangeably, but the latter is currently the more acceptable term.

Case No. 3.1: Delusional disorder, persecutory subtype

*A widowed lady aged 77 had always been a very obsessional, fastidious
person. She lost her husband when she was aged 63 and, after a normal
mourning period, appeared to adjust well. She had no children and relatively
few friends, but kept close contact with a brother and sister who lived in the
same town. She did not drink or use drugs and had always been reluctant to
take even prescription medications. At the age of 74 she developed bladder
cancer and had to have a partial removal of the bladder. Thereafter she developed some intermittent urinary incontinence which distressed her out of all
proportion to its severity.*

Apparently she suddenly woke out of a deep sleep one night and found that her bed was wet. She immediately decided that she had been raped by an intruder and that the dampness was semen, but was too afraid to get out of bed to explore the house. The next morning all the locks were secure but she remained convinced that she had been sexually assaulted. She contacted the police who came to the house and made a search but took no other action. Over the next several weeks she constantly telephoned the police, several city officials and her brother and sister. Her distress escalated and she was eventually admitted to a geriatric medicine unit in the local hospital. There she was found to be physically well, with no evidence of recurrence of her cancer. She appeared intellectually intact and could be involved at times in normal conversation, but inevitably returned to her complaints of intruders who repeatedly sexually interfered with her. She was very anxious but not clinically depressed.

A psychiatric assessment was obtained and a diagnosis of delusional disorder was made. Very reluctantly the patient accepted neuroleptic treatment and quite rapidly became calmer and less convinced about her complaints. She was discharged home but stopped taking her medication and began complaining again of being frequently assaulted. Eventually she was readmitted and restarted on the neuroleptic, with reasonable success, but once more stopped taking it when she returned home. This pattern recurred several times and the patient is now in long-term care, doing moderately well on a maintenance dose of her medication. Her cancer has not recurred.

A brief historical overview of paranoia/delusional disorder

The term 'paranoia' comes from classical Greek times, but it only very gradually attained its modern technical meaning in the second half of the 19th century. If one reviews the relevant literature from that time, it is possible to obtain a picture of paranoia which is very close to the current conceptualization of delusional disorder, especially if we consider the work of Kraepelin (1921), who crystallized many previous descriptions and added his own observations to provide the definitive definition of the disorder. Essentially, the Victorian psychiatrist's view of paranoia would have been as follows.

1   It is a primary disorder, not secondary to another psychiatric condition.
2   Paranoia is a stable disorder characterized by the presence of delusions to which the patient clings with extraordinary tenacity.
3   The illness is chronic and frequently lifelong.
4   The delusions are logically constructed and internally consistent.

5 The disorder is a monomania, with a predominant, persisting theme.

6 Despite the monodelusional aspect, the content of the delusion varies from patient to patient, though a limited number of themes predominate.

7 The delusions do not interfere with general logical reasoning (though within the delusional system the logic is perverted) and there is usually no general disturbance of behaviour. If disturbed behaviour does occur it is directly related to the delusional beliefs.

8 Many cases appear to arise in the setting of a markedly abnormal personality.

9 Hallucinations may or may not be present (there has been some dispute about this).

10 The individual experiences a heightened sense of self-reference.

At that time (as at present), the frequency of paranoia was uncertain, but it was not regarded as unduly rare. Theories about aetiology were legion but the cause of the disorder was unknown then and remains so.

Kraepelin (1921) personally described 19 cases during his career but latterly he began to have some doubts about the viability of the diagnosis. These doubts were intensified after his death when Kolle (1931) reported on 66 cases of primary paranoia originally seen in Kraepelin's former clinic in Munich, noting that approximately half had developed features of other psychiatric disorders over time. It should be stressed that the diagnosis remained stable in the other patients, but despite this, psychiatrists began to use the concept of paranoia to a decreasing extent.

That trend was accentuated by other influences. E. Bleuler (1857–1939; Bleuler 1950), renamed Kraepelin's 'dementia praecox' 'schizophrenia' and greatly widened its definition. Although he recognized paranoia as a separate disorder, he effectively blurred the boundaries between schizophrenia and paranoia/delusional disorder and many psychiatrists ceased making the distinction. At the same time, Adolf Meyer's (1866–1950; Lidz 1966) influence became very strong, particularly in the US but also among certain prominent British psychiatrists: his concept of 'reaction types' and his emphasis on the uniqueness of the individual and his or her illness tended to blur traditional diagnostic entities and to devalue descriptions of generalized syndromes, and paranoia suffered as a result. Also, Sigmund Freud (1856–1939; Freud 1950, 1958), while stating that paranoia and schizophrenia were separate conditions, promoted psychodynamic formulation as against careful nosology: wherever psychoanalysis was strong (especially in the US), traditional diagnostic habits were weakened and aetiological speculations (including a good deal on paranoia) predominated.

By the middle of the 20th century, and for a variety of reasons, the diagnosis of paranoia had become rare. Cases, it is presumed, were mostly lumped under schizophrenia, and although that was especially true of America, it also described the situation in the UK and many parts of Europe. Lewis (1970), in a perceptive historical review, 'Paranoia and paranoid', clearly regarded the concept as *passé* and very probably without validity. ICD-8 (WHO 1967) continued to recognize it, but as an extremely rare condition, while ICD-9 (WHO 1978) upgraded it somewhat to a rare chronic psychosis. Meanwhile, DSM-II (APA 1968) grouped paranoid disorders, excluding paranoid schizophrenia, under the title 'paranoid states' but queried their separateness from schizophrenia. DSM-III (APA 1980) described paranoid disorders, apparently amalgamating paranoia with paraphrenia and restricting the delusional contents in the disorders to persecution and jealousy.

In 1977, Winokur in the US returned to the Kraepelinian concept of paranoia, describing cases he had himself observed and renaming the illness 'delusional disorder'. Soon afterwards, Kendler (1980) reinforced Winokur's description. From 1975 onwards, the present author wrote on monodelusional disorders characterized by hypochondriacal delusions, then amalgamated his descriptions of so-called 'monosymptomatic hypochondriacal psychosis' with those of paranoia (Munro 1982a). By the mid-1980s, these workers' views began to be influential and by 1987, when DSM-III-R appeared, were sufficiently accepted that the description of paranoia there was, in essence, a return to Kraepelin's ideas and an affirmation that the illness was distinct from schizophrenia. DSM-IV and ICD-10 both maintain this stance.

As with any psychiatric disorder, controversies remain and despite its new-found respectability as a diagnosis, many psychiatrists are still uneasy in recognizing paranoia/delusional disorder. Why is this?

In the first instance, there are psychiatrists who trained at a time when paranoia was effectively suppressed, and therefore have no familiarity with its description. Secondly, it is relatively easy to see delusional disorder as an aberrant form of schizophrenia and simply give it the latter diagnosis. Thirdly, many delusional disorder patients remain relatively high functioning in the community and do not seek psychiatric help: to compound this, many of them show profound denial of their illness and vehemently refuse to see a psychiatrist. Strangely, the illness is better known to many outside psychiatry, including internists who see patients with somatic delusions, lawyers who deal with litigious paranoiacs, law-enforcement officers who cope with individuals who commit crimes when suffering from delusions of jealousy or erotomania, pest-control officials who receive demands for disinfestation from people with infestation delusions, and so on. Unfortunately, the awareness of paranoia is as scattered as it is widespread and the literature is extremely fragmented. Little wonder that the average psychiatrist finds it difficult to get to grips with the description of the illness, never mind actual patients who suffer from it. And, to cap it all, the terms 'paranoia' and 'paranoid' have developed such a stigma that many practitioners are not at all keen to deal with the patients whom they visualize (sometimes correctly) as difficult, demanding and, at times, dangerous.

It is hoped that the present chapter can do something to defuse this negative perception.

Illnesses associated with delusions

Although paranoia is increasingly known as 'delusional disorder', the great majority of illnesses associated with delusions do not belong to this category. Unfortunately, even here there is a degree of controversy, as some authorities regard 'delusional disorders' as all psychiatric illnesses with delusions, sub-categorizing them according to the underlying syndrome, which might be schizophrenia, severe mood disorder, or even organic mental disorder (Retterstol 1966; Berner *et al.* 1984). DSM-IV and ICD-10 restrict the term 'delusional disorder' to paranoia, but unfortunately imply that this is the only illness within the category which, as will be argued below, is overly restrictive.

When considering a possible diagnosis of delusional disorder, the other principal illnesses with delusions which must be excluded are:

- paraphrenia;
- paranoid schizophrenia;
- other schizophrenias;
- organic mental disorder, including mental disorders due to a medical condition;
- psychoactive substance-induced organic mental disorders and withdrawal disorders;
- psychotic disorders not elsewhere classified;
- mood disorders;
- misidentification syndromes;
- induced psychotic disorder (in which the beliefs are delusional though the patient is not truly deluded).

A category including several delusional illnesses?

As noted, DSM-IV and ICD-10 largely agree that 'delusional disorder' is the updated version of Kraepelinian paranoia. However, the present author has repeatedly argued that there is a group of illnesses with prominent delusional features which could readily be included in the same category as paranoia. The first of these is paraphrenia, an illness akin to schizophrenia and characterized by persistent delusions and hallucinations, but with much less disorder of affect and volition, with well-retained personality, and with striking retention of emotional rapport. (For details, see Chapter 5.)

Secondly, paranoid schizophrenia has features which link it to delusional disorder as much as to schizophrenia (Houlihan 1977). Here, symptomatology is dominated by systematized, though not encapsulated, delusions and frequently by auditory hallucinations. A family history of schizophrenia is about half as common as in other forms of schizophrenia and there is less tendency to personality deterioration. Affect is not grossly inappropriate, though preservation of affect and rapport is less than in paraphrenia, and overall deterioration is less marked than in other types of schizophrenia.

Thirdly, the delusional misidentification syndromes (DMS; Ellis & Young 1990), which currently have no place in any official psychiatric diagnostic system, are par excellence, delusional disorders. Although regarded as rare until recently, reports on the various subtypes are appearing with increasing frequency. They are generally regarded as psychiatric illnesses, but evidence is accumulating that they are frequently associated with demonstrable brain abnormalities.

McAllister (1992), basing his speculations on the work of Cummings (1985) and others, has suggested that the genesis of delusions lies in malfunction of limbic-basal ganglia mechanisms, with special emphasis on dopamine overactivity. He recognizes the contribution of right parieto-occipital abnormalities to the specific misidentification element and hypothesizes a complex interaction of cortex, limbic system and basal ganglia in generating Capgras and related DMS phenomena. Some years ago, the present author proposed a complementary theory to explain the delusions of paranoia (Munro 1982a), and more recently suggested a complex brain system whose malfunctioning would result in delusions, the nature and content of which would be determined by the specific site within the system at which abnormal activity was taking place.

I would suggest that these four disorders—delusional disorder, paraphrenia, paranoid schizophrenia and the misidentification syndromes (especially the first and last)—hang together better than they hang separately, and that they have greater similarities to each other than to other psychiatric illnesses. It is my hope that increasingly specific research will provide worthwhile back-up evidence for this assertion. However, for the moment 'delusional disorder' denotes one particular condition which will now be described.

Delusional disorder and its subtypes

As already mentioned, the essential element of this illness is the presence of a stable and well-defined delusional system which is 'encapsulated' from a relatively normal-functioning personality. The normal personality and the individual's way of life, however, become more and more overwhelmed by the dominating effect of the delusional beliefs. In many instances, the person's entire waking existence is spent dwelling, or acting upon, these delusions. Hallucinations (auditory, olfactory, coenaesthetic, etc.) may be present but are usually not prominent and are often difficult to distinguish from delusional misinterpretations or illusions (Munro 1982b).

The illness seems to affect males and females approximately equally, though data are sparse, and the age of onset can be from adolescence to extreme old age. There is some evidence that males may be at risk of earlier initiation. Many patients are unmarried, separated, divorced or widowed and the premorbid personality is said to be isolative and asocial. Even so, the condition is sometimes—perhaps often—compatible with marriage and continued employment, although many of these individuals are noted to be eccentric or fanatical.

Although it may fluctuate in intensity from time to time, delusional disorder is a very chronic condition and appears permanent in many cases. In some patients, it is possible that a long and insidious onset may result in the mimicking of a Cluster A personality disorder (e.g. paranoid, schizoid or schizotypal personality disorder), but significant premorbid personality abnormalities do seem common (Berner *et al.* 1984). Men especially appear to have a previous history of substance abuse or head-injury, suggesting the possibility of a subtle underlying organic brain abnormality in these patients.

Onset may be gradual or acute. In either instance, the patient may identify, sometimes vehemently, a precipitating factor which is difficult to confirm or deny. (For instance, patients with infestation delusions who respond well to treatment may continue to insist, 'But I *did* have scabies to begin with!') Some individuals successfully keep their delusions hidden or even utilize them: for example, grandiose apocalyptic beliefs may fit very well with the views of certain extreme religious sects, and one suspects that a small minority of the most persistent and intrusive 'community activists' are driven by delusional fervour. Other people become prominent by acting out their delusions, sometimes colliding with the authorities as a result. Erotomanic 'stalking' of women is an increasingly publicized example of such antisocial behaviour (Zona *et al.* 1993).

One of the most unique and striking features of delusional disorder is the way in which the patient can move between delusional and normal modes of thought and behaviour (Munro 1995). In the former, the individual is overalerted, preoccupied with the delusional ideas, and gives a sense of being remorselessly driven. In contrast, the normal mode is associated with relatively calm mood, reasonable range of affect, neutral conversation with an ability to be engaged in everyday topics, and some capacity for pursuit of normal activities. But the delusional beliefs are always hovering in the wings, ready to pounce and to change the person's whole attitude and demeanour. A comparison with Dr Jekyll and Mr Hyde is not totally inappropriate.

In the delusional mode, thought form is relatively normal but the abnormal thought content predominates and is associated with profound illogicality. However, the individual may be capable of marked focusing of attention and, since he or she is constantly rehearsing his or her delusional beliefs, is often able to present them forcefully and convincingly. There is no effective insight and because a delusion is held with extraordinary conviction, any attempt at contradiction is met with anger and disdain, the latter reflecting some degree of grandiosity in many cases.

Subtypes of delusional disorder are based on the particular delusional content. Historically, cases of psychiatric disorder have often been classified according to their delusional content: this is generally unacceptable, since patients with schizophrenia, severe depression, early dementia and delusional disorder may all, for example, present with similar unfounded hypochondriacal complaints. Nevertheless, once a diagnosis of delusional disorder has been made, it is legitimate to describe subcategories: in DSM-IV and ICD-10, erotomanic, grandiose, jealous, persecutory and somatic themes are distinguished. In addition, DSM-IV allows for the possibility of more than one theme existing in an individual patient—for example, erotomanic and persecutory delusions being intertwined.

Within the subcategories, further subsets can occur. For instance, the somatic (hypochondriacal) subtype includes delusions of skin infestation, of dysmorphia or of emitting a foul odour: in the persecutory subtype a proportion of the individuals becomes increasingly litigious.

Other delusional contents may occur but appear to be relatively rare. It is interesting that the repertoire of delusional beliefs in delusional disorder/paranoia is fairly limited. Some authors insist that the delusions in this illness should be 'non-bizarre'; i.e. although false, the beliefs could possibly be true (Flaum *et al.* 1991). This is a highly subjective and not very useful distinction but perhaps the number of delusional topics in delusional disorder is somewhat limited because the patient is sufficiently aware of reality to reject truly bizarre beliefs.

Certainly there is more contact with reality than in most other psychotic conditions because the patient is only partially 'insane'. It is almost pathognomonic of the disorder that the individual refuses to see a psychiatrist (Munro 1982a). Partly that seems to be the result of his incontrovertible belief in his delusions which to him are totally factual and therefore do not need any meddling from an interfering 'shrink'. He will more than readily visit a cosmetic surgeon if he thinks his physical appearance is abnormal or a lawyer if he thinks his colleagues are persecuting him, but great pressure usually has to be put on him before a psychiatric consultation can take place. But, apart from the delusional rejection of any psychiatric aetiology, there also seems to be in many cases some degree of non-delusional awareness that exposure to a psychiatrist may pose a threat to his belief system. This betokens some 'normal' insight but unfortunately it gets in the way of the patient's receiving appropriate help.

We will now go on to consider the subtypes of delusional disorder. The delusional content decides which societal area and which type of agency the patient comes in contact with, either voluntarily or involuntarily. That, in turn, often dictates the context within which the psychiatrist, if involved, has to work. Naturally, there will be differences in the way in which cases will be handled: for example, one patient may have to be seen in a forensic psychiatric setting, having already passed through law-enforcement and judicial processes, because he attacked his wife in a jealous frenzy, whereas another patient has been referred from a dermatological clinic to a psychiatric clinic in the same hospital for a diagnostic assessment. Whatever the administrative process, if a delusional disorder is diagnosed, then the illness form is relatively constant whatever the context and despite the profound differences in delusional content from patient to patient. The psychiatrist should be skilled at recognizing the illness form despite the confounding variables because the treatment approach depends on that. Essentially, the treatment is the same whatever the actual nature of the delusional belief.

Delusional disorder: the subtypes

Certain of these (e.g. somatic and persecutory subtypes) are better documented than others but there is no worthwhile evidence as to the relative frequencies of the different delusional presentations.

SOMATIC (HYPOCHONDRIACAL) SUBTYPE

Especially in the European literature, the term 'monosymptomatic hypochondriacal psychosis' (MHP; Munro 1982a) is often used to describe patients in this category. It is probably best to regard that term as obsolete and to use as an alternative the DSM-IV description, 'delusional disorder, somatic subtype'; however, the two are interchangeable.

The commonest forms of presentation are as follows.

Delusions of infestation

These are very well known to dermatologists who differentiate them from non-delusional psychiatric cases with rather similar symptoms (Lyell 1983). There are variations on the theme as follows.

1 A sensation of insects crawling over the skin. In some cases the patient claims to see the insects which may be immobile or active. Sometimes the descriptions are graphic but usually seem to be delusional misinterpretations rather than the result of visual hallucinations.

2 A complaint of worms or other creatures burrowing under the skin. The subcutaneous movements of small muscles (NB 'muscle' literally means 'a small mouse') are shown as evidence of the creatures' activities.

3 A conviction that there are foreign bodies (often described as 'like seeds') under the skin, which many patients feel compelled to dig out, thereby producing multiple excoriations. One patient of this type in the author's experience was covered in sores except between the shoulder blades, the only area she could not reach.

It is not uncommon for patients with infestation delusions to produce 'evidence' and to demand confirmation of their belief by microscopic examination. The evidence usually turns out to be skin scales or small pieces of mucus, brought in a matchbox in the UK but more often in a pill-bottle in North America.

In some cases of delusional infestation the picture is complicated by ony-chotillomania, and the damaged nails and the hair-loss are, of course, further confirmation in the patient's mind of their hypochondriacal belief. Also, in some cases, patients will use bizarre 'treatments' of their own devising, such as the use of severe heat or of caustic substances on the skin, at times causing severe lesions.

Delusions of emitting a foul odour

In these cases the patient may appear to have an olfactory hallucination since he or she can describe the odour in detail. In other individuals there is no actual perception of a bad smell but they 'know' it exists because other people show evident disgust or avoidance behaviour. There is usually a defi-nite opinion about the origin of the smell: in most instances it is either attrib-uted to leakage of flatus from the bowel (when the patient demands to see a gastroenterologist) or to abnormalities in the sweat (when he or she insists on attending a dermatologist). A subgroup of patients complain of halitosis, and are often referred to dentists or ears, nose and throat (ENT) specialists. (Another small sample of patients is also known to dentists because of a delusional belief in having an abnormal dental bite for which never-ending orthodontic treatment is demanded.)

Dysmorphic delusion

The patient believes mistakenly that he or she is grossly ugly or misshapen, usually despite all evidence to the contrary. (In some cases there may be some abnormality but the patient's complaint and incessant demands for treat-ment are out of all proportion to its severity.) Such individuals besiege cos-metic and plastic surgeons demanding treatment, sometimes threatening litigation if they do not get it. The usual view in medical circles is that surgery should be avoided in these patients since it rarely satisfies them and there are often demands for more and more procedures, but a few cases may actually benefit from operative intervention (Pruzinsky 1988). Unfortunately, it is very difficult to select out these particular cases.

Sometimes a plastic procedure will lead to bad results (such as keloid scars) and this, of course, serves to redouble the patient's complaints and importunings.

Other somatic delusional complaints

These are much less common, but there have been scattered reports of patients with monodelusional symptoms such as a conviction that one is spreading an infectious disease or that one has contracted a venereal disease (with, nowadays, acquired immune deficiency syndrome (AIDS) becoming the most favoured sexually transmitted disease). A small subgroup of anorexia nervosa patients with particularly outrageous body-image distortion may have a delusional misperception, and some individuals with complaints of severe, unremitting pain without apparent cause may have a hypochondriacal delusion. A few apparent transsexuals who make demands for mutilating operations may also be deluded. (Those who mutilate themselves extensively are more likely to be schizophrenic.)

Case Nos 3.2 and 3.3 illustrate differing hypochondriacal contents in patients with delusional disorder.

Case No. 3.2: Smell delusion

A 42-year-old unmarried man was admitted to a psychiatric in-patient unit saying that if he did not get help he would kill himself. He said that, 6 months previously, he had become convinced he was emitting an unpleasant smell. He himself had never noticed the smell but he knew it was there because workmates had started to avoid him, look at him oddly and make sotto voce comments about him. The patient believed the smell was due to leakage of flatus from his bowel and he had attended several gastroenterologists who were unable to find a physical problem and could not help him. His family physician had prescribed a benzodiazepine with no benefit. The patient now spent virtually all his time at home, hiding from other people, and could not even visit his local tavern because he felt that people there were also watching him and showing disgust.

He had always been rather solitary, but there was no previous or family history of psychiatric illness. He had had chronic mastoiditis as a child, had a significant head injury at the age of 32, and had been a heavy drinker for many years though he now drank moderately. At the time of admission to hospital he was distressed, anxious and unhappy, but not clinically depressed. He had a single, fixed, unshakable delusion about giving off a smell which was not apparent to anyone else, but his general personality appeared virtually unimpaired. His physical health was normal.

Several phenothiazines were initiated but provided no benefit. Then pimozide was started and the delusion rapidly faded. The patient became much happier and after discharge he returned to normal activities. Five months later his delusion returned apparently because he had stopped his medication: when it was restarted the delusion again disappeared and he felt well. Over the next 3 years he continued to do well except that he had two episodes of postpsychotic depression which required antidepressant treatment concomitant with the antipsychotic treatment. When last seen he remained on pimozide and a maintenance tricyclic antidepressant under the care of his family physician.

Case No. 3.3: Dysmorphic delusion

Information on this patient is limited because of his marked secretiveness. He was a young man, aged 20 and unmarried. He was referred for a psychiatric opinion by a plastic surgeon who was becoming alarmed at the patient's importunate demands for cosmetic surgery. Ever since childhood he had been a 'loner' and at the age of 15, he had become totally convinced that people were looking at his nose and his whole life became centred on this belief. He began to demand corrective surgery, although there was no obvious abnormality and finally, at age 18, he had a cosmetic rhinoplasty. He was pleased for about a year, then began to be haunted again by the belief that his appearance was odd, but this time he thought his neck was unduly long. For the past year he had been making demands for operations on an increasingly frustrated surgeon who repeatedly told him his request was impossible, but without effect.

The patient would not permit us to obtain collateral information from relatives, and the family history of psychiatric illness was uncertain. His physical health was normal and his physical appearance was in no way unusual. Apart from his one unshakeable hypochondriacal belief, the patient's mental state appeared normal, although several observers commented on a slight, undefinable oddness of manner. He denied any abuse of alcohol or drugs at any time.

He had been treated with a benzodiazepine with absolutely no effect and somewhat reluctantly agreed to take a neuroleptic. After approximately 2 weeks he felt more cheerful, said he still felt his neck was overlong but thought he could defer surgery for the time being, and was able to concentrate much more on mental topics. He did not wish psychiatric follow-up, but was referred back to his family physician with a recommendation that the neuroleptic be continued.

It will be noted that both these individuals were solitary people who developed single hypochondriacal concerns for which no underlying causes could be found. In both cases distress was very marked and demands for help were increasingly importunate. The older man had a previous (but not recent) history of alcohol abuse and had had a serious head injury in the past. Information on the younger patient was sparse, but neither substance abuse nor head injury seemed to be factors in his case. The family history of psychiatric illness was negative in one and uncertain in the other. The older man developed his illness at age 41, the younger possibly in his mid-teens.

Despite the detail differences and the different delusional contents, both patients were regarded as suffering from delusional disorder and both responded rapidly and well to neuroleptic treatment. The patient with the smell delusion suffered two bouts of postpsychotic depressive illness while under treatment and this phenomenon will be mentioned later.

PERSECUTORY SUBTYPE

In this, the archetypal presentation of classical paranoia, the patient develops severe delusions of reference, is convinced that the environment is threatening towards him or her, and may become certain that certain individuals or organizations are pursuing him or her. These may be specifically identified or may remain as 'them'. These patients show the phenomenon of 'centrality': they are often aware that there is no logical reason for the persecution and cannot explain why they have been picked out—they often indeed acknowledge that they are not important enough for this. Yet they remain convinced that the persecution exists and is becoming increasingly elaborate, and can shrug off the fact that such an operation must cost inordinate amounts of money, and the equal fact that, despite continual surveillance and threat, they are unharmed. An element of grandiosity enters here, making it possible for the patient to accept that such unlikely things are happening.

Case No. 3.1 illustrates one such presentation, in this case an elderly lady of very rigid personality type who developed mild incontinence after an operation and who developed an elaborate delusional system thereafter. It seems likely that the incontinence provided the content of her delusional beliefs, but in our present state of knowledge there is nothing in her history to tell us why she developed her delusional illness or why it occurred at the time it did.

A variation on the persecutory subtype occurs when the individual goes to court seeking redress for imagined wrongs, often presenting his case in an overintensive, unbalanced way, and quite possibly ignoring his lawyer's advice when that runs counter to his own agenda. When he loses, as he frequently does, he is distressed but undiscouraged, and straightaway goes on to reopen his case. In Case No. 3.4, the man who is the constant plaintiff can afford to hire lawyers to represent him, and can spend much of his time in court. Less well-endowed individuals with this type of delusionally impelled behaviour may be undeterred by lack of affluence and may be a considerable cost to the legal aid system.

Case No. 3.4: Litigious paranoia

A single man of 32 received a parking ticket some 5 years ago. He had never had any sort of trouble with the authorities before and had always led a very circumscribed, law-abiding life. He was enraged at being accused of a parking offence and insisted on going to court to plead not guilty. When it was pointed out to him that he certainly was guilty, he tried to argue the point with the magistrate and had to be led from the court, still arguing.

Since then he has consulted several lawyers and has persuaded a small number to pursue his case: usually he never reaches court but whether or not he does, he always loses. This does not in the least discourage him. When questioned, he will admit that originally he parked his car longer than was allowed, but he then produces a series of convoluted arguments as to why he should not have been found guilty. Any attempt to argue with him is met with scorn and derision.

He has led a kind of double life for several years, continuing to work efficiently as an office clerk though with a reputation for being self-absorbed and unsociable. After hours he spends all his time reading legal texts and drawing up complicated proposals for further legislation. He has been warned by one judge that he may be charged with mischief for wasting the court's time, but is totally undeterred. He has spent very large sums of money despite having a modest income.

Attempts have been made to obtain a psychiatric assessment which he has always spurned. A mutual acquaintance arranged for the author to meet with the patient relatively informally, making no secret of the former's profession. The patient was amiable enough but refused to discuss his legal case, hinting that it was at an important stage and therefore sub judice. On other topics he appeared at ease and showed no obvious mental abnormality. He declined any psychiatric help. So far as is known, he still continues to pursue his case.

EROTOMANIC SUBTYPE

This subtype is sometimes known as de Clérambault's syndrome (Segal 1989), in which the deluded individual is convinced that some other person is deeply in love with him or her (also see Chapter 7). In textbooks it is said that the other person (who is usually totally unaware of the situation) is most often someone who is prominent in society, and that does occur. However, quite often the other person is an ordinary citizen who, for some reason, arouses deep feelings in the patient. At one time the disorder was regarded as being restricted to lonely middle-aged spinsters (Retterstol & Opjordsmoen 1991), but in fact it can affect both sexes and all ages. The feelings are generally heterosexual but in a proportion of cases are homosexual.

Many of the patients never make any contact with the other individual and they often have unlikely rationalizations as to why the other does not contact them. Sometimes they write letters or tape-record messages, but do not send them. On the other hand, there are those who act out their fantasies and men seem more likely to do this than women (Buchanan 1993). They may follow the other person, and some of them become 'stalkers' (Zona *et al.* 1993). They may confront the other person and demand to know why he or she does not declare feelings of love, frequently to the very considerable astonishment of the person confronted. Occasionally they will display anger and even violence towards him or her: this can be very frightening, as the patient is undeterred by denial of any love-feelings, by rational argument or even by legal deterrent.

In Case No. 3.5, the patient was a middle-aged woman, but equally could have been a male, young or old. She found it impossible to communicate her feelings to anyone, either the victim or her husband, and chose to attempt suicide as a way out of her unremitting distress. It should be noted that she was not clinically depressed, but in all the subtypes of delusional disorder, the illness is so persistent and insistent that many of the patients become extremely anxious, unhappy and chronically desperate and this wretchedness may persist for many years, indeed permanently.

Case No. 3.5: Erotomania

A married but childless woman of 62 took a small overdose and was psychiatrically assessed in the Emergency department after she had been physically cleared. At first she was very reluctant to discuss her problems, but finally told a female psychiatrist that she had taken the overdose in desperation because she was afraid a male elder in her church was trying to break up her longstanding marriage. She said that, about a year before, she became aware that when he was greeting her and her husband at the church door, the elder was showing much more interest in her than he should. This had steadily got worse, but her husband did not notice and she could not broach the subject with him or with the man himself.

She found herself becoming increasingly anxious as each Sunday approached. The elder never said anything specific to her, but she knew by his manner that he was sexually propositioning her. She felt that if the rest of the congregation learned about this she would be condemned as a 'loose woman' and this preyed on her mind continuously. Finally, in her distress, she decided suicide was the only way out. However, at interview she had no clinical symptoms of depression. She was very anxious, cognition and memory were normal, and she was totally preoccupied with her problem. She denied herself having any feelings of attraction towards the man in question.

She gave permission for her husband to be interviewed and when he heard the story for the first time, he ridiculed the possibility that the elder had any secret intentions towards his wife. Apparently he was a very elderly individual in poor physical health: an independent source of information later confirmed that the husband's attitude was almost certainly correct.

The patient proved to be very compliant with treatment and accepted a neuroleptic drug which rapidly reduced her distress and then her preoccupation. After 2 months she continued to do well and was referred back to her family physician for continuing treatment.

JEALOUSY SUBTYPE

Pathological jealousy need not be delusional, but in this form the individual's belief is fixed, often associated with passionate feelings including intense anger, and is not amenable to discussion or reasonable disproof. The suspicions are usually fixed on the sexual partner (heterosexual or homosexual) and tend to escalate, making his or her life an increasing misery. Unrelenting accusations are made, violence is common and murder is not unknown.

The deluded individual will often seek for 'proof' of his suspicions, searching repeatedly for such things as seminal stains on clothing, lipstick smears, love bites and so on. He or she may follow the victim who, in any case, dare not be out of sight for fear of repeated accusations. In one case in the author's experience the husband would even tape his wife's slippers to the floor at night, and then accuse her if he thought they had been moved to the slightest degree.

The accused person is often afraid to leave because of threats that he or she will be followed and coerced to return. Not surprisingly, some of them become housebound because they simply cannot face the stress of being bombarded with accusations or being assaulted when they return from even the briefest of outings. Case No. 3.6 demonstrates some typical aspects.

Case No. 3.6: Jealousy

A married woman of 39 sought psychiatric help because of severe anxiety symptoms. At the first interview she was very guarded but subsequently poured out a story with great intensity, the burden of which was that her husband had been frequently and flagrantly unfaithful to her for at least 3 years. She said that he totally denied her accusations but she knew from his manner that he was an insatiable lecher.

The husband reported that, for the past 4 or 5 years, he had increasingly had to restrict his life-style because of his wife's belief in his infidelity, which he totally denied. Each morning when he arrived at work he had to telephone her to say that he was there, then she had to telephone back to confirm that he actually was at work. If his arrival was delayed to the slightest extent she would harangue him endlessly. She would repeatedly call him during the day to check on him and he had to phone her just before he left his office. He took sandwiches for lunch so that he could not be accused of having assignations, though he said his wife accused him anyway. At weekends he spent all his time with his wife, and he had given up all social activities in which she was not involved. Despite all of this—and he gave the impression of being extraordinarily tolerant—she continued to accuse him, often in an unpleasant and sometimes public way. From time to time she had physically attacked him. He said that their two children, aged 15 and 12, were becoming very distressed with their mother's behaviour. At first they had believed her but no longer did.

When asked why he put up with her behaviour the husband said the patient had been an extraordinarily pleasant person, quiet and shy but with a sense of humour. She came from a family with severe alcoholism problems and she herself had abused alcohol and drugs as a teenager, but had not done so since her marriage. On occasions when she was somewhat less agitated, he said that even now there were glimpses of her normal personality and although she never retreated on her accusations, she sometimes expressed regret for upsetting him and the children.

The patient continued to believe in her husband's infidelity, but accepted neuroleptic medication because she was afraid her marriage might break up if she did not do something. After several weeks the abnormal beliefs were considerably mitigated but did not completely disappear. Both husband and wife said life was now tolerable and she agreed to continue taking a maintenance dose of her medication.

GRANDIOSE SUBTYPE

One of the first psychiatric patients the present author saw as a medical student was an elderly lady who had been in hospital for almost 50 years, who was penniless and yet believed that she owned the city in which she lived. She also believed that her psychiatrist was her financial agent and she could discuss her 'business affairs' in what at first appeared to be a sensible and reasonable manner. Although I knew the facts of her case, in my inexperience I found it very hard not to believe her as she was talking about her supposed wealth and influence and many years later she still stands out in my memory. She was suffering from 'grandiose paranoia' and was in no way manic. Her condition was extremely chronic and was totally unchanged by the limited treatments of the time.

Psychiatrists see relatively few patients with grandiose delusional disorder. In the first instance the patient is usually happy, so why would he want to see a psychiatrist whose aim would be to make him less happy? It is usually only if the individual acts out his delusion in a way that offends society (e.g. spending money he does not possess, interfering inappropriately in public affairs, or promulgating apocalyptic ideas which interfere with societal mores or behaviours) that he will come to attention, and may possibly be required to undergo psychiatric examination. In a few cases, the person does no harm but is so wrapped up in his grandiose beliefs that he completely loses touch with reality and neglects himself, thereby ending up in an institution.

It is fascinating how such patients can ignore the incongruity of their delusions and the incompatibility of their deluded state with their actual circumstances, something which has been described as mental double-book-keeping. This is particularly true when one observes the patient in his or her 'normal' mode when conversation can be perfectly mundane.

A frightening possibility in grandiose delusional disorder is that some individuals may act out their delusions within malignant cults or extreme religious sects in which violence and even terrorism may play a part.

Case No. 3.7: Grandiosity

The patient was a young married woman who had had a very abusive and emotionally deprived childhood. During her adolescence she had severe eating problems, both anorexia and bulimia, and although these were less marked now, they still recurred to some extent under stress. Her marriage had obviously been a flight from her highly dysfunctional family and she had impossible expectations of her husband. There appeared to be real affection between them but there were sexual problems and frequent quarrels, often generated when she felt she was not being shown affection. She had no history of alcohol or drug abuse and her physical health was good.

Gradually, over a period of about a year, she became increasingly convinced without evidence that her husband was heavily abusing drugs. Then she began to believe that he was trading in drugs, first locally then eventually internationally. Finally she was convinced that he was a drug czar with connections worldwide, and because his work involved some travel she was sure that he was meeting contacts or collecting consignments of drugs when he was away from home. The husband's behaviour gave rise to no obvious cause for suspicion, but ultimately she was repeatedly telephoning Interpol, the FBI and other crime agencies to report on her husband's movements. Presumably she got no confirmation from these organizations but this did not deter her.

Her husband eventually persuaded her to have a psychiatric assessment. At interview she was restless, exalted and grandiose, but otherwise she had none of the features of mania. When she was persuaded to talk about a neutral topic she was much calmer and relatively reasonable, but inevitably returned to her preoccupation, when her restlessness and exaltation returned. She could not be persuaded her beliefs were wrong but rather surprisingly accepted neuroleptic medication. Her delusions rapidly resolved, her mood settled to normal and she developed reasonably good insight.

Interestingly, about 3 years after treatment was initiated, she said on one occasion, 'Life was never so interesting as when I was crazy!'

As an aside, it should be noted that in the seven cases presented in this chapter, outcome is good in four, fair in two and poor in one (who refused treatment). This is not inconsistent with overall treatment results in delusional disorder (Munro & Mok 1995) and should dispel undue gloominess about therapeutic responsiveness in this illness, a point that will be re-emphasized when treatment is considered in more detail. Persuading the patient to comply with therapy is possibly the greatest challenge for the psychiatrist who wishes to treat delusional disorder.

Non-delusional illnesses which may mimic delusional disorder

Earlier, we have considered other illnesses characterized by delusions which have to be distinguished from paranoia. It is also important to mention other, non-delusional disorders which may bear a superficial resemblance to some of the subtypes of delusional disorder.

The most important of these is body dysmorphic disorder (BDD), an illness formerly known as dysmorphophobia, which is now an obsolete term (Munro & Stewart 1991). BDD is a chronic, non-psychotic somatoform disorder in which there is a persistent subjective belief of bodily abnormality. The patient is convinced that the abnormality is obvious to others: in some cases a relatively minor physical abnormality does exist but this is totally insufficient to warrant the serious concern shown by the sufferers. The complaint is usually very specific and there is intense importuning for care from the specialists perceived by the patient as appropriate.

The appearances are very like those of delusional disorder, somatic subtype, but the complaint is not delusional: rather, it takes the form of an overvalued idea. It has been suggested that BDD has features similar to obsessive-compulsive disorder, a similarity enhanced by the response of both illnesses to serotonergic antidepressants. Certain workers have claimed that a minority of BDD cases may temporarily become psychotic and in this state may be indistinguishable from cases of delusional disorder (McElroy *et al.* 1993; Phillips & McElroy 1993). The present author has argued that this is not the case, since the descriptions are more suggestive of brief psychotic episodes and the patients appear to respond to serotonergic antidepressants, whereas delusional disorder cases appear to improve only with neuroleptic drugs. Nevertheless, in our present state of knowledge we cannot be certain that a spectrum from BDD to the somatic subtype of delusional disorder does not exist and the topic is worthy of more focused research.

Other forms of somatoform disorder, notably somatization disorder and conversion disorder, may also superficially resemble delusional disorder, somatic subtype. As has been mentioned, a small number of apparent cases of eating disorder may actually be suffering from delusional disorder, but true eating disorder cases may present with beliefs about physical appearance that are so bizarre that it is easy to mistake them for delusions. Careful history-taking and differential diagnosis are essential here.

Equally, some cases of obsessive-compulsive disorder may have extremely persistent, quasi-delusional thoughts and fears regarding cleanliness, imagined physical illness, infidelity fears and so on. Usually, however, the patient has insight and resists the thoughts while, in contrast, delusional disorder patients are in total consonance with their beliefs.

From time to time there are reports of pathological jealousy of non-psychotic type (Stein *et al.* 1994). The jealousy may be exceedingly severe and lead to profound limiting behaviour and even aggression towards the sexual partner. An obsessional element may again be important here.

Finally, certain personality disorders can have features reminiscent of delusional disorder, especially the paranoid, schizoid and schizotypal varieties. In these, patients can show features such as suspiciousness, ideas of reference, isolated and withdrawn behaviour, highly eccentric beliefs (e.g. about health and non-traditional treatments), marked interpersonal difficulties and difficulty with reality-testing. Despite all of these, the patients are not psychotic and their ideas are not delusional.

It is extremely important to make careful diagnostic distinctions since it is rarely appropriate to prescribe neuroleptic drugs to any of the foregoing disorders. In fact, it has been the present author's unfortunate experience in the past to have to rediagnose several cases labelled as 'paranoid' or 'delusional' illness who were actually suffering from obsessive-compulsive disorder. The unhappiest aspect of this was that all of the patients had been prescribed long-term neuroleptics and some of them had developed tardive dyskinesia.

Treatment aspects of delusional disorders

When psychiatry lost interest in Kraepelinian paranoia in the first half of the present century, there were no specific treatments for it (or for most other psychiatric illnesses either). Subsequently, if the disorder was mentioned at all it was usually dubbed untreatable. Now that delusional disorder has been rehabilitated, this pessimistic attitude still often prevails, which is unfortunate. The illness proves to be readily treatable, the greatest limiting factor being the difficulty in getting many patients to comply with medication.

In 1975, the present author and a colleague reported on the successful response of five cases of monosymptomatic hypochondriacal psychosis (i.e. delusional disorder, somatic subtype) to a diphenylbutylpiperidine neuroleptic, pimozide (Riding & Munro 1975). Since then many, mostly anecdotal, reports have appeared in the world literature, describing the treatment of this subtype with psychotropic drugs, pimozide being the commonest drug of first choice. More recently, reports on the treatment of jealousy, erotomanic and persecutory subtypes have also started to appear. Unfortunately, the literature is very scattered and often difficult to interpret, but there is a growing consensus that treatment is frequently successful.

The present author and a colleague recently reviewed approximately 1000 articles on paranoia/delusional disorder, the earliest from 1961 but the great majority from 1980 onwards, and we were eventually able to report on treatment in 209 cases (Munro & Mok 1995). Prior to 1980, a variety of neuroleptics was used in treatment but since then pimozide has become the most popular medication. We found that, combining results from all the neuroleptic drugs, 52.6% of patients were regarded as recovered and 28.2% were reported as having partially recovered: in other words, 80.8% of patients made a complete or partial recovery from this severe, chronic and reputedly 'untreatable' disorder. Of the 19.2% of patients who showed no improvement, a proportion failed to respond because they covertly or overtly failed to take their medication.

Comparison of efficacy of pimozide with other neuroleptics indicated that pimozide had a significant advantage. This has to be accepted with caution since the reports on the other neuroleptics tended to be older and less detailed, but three small-scale drug trials do seem to support pimozide's effectiveness and it is interesting that many dermatologists now use it to treat cases of delusional parasitosis.

There is a great need for more systematic treatment studies in delusional disorder but the exciting news is that, if one can persuade the patient to accept the appropriate treatment, the outcome results are at least as good as in any other major psychiatric disorder. Not only that, recovery is very complete in many cases and residual disability is often minimal. Unfortunately, medication does not cure the condition and the majority of patients have to be maintained indefinitely on neuroleptic treatment.

One point to add: in a proportion of cases (12% in the author's own series; Munro 1982a) of treated delusional disorder the patient develops a significant degree of postpsychotic depression. This is analogous to the postschizophrenic depression which DSM-IV mentions but does not classify.

It is important to recognize this phenomenon, as the depression may be of severe degree and is apparently not simply a side-effect of the psychotropic medication. Treatment is by administration of an antidepressant in adequate dosage in addition to the neuroleptic.

Folie à deux

Before bringing this chapter to its conclusion it is important to introduce this phenomenon which may accompany illnesses like delusional disorder, schizophrenia and major mood disorder (Sacks 1988). This is discussed in detail by Hughes and Sims in Chapter 8. It has been known by a variety of names (currently 'shared psychotic disorder' in DSM-IV and 'induced delusional disorder' in ICD-10), it used to be regarded as rare but is not: for example, the present author found nine instances in relation to 50 cases of delusional disorder (Munro 1982a).

Folie à deux occurs when mental symptoms, usually delusions, are communicated from a fanatically insistent psychiatrically ill individual to another individual, who accepts them as true. Obviously the individuals are usually closely associated and social isolation is common. The content of the transmitted belief varies from case to case, and one may see shared delusions of persecution, of grandeur or of physical abnormality.

The majority of individuals who adopt another's delusional beliefs are not themselves psychotic, despite the implications in the DSM-IV and ICD-10 names. They tend to be impressionable people who accept the delusions as the result of long and overclose association with the primary patient. Social isolation reduces the opportunity for reality-input and reality-testing. In this type of case the so-called '*folie imposée*' will usually fade spontaneously when the two people are separated or if the primary patient is successfully treated. It is usually inappropriate to treat the secondary case with anti-psychotic medication unless the beliefs there have also evolved into delusions (a phenomenon known as *folie simultanée*) (Lazarus 1985).

In some instances, treatment of the situation may be very difficult. If the primary individual refuses medication, it is not uncommon for the secondary individual to collude and equally to resist help. Much time and tact may be required to deal with this. (Treatment is discussed in Chapter 8.)

Folie à deux is often overlooked and physicians may be extremely perplexed if a patient expresses ideas which seem clearly delusional but which are supported by a seemingly rational relative. As an example, the present author had to deal with a patient who wrongly believed that he emitted a foul smell (see Case No. 3.2). To the dismay of staff, his two sisters insisted that he did indeed give off a bad smell: they seemed good witnesses, and we wondered whether we were mistaken about the nature of the case. Eventually, after careful questioning, both sisters agreed that neither had ever experienced the smell, but said that they fully believed their brother because he was always such an honest man. When a doctor doubts his clinical judgement in a circumstance like this, it may lead to much unnecessary investigation and inappropriate treatment. Awareness of the condition can usually prevent this.

Conclusions

Kraepelin (1921), almost a century ago, clearly differentiated between mood disorders, delusional disorders, schizophrenia and organic brain disorders, although he recognized that all of these illnesses had certain features in common, including delusions. Nevertheless, he emphasized their individually distinctive characteristics as well as their different natural histories and outcomes. To an increasing extent we can add nowadays the differential responses to specific treatments. For many years after his time, the nosological scene in psychiatry was a desert, especially in the US, where diagnostic precision was largely swept away and virtually everything 'bizarre' became schizophrenic. Paranoia/delusional disorder, because of a superficial resemblance to schizophrenia, was confused with that illness and psychiatrists mostly ceased to be aware of it, though they still used terms like 'paranoia' and 'paranoid' without bothering to define them.

Schizophrenia, like Yugoslavia, is breaking up, and delusional disorder is one of the first disorders to secede from an overinclusive category. It is rewarding to see that the conceptualization and description of delusional disorder are now being advanced and it is safe to say that there is a fruitful field of research here for the coming generation. It is equally gratifying to report that treatment of this prolonged and wretched illness has assumed a much more optimistic aspect in the recent past.

References

American Psychiatric Association (1968) *Diagnostic and Statistical Manual of Mental Disorders*, 2nd edn (DSM-II). American Psychiatric Association, Washington, D.C.
American Psychiatric Association (1980) *Diagnostic and Statistical Manual of Mental Disorders*, 3rd edn (DSM-III). American Psychiatric Association, Washington, D.C.

American Psychiatric Association (1987) *Diagnostic and Statistical Manual of Mental Disorders*, 3rd edn, revised (DSM-III-R). American Psychiatric Association, Washington, D.C.

American Psychiatric Association (1994) *Diagnostic and Statistical Manual of Mental Disorders*, 4th edn (DSM-IV). American Psychiatric Association, Washington, D.C.

Berner, P., Gabriel, E., Kronberger, M.L. *et al.* (1984) Course and outcome of delusional psychoses. *Psychopathology* 17, 28–36.

Bleuler, E. (1950) *Dementia Praecox or the Group of Schizophrenias* (transl. J. Zinkin). International Universities Press, New York.

Buchanan, A. (1993) Acting on delusion: A review. *Psychological Medicine* 23, 123–134.

Cummings, J.L. (1985) Organic delusions: Phenomenology, anatomical correlations and review. *British Journal of Psychiatry* 146, 184–197.

Editorial (1980) Paranoia and immigrants. *British Medical Journal* 281, 1513–1514.

Ellis, H.D. & Young, A.W. (1990) Accounting for delusional misidentifications. *British Journal of Psychiatry* 157, 239–248.

Fish, F. (1962) *Schizophrenia*. J. Wright and Sons, Bristol.

Flaum, M., Arndt, S. & Andreasen, N.C. (1991) The reliability of 'bizarre' delusions. *Comprehensive Psychiatry* 32, 59–65.

Freud, S. (1950) *Aus den Anfängen der Psychoanalyse (1887–1902); Briefe au Wilhelm Fliess*. Fischer, Frankfurt.

Freud, S. (1958) The case of Schreber. In: *Complete Works* (ed. J. Strachey), Vol. 12, pp. 3–84. Hogarth Press, London.

Gregory, I. & Smeltzer, D.J. (1977) *Psychiatry*, pp. 186–187. Little, Brown & Co., Boston, Mass.

Houlihan, J.P. (1977) Heterogeneity among schizophrenic patients: Selective review of recent findings (1970–75). *Schizophrenia Bulletin* 3, 246–258.

Kendler, K.S. (1980) The nosologic validity of paranoia (simple delusional disorder). *Archives of General Psychiatry* 37, 699–706.

Kendler, K.S. (1984) Paranoia (delusional disorder): A valid psychiatric entity. *Trends in Neuroscience* 7, 14–17.

Kendler, K.S., Masterson, C.C., Davis, K.L. (1985) Psychiatric illness in first-degree relatives of patients with paranoid psychosis, schizophrenia and medical illness. *British Journal of Psychiatry* 147, 524–531.

Kolle, K. (1931) *Die Primäre Verücktheit: Psychopathologische, Klinische und Genealogische Untersuchungen*. Thieme, Leipzig.

Kraepelin, E. (1921/1976) *Manic Depressive Insanity and Paranoia* (transl. R.M. Barclay, ed. G.M. Robertson). Livingstone, Edinburgh; Arno Press, New York.

Lazarus, A. (1985) Folie à deux: Psychosis by association or genetic determinism? *Comprehensive Psychiatry* 26, 129–135.

Lewis, A. (1970) Paranoia and paranoid: A historical perspective. *Psychological Medicine* 1, 2–12.

Lidz, T. (1966) Adolf Meyer and the development of American psychiatry. *American Journal of Psychiatry* 123, 320–332.

Lyell, A. (1983) Delusions of parasitosis. *British Journal of Dermatology* 108, 485–499.

McAllister, T.W. (1992) Neuropsychiatric aspects of delusions. *Psychiatric Annals* **22**, 269–277.

McElroy, S.L., Phillips, K.A., Keck, P.E. *et al.* (1993) Body dysmorphic disorder: Does it have a psychotic subtype? *Journal of Clinical Psychiatry* **54**, 389–395.

Munro, A. (1982a) *Delusional Hypochondriasis.* Clarke Institute of Psychiatry Monograph Series, No. 5, Toronto.

Munro, A. (1982b) Paranoia revisited. *British Journal of Psychiatry* **141**, 344–349.

Munro, A. (1995) The classification of delusional disorders. *The Psychiatric Clinics of North America* **18**, 199–212.

Munro, A. & Mok, H. (1995) An overview of treatment in paranoia/delusional disorder. *Canadian Journal of Psychiatry* **40**, 616–622.

Munro, A. & Stewart, M. (1991) Body dysmorphic disorder and the DSM-IV: the demise of dysmorphophobia. *Canadian Journal of Psychiatry* **36**, 91–96.

Phillips, K.A. & McElroy, S.L. (1993) Insight, overvalued ideation and delusional thinking in body dysmorphic disorder: theoretical and treatment implications. *Journal of Nervous and Mental Disorders* **181**, 699–702.

Pruzinsky, T. (1988) Collaboration of plastic surgeon and medical psychotherapist: Elective cosmetic surgery. *Medical Psychotherapy* **1**, 1–13.

Retterstol, N. (1966) *Paranoid and Paranoiac Psychoses.* Thomas, Springfield, Ill.

Retterstol, N. & Opjordsmoen, S. (1991) Erotomania: Erotic self-reference psychosis in old maids. A long-term follow-up. *Psychopathology* **24**, 388–397.

Riding, J. & Munro, A. (1975) Pimozide in the treatment of monosymptomatic hypochondriacal psychosis. *Acta Psychiatrica Scandinavica* **52**, 23–30.

Sacks, M.H. (1988) Folie à deux. *Comprehensive Psychiatry* **29**, 270–277.

Segal, J.H. (1989) Erotomania revisited: From Kraepelin to DSMIII R. *American Journal of Psychiatry* **146**, 1261–1266.

Stein, D.J., Hollander, E. & Josephson, S.C. (1994) Serotonin reuptake blockers for the treatment of obsessional jealousy. *Journal of Clinical Psychiatry* **55**, 30–33.

Winokur, G. (1977) Delusional disorder (paranoia). *Comprehensive Psychiatry* **18**, 511–521.

World Health Organization (1967) *International Statistical Classification of Diseases*, 8th revision (ICD-8). World Health Organization, Geneva.

World Health Organization (1978) *International Statistical Classification of Diseases*, 9th revision (ICD-9). World Health Organization, Geneva.

World Health Organization (1992–1993) *The ICD-10 Classification of Mental and Behavioural Disorders.* World Health Organization, Geneva.

Zona, M.A., Sharma, K.K. & Lane, J. (1993) A comparative study of erotomanic and obsessional subjects in a forensic sample. *Journal of Forensic Sciences* **38**, 894–903.

CHAPTER 4

Reactive Psychoses

GABOR S. UNGVARI AND
PAUL E. MULLEN

Introduction

The concept of reactive psychosis was elaborated in European psychiatry. The core concept is of a state of severe disturbance in the mental state with an abrupt onset which usually lasts from a few days to a few weeks and which is resolved by a complete clinical recovery. As the name implies, the disorder emerges in the context of a stressful life situation to which the disorder can be understood as a reaction. The occurance of phenomenologically similar episodes without obviously stressful antecedents (as with the *bouffée délirante* of French psychiatry) has led to the propogation of terms which attempt to encompass both the reactive and spontaneous, such as the acute and transient psychotic disorders (ATPD) of ICD-10 (World Health Organization (WHO) 1992) and the brief psychotic disorder of DSM-IV (American Psychiatric Association (APA) 1994). These diagnostic groupings attempt to draw together reactive psychosis and a ragbag of descriptions of psychiatric episodes which share a sudden onset, dramatic symptomatology and rapid and complete resolution. This chapter will concern itself with those disorders which emerge as a reaction to life situations, most of which are of a type which would be markedly stressful to most people though some are threatening for the patient because of their highly personal import.

A couple of clinical examples at the outset may assist.

Case No. 4.1

A 19-year-old student presented at the emergency room in a distressed state. She was speaking rapidly and constantly repeating that something dreadful would happen to her. She had a perplexed air and was disorientated in time but not place. She reported auditory hallucinations accusing in nature. She was admitted and given night sedation. The next day she was less agitated but still expressing fears of being in danger though the source of the threat was ill defined. She was markedly self-referential and clearly puzzled by the meaning of even the most innocent remark or mundane occurrences. A history was obtained from her mother and later amplified by the patient.

She was an academically able young woman, though somewhat shy and oversensitive. She had become involved at university in a relationship with a fellow student who though reputedly talented was erratic and known to be abusing a range of drugs. She had become pregnant and, under pressure from the young man and her parents, had had an abortion 2 months previously. A week prior to her admission the young man had died as a result of what was presumed to be an accidental overdose of opiates. Prior to the admission, her parents had been astonished at how well she had coped with these events.

She remained hallucinated and self-referential over the next week but with a gradual decrease in the intensity of the distress and psychotic symptomatology. Ten days after admission, she showed no continuing abnormalities of mental state but was able to express understandable sadness and anger about the recent losses.

Brief psychotic episodes are encountered not infrequently in prison where vulnerable men and woman may be exposed to a threatening environment not mitigated by much support or sympathy.

Case No. 4.2

A 27-year-old man 3 years into a sentence for killing an acquaintance in a drunken brawl was transferred to a new prison. A rumour circulated that he was, in prison parlance, a 'dog'—that is, an informer. He knew none of his fellow prisoners. He was subjected to a campaign of silence during the day and the calling of threats at night after lock down. Two weeks after transfer, he refused to leave his cell at morning muster. He accused prison officers of having poisoned his food and, when approached, became violently resistive. On examination he described an elaborate plot against him involving prison authorities and a supposed prison drug ring (there may well have been a drug ring but not with the membership and characteristics of the one described by the patient). He believed gas was being surreptitiously pumped into his cell and his food poisoned. He described hearing conversations and orders being issued with reference to his execution. He was in a state of extreme agitation with a suspicious manner which erupted intermittently into denunciations of us for involvement in the plot. He was transferred to a psychiatric unit at a different prison. On arrival he immediately withdrew to a corner of his cell, remaining curled up but visibly alert. He was observed over a 24-hour period in which, though he rarely moved, he remained apparently awake with his eyes constantly darting around the room presumably searching for signs of danger. He was eventually induced to take medication. His state gradually resolved over the next 3 weeks but even when he accepted he was no longer the object of the murderous attentions of staff and fellow prisoners, he still remained uncertain whether at the outset there had not been an attempt to gas and poison him. He remained a rather suspicious individual who kept very much to himself, spending nearly all his waking hours working with a computer. Further enquiries revealed he had always been a shy, reclusive individual with no close friends and few if any social outlets.

Both the patients made a complete recovery and there were no known recurrences, the first patient being followed up for 3 years and the second seen intermittently over the term of his sentence and for some 18 months following release.

The precipitating life event in a reactive psychosis will usually have an appreciable bearing on the development, course and content of the ensuing psychosis. In the pathogenesis of the reactive psychosis, premorbid personality, life history and somatic predisposition are inextricably interwoven with the situation which has overwhelmed the individual. Reactive psychoses may occur in previously apparently healthy individuals or against the background of chronic somatic or psychiatric conditions, such as personality disorders or mental retardation. As with all major psychiatric disorders, the *psychogen* (psychologically generated), the *situagen* (the stressful life situation), and the *somatogen* ('extra-conscious' according to Jaspers, 1948/1963) mechanisms and their interconnections play a part in pathogenesis. The primary aetiologies in reactive psychoses are the situational and psychological elements with traumatic life events becoming pathogenic in such disorders primarily through the psychological vulnerabilities of the individual.

The undeniable weakness of the classical notion of reactive psychoses is the strong subjective component in their diagnosis since they are defined more on the basis of a causal hypothesis based on psychopathological principles (see sections on Jaspers and precipitating events) than by a set of easily identifiable symptoms. In fact, one of the major stumbling blocks hindering wider acceptance of reactive psychoses has been the difficulty in 'translating' the general psychopathological principles laid down by Jaspers into easily applicable clinical criteria.

Reactive psychoses lie at the crossroads of a number of unresolved theoretical and clinical problems in psychiatry including psychogenesis, the relationship between life events and psychosis, the concept of psychosis, the nature of vulnerability to psychosis and the nosological position of the so-called 'third psychosis'.

Since the inception of the term (Sommer 1894), the broad issues of psychogenesis and the role of life events in the genesis of psychoses have been extensively discussed in the literature. An exhaustive account from an historical perspective on psychogenesis can be found in Faergeman's (1963) monograph and Lewis' (1972) seminal paper. Psychogenesis has been interpreted from several viewpoints (Dahl 1987). In this chapter we follow Jaspers' standpoint because he laid the psychopathological foundation for constructing the concept of reactive psychoses. According to Jaspers (1913, 1948/1963), psychogenesis applies if a psychic reaction has its origin in experiences, it is rationally and emotionally understandable, and 'empathizable' without the aid of a specific theoretical construct such as, for instance, psychoanalysis.

In addition to the different interpretation of psychogenesis, the other reason for the discrepancy, and discontinuity, between classical and modern studies on reactive psychoses is the changing concept of psychosis in general. Current definitions tend to emphasize only impaired reality testing as manifested by delusions, hallucinations, disorganized speech or catatonic behaviour (Edgerton & Campbell 1994). This conceptualization is more restrictive than classical attempts to define the essence of psychosis which depended on notions of a disturbance in mental functioning severe enough to disrupt the continuity of the individual's customary way of experiencing and acting in their world (their praxis) (Dahl 1986). Jaspers' approach was even broader. He wrote: 'those psychic deviations which seize upon the individual *as a whole* are called psychoses . . . psychoses are mental and *affective illnesses*' (Jaspers 1948/1963, p. 575, emphasis added). Owing to the differences in conceptualizing psychosis, modern nosologies (e.g. ICD-10, DSM-IV), and even modern Scandinavian studies (e.g. Jorgensen 1985; Jorgensen & Jensen 1988), acknowledge only the paranoid forms of reactive psychosis, while excluding reactive emotional syndromes and those with disturbance of consciousness.

Most of the studies on reactive psychoses were conducted before modern methodological principles were introduced into psychiatric research. As a consequence, the findings reported are not always comparable to each other due to different sample selection and varying diagnostic criteria. The concept of a group of reactive psychoses did, however, emerge from the work of experienced clinicians struggling to come to terms with the clinical realities which they had to confront, rather than from systematic studies which pre-ordain the nature of the reality to be studied.

This chapter aims to provide a brief overview of the history and development of the concept of reactive psychoses and summarize the most important studies. For further details interested readers may consult a number of comprehensive reviews from the European (e.g. Faergeman 1963; Stromgren 1974, 1986; McCabe 1975; Degkwitz 1985; Dahl 1987; Retterstol 1987) and American perspectives (Stephens *et al.* 1982; Jauch & Carpenter 1988a, 1988b; Menuck *et al.* 1989; Remington *et al.* 1990).

There is some terminological confusion with respect to reactive psychoses mirroring differing scientific principles and clinical traditions. For example, 'constitutional psychoses' was a term employed when primacy was ceded to the aetiological role of disordered personality (Refsum & Astrup 1980), and psychogenic psychoses was used when placing emphasis on the psychological impact of the precipitating stress (Astrup *et al.* 1959). Nowadays most authorities agree that the rather neutral term of reactive psychoses is the most appropriate (e.g. Arentsen 1968; Stromgren 1986) which usage will be adhered to in this chapter. We prefer the plural psycho*ses* since we are dealing with a group of psychotic disturbances.

Notes on the conceptual history of reactive psychoses

Although there have been pioneering efforts (e.g. Faergeman 1963; Odegaard 1968; Lewis 1972; Stromgren 1974; Degkwitz 1985; Stromgren 1986; Dahl 1987; Retterstol 1987; Jauch & Carpenter 1988a, 1988b), the comprehensive conceptual history of reactive psychoses has yet to be written. Here we attempt only to outline the main trends of the development of the concept.

Jaspers (1913) and Wimmer (1916) are usually credited with establishing the category of reactive psychoses. This commonplace is, however, only partly true because there had been several previous contributions. The history of the term 'psychogenesis' goes back to, among others, Esquirol and Heinroth in the early 19th century. Sommer (1894) elaborated on psychogenesis in relation to hysterical phenomena without focusing on psychogenic (reactive) psychoses. A more important antecedent was Morel's theory of degeneration (Pichot 1986) which had a major impact on Wimmer's views (Faergeman 1963) and formed the theoretical basis of the 'constitutional psychoses' as reactive psychoses were called in Norway up to the early 1960s (Odegaard 1968). Kleist's (1921) reactive and autochton degeneration psychoses also hark back to Morel's idea.

From the turn of the century, and particularly during World War I, several psychoreactive illnesses surfaced in the literature. They were named after the situation in which they occurred (*'Situationspsychosen'*; Lewin 1917); for instance, prison psychosis (e.g. Rudin 1901), war (battle)-psychosis (e.g. Bunse 1918), and fear psychosis (e.g. Kleist 1918). Basically all these situational psychotic reactions depicted very similar situations and clinical presentations. Baetz (1901) described his own experience during an earthquake in Tokyo which became known as *Emotionslahmung* (emotional paralysis). Kraepelin (1915) called attention to the paranoid reaction of deaf people. Allers (1920) reported three brief case histories of psychotic reactions in soldiers treated in military hospitals who were isolated due to a language barrier which were characterized by short-lived paranoid episodes which resolved as soon as native speaker translators became available. Similar clinical pictures were later reported as 'immigrant psychoses' (e.g. Frost 1938; Eitinger 1959).

It is worthy of note that many such descriptions have been annexed to what we now term post-traumatic stress disorders (PTSD). At first glance PTSD appears, other than in terms of its precipitation, to occupy an entirely separate realm from reactive psychosis, it being an extended non-psychotic disturbance with marked affective and dissociative symptoms. In clinical practice, however, some of those quite properly described as having PTSD have an initial reaction to the trauma which could be regarded as amounting to a reactive psychosis. If one accepts the notion of reactive psychoses which extend beyond clinical pictures dominated by delusions and/or hallucinations to incorporate disturbances of consciousness (e.g. fugues), disturbances of volition (e.g. stupor) and disturbances of affect (emotional paralysis), then the potential overlap with cases currently classified as PTSD becomes clear.

In a seminal paper, Bonhoeffer (1911) asserted that there are psychogenic states other than hysteria and brought together several forms of reactive psychoses (e.g. reactive depressive and manic syndromes, paranoid and twilight states). Bonhoeffer had also mentioned most of the psychopathological principles with which Jaspers characterized his *genuine reaction*. The legitimization and widespread acceptance of reactive psychoses came, however, with Jaspers' and Wimmer's efforts to synthesize the diverse descriptions into a meaningful psychopathological and clinical entity.

JASPERS' VIEWS ON REACTIVE PSYCHOSES

Jaspers, a theoretician, never produced clinical criteria for diagnosing reactive psychoses. He formulated the psychopathological concept of genuine reactions, being more concerned with the science of psychopathology and the theoretical underpinnings of reactive states in general. The unsurpassable lucidity of Jaspers' concept is mainly attributable to the introduction and consistent application of basic methodological principles to psychopathology. Jaspers distinguished between meaningful connections and causal effects and also between the understandable psychic phenomena than can be grasped by empathy and the non-understable, which are only explainable by appeal to extra-conscious mechanisms, in the form of the functions and dysfunctions of brain. The latter are exclusively the subject of objective, scientific inquiry. Jaspers postulated that the particular form of many psychiatric disorders (e.g. autochthonous delusions, and obsessive-compulsive phenomena) would only be explored and explained with the advance of science, while the theme, or content, was at least partly derived from the individual's life experience, and therefore in principle understandable in terms of meaningful connections.

From a psychopathological perspective Jaspers (1948/1963) distinguished three basic forms of psychiatric disorders as 'ideal types': *processes*, subsuming endogenous psychoses and organic conditions; *developments*, comprising among other things most of what we would now call personality disorders; and *genuine reactions*. They are ideal types in the sense that they do not exist in pure form in any individual case and usually a thorough psychopathological analysis would reveal elements from each in a single patient.

Jaspers (1948/1963) defined the characteristics of reactions as:

1 following a precipitating factor which is in a close time relationship with the reactive state and which we can accept as adequate to provoke the subsequent disorder;

2 a meaningful connection between the contents of the precipitating experience and those of the abnormal reaction;

3 the abnormal reaction usually comes to an end when the primary cause for the reaction is removed.

Jaspers felt that 'in all psychogenic reactions (*Erlebnisreaktionen*) it is the meaning of the experience which is the decisive factor in precipitating the state' (p. 365). 'In reactive psychosis we observe either an immediate reaction to some incisive experience or some kind of explosion following a long period of unnoticed growth and meaningfully connected with the life-history and recurrent impressions of every day' (p. 385). In distinction to *process*, in *reaction proper* 'the content is meaningfully connected with the experience. The reaction would have never occurred without the experience and throughout its entire course remains dependent on the experience and what is connected with it' (p. 384). Reactive psychosis 'springs from a conflict with reality which has become intolerable. The psychosis manifests all the individual's fears and needs as well as their hopes and wishes in a motley procession of delusion-like ideas and hallucinations. It serves as a defence, a refuge, an escape, as a wish-fulfilment' (p. 389). By the nature of the reactive psychosis, when it resolves there should be full insight and Jaspers noted: 'When the psychosis is over the patient may be able to assess the psychosis unreservedly as an illness.' He continued, however, that 'After every reaction, it is true, there is return to the "status quo ante" as regards the specific psychic mechanisms and functions, the capacity to perform, etc. But the various contents may continue to exert an influence' (p. 385).

Jaspers clearly distinguished the aspects of meaningfulness in terms of the precipitating event, the purpose and the content of the psychosis from that of causality in the pathogenesis of the reactive psychoses. He emphasized that 'however well we understand the experience, its shattering significance and the content of the reactive state, the actual translation into what is pathological remains nevertheless incomprehensible' (p. 384).

Jaspers classified reactive states from three aspects. According to the *precipitating factors* he listed 'prison psychosis', 'battle psychosis', 'psychoses of isolation' and 'reactions of homesickness' (p. 389). As for the *clinical manifestations*, Jaspers realized that distinct entities cannot be delineated so he spoke of *types* of reactions such as reactive depression, explosive reactions (essentially Kretschmer's primitive reactions), clouding of consciousness, Ganser syndrome, hysterical delirium and stupor, persecutory and querulant ideas and 'reactions with hallucinations and delusions' (p. 391). Manifest personality disorders and somatic illnesses, malnutrition, exhaustion, and the whole variety of psychiatric disorders could constitute *predisposing factors* rendering the individual vulnerable to react to an overwhelming stressful situation with the emergence of such psychotic phenomenology.

We quoted extensively from Jaspers because his comprehensive discourse on reaction still serves as the basis for the concept of reactive psychoses. Interestingly, another of Jaspers' (1913) seminal papers, half of which was devoted specifically to reactive psychoses, is hardly ever cited in the literature. In this article, two brilliant case histories of reactive psychosis, one grafted onto alcoholism and the other to schizophrenia (superimposed psychosis, or comorbidity, in contemporary terms), illustrated his theoretical position. Jaspers further refined his concept in this paper noting in reactive psychoses an abnormal constitution reacts to an exogenous situation of stress in an abnormal fashion followed by full recovery, i.e. a return to the original (premorbid) condition. This implies that the disposition ('extra-conscious mechanisms') was inherently vulnerable and was an important aspect in the pathogenesis. (Contrast with our modern concept of PTSD which, rightly or wrongly, posits a normal person in an abnormally stressful situation.) Thus, in reactive psychoses a hypothetical causal predisposition and a real understandable connection exists between the experience and the ensuing psychosis. According to Jaspers, the symptoms of the psychosis themselves offer few diagnostic clues, but the diagnosis depends on the evaluation of the genesis and course of the disorder. In practice the diagnosis of reactive psychosis is considered when there is a sudden onset of a florid psychotic state which resolves rapidly, usually in response to removing the patient from a situation of stress or when that stress is otherwise relieved.

Jaspers acknowledges that there are transitional and mixed cases where causal and understandable factors cannot be teased out. To link experience with content is not always possible. What Jaspers never mentioned was that the capacity of the given clinician to empathize, understand and reconstruct the patient's life and relate it to psychopathology varies widely, which brings in an unavoidable subjective element into the concept. This explains in part its unpopularity in modern diagnostic systems. In one of his many side-swipes at psychoanalysis, he did call for modesty in the exhibition of empathy and warned against the hubris and simplicity which assumes our own internal world is a sufficient guide to grasping all and every psychopathological experience.

In clinical practice, the search for Jasperian criteria in series of reactive psychoses has yielded inconclusive, and mainly disappointing, results. Many (e.g. Astrup *et al.* 1959; Faergeman 1963) found them rare in their patients and Opjordsmoen (1987) found only five patients fulfilling Jaspers' criteria out of 125 paranoid psychoses, but these 'Jaspers-positive' patients all showed symptomatic recovery, no relapse and an excellent social outcome. In Jorgensen's (1986) series, however, 54% of those with reactive paranoid psychoses met Jaspers' criteria but they had no prognostic significance. In McCabe's (1975) prospective study, Jaspers' criteria were not prerequisites of inclusion. Yet, in 82% of them a temporal relationship between trauma and psychosis could be established, 85% had a trauma regarded as adequate to precipitate the psychosis and in 82% the content of the psychosis reflected the stressful event. The meaning of the psychosis (e.g. escape, wish) was clear to the clinicians in every case. Altogether, 60% of the subjects fulfilled all Jaspers' criteria while 90% met at least three of the four.

It might of course be wondered why those who did not meet the basic psychopathological principles of Jaspers were given the diagnosis of reactive psychosis in the first place. (See also the section on precipitating event where the lack of the salient feature of the concept, the traumatizing event, is discussed.) We would echo Frey's (1968) opinion that: 'Although a certain amount of lip service is paid to Jaspers' criteria and teleological explanations, it seems to be a fact that what really matters, when it comes to diagnosing reactive psychosis, is if the disease in question cannot be labelled schizophrenia, manic-depressive or an organic psychosis' (p. 1).

SCHNEIDER AND THE GERMAN VIEW OF REACTIVE PSYCHOSES

It was Kurt Schneider, trained in the same Heidelberg school of psychiatry as Jaspers, who succinctly summarized Jaspers' theoretical position from a clinical point of view. Schneider's (1927) criteria for 'abnormal psychic reactions' ('*Die abnormale seelische Reaktionen*') were, by and large, identical with those of Jaspers. However, Schneider's contribution was controversial. Like his many contemporaries (e.g. Kretschmer 1918; Birnbaum 1928), Schneider applied the term 'psychosis' only to psychiatric disorders having a proven or possible organic aetiology. By diminishing the role of somatic ('extra-conscious' as Jaspers put it) factors in the pathogenesis of reactive psychoses, Schneider excluded them from the group of psychoses. Thus, despite his ingenious description of their clinical manifestations, namely emotional syndromes, disorders of consciousness and paranoid states, he did not recognize reactive psychoses as a distinct entity. Owing to Schneider's high reputation and influence, the clinical category of reactive psychoses slowly faded away in Germany (Degkwitz 1985). However, the German contributions, particularly those of Jaspers, Schneider, Kretschmer and Birnbaum, were utilized by Scandinavian schools of psychiatry (Stromgren 1974, 1986).

WIMMER, STROMGREN AND THE SCANDINAVIAN SCHOOL

Despite all the controversies, through most of this century Scandinavian psychiatric schools have kept the clinical concept of reactive psychoses alive. In fact, the first monograph on the topic was written by a Danish psychiatrist, August Wimmer (1916), based on a lecture he gave in 1913 (Schioldann-Nielsen 1993). Wimmer's criteria for reactive (psychogenic) psychoses were:

1   they are 'clinically independent psychoses';
2   they develop 'usually on a definite predisposed foundation';
3   they are 'caused by mental agents [which] determine the moment for the start of the psychosis, the fluctuations (remissions, intermission, exacerbations) [and] very often its cessation';
4   'the *form* and the content of the psychosis are, more or less directly and completely ('comprehensibly'), determined by precipitating mental factors';
5   they have a 'predominant tendency . . . to recovery and . . . they never end in deterioration' (italics added).

Wimmer (1924/1993) held on to his view in a later paper (the only one of his writings available in English): 'these hysterical or psychogenic mental disorders appear on a predisposed substrate and through the influence of psychological factors in such a way that, at the same time, these psychic factors are *pathogenic* and *pathoplastic*' (p. 429). Wimmer's clinically oriented formulation established what is frequently mentioned as the Scandinavian concept of reactive psychoses. Wimmer postulated reactive psychoses as independent entities whereas Jaspers left their nosological position open. Jaspers' German contemporaries and successors treated them as reactions and not as a putative disease entitity. More importantly, according to Jaspers only the *content* is determined by the mental trauma while in Wimmer's understanding its causative role is much broader in so far as the *form*, i.e. clinical manifestations, of the psychosis is also defined by it. Thus, Wimmer altered the concept by assuming that understanding why the psychosis emerged at that time and why it took this particular form amounted to explaining its causation.

While Wimmer's great achievement was to establish reactive psychoses as clinical entities, the price paid for the extension of psychogenesis to a total causal explanation tended to blur the boundaries of the concept. Wimmer's interpretation paved the way for psychological, mostly psychoanalytical, deliberations. The shift of balance to a purely sociopsychological conceptualization has hindered the development of a comprehensive research strategy aiming at a biopsychosocial synthesis.

Wimmer's work was continued by Faergeman (1963), whose monograph made the concept accessible to Anglo-Saxon psychiatry. Driven by his training in psychoanalysis, Faergeman further extended the limits of psychological understanding and interpretation and re-emphasized Wimmer's conviction that not just the content but the form of psychosis was understandable in these terms. Furthermore, he excluded what he termed formal thought disorder from the criteria, which is obviously contradictory, given that reactive psychoses present mostly with acute syndromes characterized by disintegration of thought processes and/or clouded consciousness. Despite these conceptual problems, Faergeman was a brilliant clinician and his eloquently written book is still a rich source of information on the subject. Faergeman's other major contribution was that he conducted the first well-organized follow-up of reactive psychoses.

The most influential proponent of the Scandinavian concept of reactive psychoses was Erik Stromgren, who had a major role in getting international, including Anglo-American, psychiatry to notice and, to a certain extent, to accept reactive (psychogenic) psychoses as distinct clinical entities. Stromgren's views compiled from his paper (Stromgren 1974, pp. 100–101) can be summarized as follows.

1   The mental trauma must be of such a nature that the psychosis would not have arisen in its absence.
2   There is a predisponding vulnerability in the individual's personality, but such a predisposition is certainly not an obligatory condition for the start of the psychosis.
3   There is a close temporal correlation between the trauma and the start of the psychosis.
4   The mental trauma plays an important, and even dominant, part in the clinical picture and it usually largely determines the content of the psychosis.
5   If the precipitating situation resolves, the psychosis will usually also resolve, though even if the situation persists the psychosis will not go on for ever.
6   It is not the 'objective' force of the trauma which determines the reaction of the patient; it is the subjective experience determined by the special sensitivity of the patient to the trauma.
7   However, even if the mental trauma cannot be ascertained, *this is not a sufficient cause for discarding the diagnosis of psychogenic psychosis.*

With the exception to the last, theoretically untenable criterion, Stromgren actually moved back to Jaspers' original formulation, largely abandoning Faergeman's psychoanalytic standpoint. Stromgren (1974) postulated that mental trauma tarnishing the self-image of the individual could lead to a paranoid reaction, examples of paranoid reactions being Kretschmer's (1918) sensitive delusions of reference, litigious paranoia, and the paranoid reactions of prisoners. Reactive paranoid syndromes may also emerge in response to social isolation (including that provided by deafness, immigration and sensory deprivation). Disorders of consciousness could follow a 'sudden disruption of the patient's *image of the environment*' (Stromgren 1974, p. 109; italics in original), as after an earthquake. The clinical picture can include confusional, clouded and delirious states. Finally, emotional reactions could be triggered by '*simple situational conflicts* . . . which, however unpleasant and undesirable they may be are not wholly unforeseen' (p. 109; italics in original). These consist predominantly of reactive depressions and manic-like excitations (e.g. funeral mania). In clinical practice, like the different clinical forms, the stressful situations are partially overlapping. It should also be noted that these reactive psychoses could last from a few days, as with funeral mania, to months or years as with litigious paranoia.

Most authors (e.g. Astrup *et al.* 1959) were sceptical towards Stromgren's hypothesis with regard to specific types of trauma generating specific types of psychoses. Faergeman (1963) could not confirm the relationship concerning the type of trauma and the form of psychosis except for the paranoid subtype. Stromgren's hypothesis was most thoroughly tested by McCabe (1975), who found that a statistically significant number of patients presented the syndrome predicted by the type of trauma, a finding which still requires replication.

It is questionable whether it was useful to give such prominence to the emotional syndromes and in particular the reactive depressions, characterized as they are by neurotic premorbid traits, normal motor activity, initial rather than terminal insomnia and guilt feelings about past events. It is not that such conditions are not seen clinically—they most certainly are, forming probably the largest group of mood disorders in the community — the problem is that these are not psychotic by current standards and arguably not psychotic even by the criteria which rely on a clear break in the continuity of mental life.

With some modifications, Wimmer's, Faergeman's and Stromgren's views have prevailed in all Scandinavian countries up to the present day, although there have been at least four, partly overlapping, interpretations of the concept (for details see Dahl 1987; Guldberg *et al.* 1996). Recently an attempt has been made to improve the reliability of the diagnosis of reactive psychoses across the Nordic countries (Hansen *et al.* 1992). Improved reliability will certainly give further impetus to clinical and, presumably, biological research.

The first operationalized criteria for reactive psychoses have been published (Opjordsmoen 1987; Jorgensen & Jensen 1988). Both papers focus exclusively on the paranoid (delusional) subtype and omit reactive emotional (affective) syndromes and disorders of consciousness. More recently, Guldberg *et al.* (1996) attempted to operationalize reactivity by developing the reactivity of psychosis rating form (RPRF). The RPRF has 10 variables encompassing all the relevant features of reactive psychoses (e.g. onset of stressor, meaning of psychosis) and it was found to have good interrater reliability and construct and discriminant validity (Guldberg *et al.* 1996).

Nosological considerations

In search of a 'third psychosis', several more or less similar acute psychoses have been described to overcome the deficiencies of Kraepelin's dichotomy of the so-called endogenous psychoses (Pull 1995). Many of these show similarities to the reactive psychoses in one or more aspects of their clinical manifestations. In the following paragraphs some of the acute psychoses more frequently occurring in the literature will be briefly reviewed only in their relation to reactive psychoses. In addition, the 'culture-bound' syndromes will be mentioned here with reference to their link with reactive psychoses.

HYSTERICAL PSYCHOSIS

Never part of official classifications, the term 'hysterical psychosis' has haunted psychiatric nosology over the past hundred years. Its history is reviewed by Mentzos (1973) and Refsum and Astrup (1982). The diagnostic criteria proposed by Hollender and Hirsch (1964) cover those of the classical reactive psychoses with the restriction that the premorbid personality is 'hysterical' and the 'acute episode seldom lasts longer than one to three weeks' (Hollender & Hirsch 1964). Evaluating blindly the case notes of patients with hysterical psychosis, non-hysterical reactive psychosis and schizophrenia for a number of demographic and clinical variables, Modestin and Bachmann (1992) found no difference between hysterical and reactive psychoses while patients with schizophrenia differed significantly from both groups. Their conclusion, shared by many authors (e.g. Langness 1967; Cavenar *et al.* 1979), was that hysterical psychosis is essentially a reactive psychosis occurring against the background of hysterical character traits.

ACUTE SCHIZOAFFECTIVE PSYCHOSIS

A careful reading of Kasanin's original paper (Kasanin 1933) reveals that his acute schizoaffective psychosis shares many features of reactive psychoses. Kasanin observed a stressful life event prior to the acute onset of the psychosis: 'Preceding the attack there was, however, a difficult environmental situation which served as a precipitating factor' (p. 101). Premorbid personality was 'very sensitive, critical of themselves, introspective, very unhappy and preoccupied with their own conflicts' (p. 101). More importantly, personality, situation and psychosis form a meaningful entity: 'The interesting thing about the psychoses is that one is able to reconstruct them psychologically when one reviews the various symptoms and behaviour . . . Their reaction is one of a protest, or a fear without the ready acceptance of the solution offered by the psychosis' (p. 101). In line with the meaningful connections characterizing these psychoses, symptomatologically 'there is comparatively little of that extremely bizarre, unusual and mysterious' (p. 101). The psychosis ends in complete recovery with full insight. Since Kasanin's original description, the conception of schizoaffective psychoses has undergone several transformations and its current usage bears little resemblance to reactive psychoses, though whether these developments have enhanced its clinical relevence is open to question.

CYCLOID PSYCHOSES

Despite similarities in their clinical presentation (acute onset, confusion, aetiologically charged psychotic symptoms, excellent short-term prognosis), cycloid psychoses are not related aetiologically to reactive psychoses (Leonhard 1957). According to Leonhard, stressful life events may precipitate the onset of cycloid psychoses but the content does not reflect the traumatic situation, if there was any, and their course and outcome are unrelated to environmental changes.

SCHIZOPHRENIFORM PSYCHOSES

On the basis of a personal follow-up, Langfeldt (1939) distinguished process schizophrenia characterized by typical schizophrenic symptoms and poor prognosis from a group of psychoses with good prognosis but similar to schizophrenia in their presentation which he called schizophreniform states. Two of the five subtypes of these schizophreniform psychoses he described as 'psychogenically comprehensible' (Langfeldt 1982) which in effect makes them indistinguishable from reactive psychoses. In Retterstol and Dahl's (1983) opinion, the term schizophreniform psychosis, as used nowadays, expresses diagnostic uncertainty between schizophrenia and reactive psychosis.

SCHIZOPHRENIA-LIKE EMOTION PSYCHOSIS

Schizophrenia-like emotion psychosis (*schizophrenieähnliche Emotionspsychosen*) was originally developed by Straehelin and elaborated by Labhardt (1963). Its criteria, based on Jaspers' principles, are basically identical with those drawn up by Wimmer (1916) for reactive (psychogenic) psychoses (Labhardt 1963).

BOUFFÉE DÉLIRANTE

Bouffée délirante is a French concept of remarkable stability over more than a hundred years (Pull *et al.* 1987), denoting an acute, brief, non-organic psychosis with sudden onset, ever-changing (polymorphous) delusions and hallucinations, clouded consciousness and rapidly fluctuating affective states. *Bouffée délirante* remits spontaneously but tends to recur (Pichot 1986). In Magnan's classical interpretation (see Pichot 1986), a fragile premorbid personality ('degeneracy') confers the vulnerability to *bouffée délirante* patients, while traumatizing events play minimal, if any, part in its pathogenesis. In the official French classification (INSERM) (see Pichot 1982), a reactive variant of *bouffée délirante* is entertained, which is clinically the same as the classical type but occurs in response to a stressful situation. The reactive type is said to take up approximately 15% of all *bouffée délirante* cases, and corresponds to the reactive paranoid psychosis (Pichot 1986). The INSERM classification also has a separate rubric for reactive confusional states overlapping with the reactive psychosis, confusional type (Pichot 1982).

CULTURE-BOUND SYNDROMES

This hotly debated term is applied to a wide array of clinical presentations thought to occur more or less exclusively in particular cultures (for a recent review, see Levine & Gaw 1995). From our point of view, particularly interesting are the brief, acute psychoses with good prognosis reported from many developing countries (Stevens 1987). Yap (1967), who was among the first to realize the nosological importance of 'culture-bound' syndromes, noticed the similarities between them and reactive psychoses, coining the term 'culture-bound reactive syndromes'. Although a consensus has not been reached as to their nosological position, agreeing with Yap's notion, many authorities regard syndromes like *windigo*, *amok*, *latah*, *pibloktoq* and *qi-gong* as essentially psychoreactive disorders (Langness 1967; Friedmann 1982; Levine & Gaw 1995; see Chapter 15). According to Ruiz and Gomez (1984), many culture-bound reactive syndromes are hysterical (reactive) psychoses 'which usually have a problem-solving effect' and 'are exaggerated caricatures of culturally sanctioned communications' (p. 37). Wig (1990) felt that 'most of the culture-bound symptoms can be classified under the standard diagnostic group of . . . acute psychotic disorders or neurotic and stress-related disorders' (p. 205). In Wig's (1983) opinion, brief reactive psychosis (DSM-III) comprised 'hysterical psychosis', possessions syndromes and other culture-bound psychotic disorders' (p. 85). In contrast to clinical pictures encountered in Western cultures, the form and content of 'culture-bound' reactive psychoses are patterned, i.e. being more determined by the beliefs, traditions and habits of local culture. Only systematic comparative studies (e.g. Pierloot & Ngoma 1988) will determine whether the European criteria of reactive psychoses can be applied to all of the 'culture-bound' acute psychoses.

Reactive psychoses in international classifications

ICD-8, ICD-9 AND ICD-10

Reactive psychoses first appeared in ICD-8 (WHO 1967) under the heading of 'Other Psychoses' (298) as 'reactive depression' (298.0), 'reactive excitation' (298.1), 'reactive confusion' (298.2), 'acute paranoid reaction' (298.3) and 'unspecified reactive psychosis' (298.9) although users were cautioned to apply them sparingly. A similar note warns the clinician in ICD-9 (WHO 1978) where the classical clinical forms of reactive psychoses are accommodated under the headings of 'Schizophrenic Reaction' (295.9) and 'Other

Non-organic Psychoses' (298.0–8) comprising depressive and excitative types, reactive confusion, acute paranoid reaction, psychogenic paranoid psychosis and non-specified reactive psychoses. A separate rubric, 'Neurotic and Reactive Depression' (300.4) contains reactive depressive psychoses while 'Hysteria' 'dissociative reaction and Ganser syndrome' (300.1) would cover part of the reactive psychoses presenting with clouded consciousness. Psychiatrists familiar with the concept of reactive psychoses found enough diagnostic rubrics but the fragmented arrangement of different subtypes did not encourage the uninitiated clinician to use them.

The approach taken by ICD-10 represents a radical departure from the original European interpretation of reactive psychoses. Unlike its predecessor, ICD-10 does not recognize reactive psychoses as an independent category. Driven by the twin goals of rationalization, i.e. avoiding any aetiological assumptions (Cooper 1994), and worldwide consensus, i.e. to incorporate benign acute psychoses frequently encountered in developing countries (Wig 1990; Okasha *et al.* 1993; Susser *et al.* 1995b), ICD-10 created a new composite diagnostic class, 'Acute and Transient Psychotic Disorders' (ATPD) with the aim of embracing different types of acute psychoses described in the classical European literature such as the *bouffée délirante*, the cycloid psychoses, schizophreniform states, the reactive psychoses and even acute schizophrenia of short duration. Three of the six subtypes of ATPD (F23) are basically wastebasket categories (F23.3, F23.8 and F23.9). 'Acute polymorphic psychotic disorder without symptoms of schizophrenia' (F23.0) is compiled from the characteristic symptomatology of *bouffée délirante* and the cycloid psychoses. The remaining two categories, F23.1 and F23.2, are defined by two sets of symptoms: one identical with schizophrenia but lasting less than 1 month, the other are those of the acute polymorphic psychotic disorders. Any of the subtypes may occur with or without the modifier 'associated acute stress' but there is no requirement to link any features of the psychosis to the stressful life situation which has been a principal component of the definition of reactive psychoses. In keeping with the findings of the classical literature, the 'allowed' duration for ATPD is 3 months.

Further research is needed to justify fusing reactive and non-reactive psychoses into one category. The only study to compare these two groups of psychoses is that of Kapur and Pandurangi (1979) from India. These authors found significant differences between the two types of brief psychoses in terms of the presence of hysterical and affective features and less disturbed behaviour, and also more dependency and anxiety traits in the premorbid personality, all in the reactive form.

The division of acute psychoses in ICD-10 is deliberately simplistic (Cooper 1994) and seductively logical. Because of its practical layout, ATPD will predictably have a satisfactory reliability. However, the inherent danger of its simplicity is that it may reduce mental health professionals not trained in classical descriptive psychiatry to count individual symptoms and catalogue stressful events separately from each other; in short, there is encouragement to pursue a multi-axial classification which fails to recognize the interaction of theoretically distinct axes in giving rise to both the form and the content of psychoses.

DSM-III, DSM-III-R and DSM-IV

Until DSM-III (APA 1980) most reactive psychoses were diagnosed as acute schizophrenia in North America (Allodi 1982). Hysterical psychosis (Hirsch & Hollender 1969) was also used, mostly by academic psychiatrists (Allodi 1982). DSM-III and its successive revisions are the result of compromise and consensus reached by a panel of experts rather than the operationalization of the pre-existing rich clinical experience accumulated by classical descriptive psychiatry.

In DSM-III-R (APA 1987), the diagnostic criteria for brief reactive psychosis are based on some, albeit not all, of Jaspers' criteria of abnormal reaction. In an attempt to bring DSM-III-R closer to the Scandinavian concept of reactive psychoses (Kendler *et al.* 1989), the restrictive DSM-III criteria were modified significantly. The maximum duration of psychosis was extended to 1 month. More importantly, DSM-III-R states that the psychosis occurs not simply after, but in response to the stressful life event(s), i.e. the interaction between the event(s) and the psychosis is emphasized, thus giving Jaspers' notion more prominence. The balance is further shifted to Jaspers' direction by permitting a chain of events, instead of one, to contribute to the pathogenesis of reactive psychosis. The importance of confusion and perplexity in the clinical picture are underscored, basically acknowledging the existence of the disorders of consciousness, a classical category of reactive psychoses. The relationship between reactive and organic conditions is more sensibly worded by not ruling out chronic organic conditions as a predisposing factor, provided they do not initiate or maintain the reactive disturbance.

Nevertheless, the American concept was still more restrictive than the classical one for four main reasons (Jauch & Carpenter 1988b). First, it excludes patients with premorbid schizotypal personality disorder or prodromal symptoms of schizophrenia, which is an arbitrary decision not supported by empirical evidence. In the European tradition, reactive psychoses may occur independently or may be superimposed on any chronic organic or even non-organic psychiatric conditions (Bleuler 1911/1950; Jaspers 1913). This ubiquitous character is the core feature of reactivity. Secondly, like ICD-10, DSM-III-R ignores reactive affective psychoses, i.e. emotional reactions, which constitute a substantial part of reactive psychoses in classical series (e.g. Faergeman 1963; McCabe 1975; Andersen & Laerum 1980). It seems to be an illogical decision to differentiate between reactive and non-reactive paranoid disorders but to insist on the unitary nature of mood disorders. Thirdly, the maximum duration of brief reactive psychosis is limited to 1 month, an extension of the 2-week criterion in DSM-III, which is still far too short in light of several classical and recent studies (e.g. Faergeman 1963; McCabe 1975; Andersen & Laerum 1980; Pandurangi & Kapur 1980; Munoz *et al.* 1987; Opjordsmoen 1987; Jorgensen & Jensen 1988). Fourthly, emphasizing the severity of stressor(s), DSM-III-R pays no heed to individual vulnerability, another salient constituent of the original concept (Birnbaum 1928; Jaspers 1948/1963; Stromgren 1974; Dahl 1987).

Although DSM-III-R represented an improvement over its predecessor, it still fell short of reflecting the fertile clinical traditions of the European, particularly German and Scandinavian, schools of psychiatry (Dahl 1986; Jauch & Carpenter 1988b). For this reason Jauch and Carpenter (1988b) suggested a return to the traditional concept of reactive psychoses. Instead, and similarly to ICD-10, DSM-IV did not even retain (brief) reactive psychosis as a separate entity. In DSM-IV the 'acute stressor' serves only as a specifier to a new, composite category, 'Brief Psychotic Disorder' (298.8). Apart from collapsing good-prognosis reactive and non-reactive brief psychoses into one category, DSM-IV has not brought about significant changes with respect to the individual criterion of reactive psychoses. Unfortunately, the 1-month duration criterion was not changed despite criticism (e.g. Munoz *et al.* 1987, Remington *et al.* 1990) and ample empirical evidence that it is too restrictive. As mentioned earlier, in the experience of Scandinavian authorities reactive psychoses last from weeks to months (Stromgren 1974; Jorgensen & Jensen 1988). In Opjordsmoen's (1987) experience, full remission was seen even after 4 months and the psychosis had lasted 1–4 weeks at admission. Similarly, Pandurangi and Kapur (1980) found the average duration of illness was already 31 days at the first consultation.

Although there is preliminary evidence that Scandinavian and American viewpoints on functional psychoses are converging (Dahl *et al.* 1992), a coherent representation of the European concept of reactive psychoses does not exist in the successive editions of DSM (Stromgren 1994). Just like in its predecessors, in addition to 'Brief Psychotic Disorder' there are several diagnostic categories in DSM-IV to accommodate the traditional subforms of reactive psychoses, e.g. 'Shared Psychotic Disorder' (297.3), 'Psychotic Disorder NOS' (298.9) and 'Adjustment Disorder with Depressed Mood' (309.0) (Stromgren 1994).

The creation of the 'Brief Reactive Psychosis' category in DSM-III stimulated little research interest. Due to its sterile and restrictive criteria and, perhaps, American clinicians' ignorance of the concept, brief reactive psychosis was rarely found in hospital admission series, comprising less than 0.5% of all psychoses (Jauch & Carpenter 1988b). Astrup, a Norwegian psychiatrist, performed a chart review of 283 first admission psychotic patients in a teaching hospital in Baltimore without knowing the results of their 5- to 16-year follow-up (Stephens *et al.* 1982). None of the 91 patients with reactive psychoses according to Astrup were rediagnosed as having brief reactive psychosis by an experienced American clinician who was unaware of Astrup's diagnoses or the follow-up results. However, a substantial proportion of reactive psychoses turned out to be 'Atypical Psychosis' according to DSM-III, a finding replicated in a similar diagnostic exercise (Dahl *et al.* 1992). In both studies, comparing European and DSM-III-based American diagnostic practices, American clinicians preferred the aetiologically neutral diagnosis of 'Atypical Psychosis' rather than that of 'Brief Reactive Psychosis.'

Notwithstanding occasional case reports (e.g. Weiss & Rhoads 1979; Krieger & Zussman 1981; Harry & Favazza 1984; Steiner 1991), the paucity of studies attests to the reluctant acceptance of brief reactive psychosis by North American psychiatrists. A systematic chart review performed by Munoz *et al.* (1987) casts doubt on the validity of brief reactive psychosis as defined by DSM-III. The weaknesses of the DSM-III concept of brief reactive psychosis and the mechanical, symptom-by-symptom application of its faulty criteria resulted in these discouraging results. In contrast, Beighley *et al.* (1992) found DSM-III-R criteria useful and easily applicable. They reported a small series of (DSM-III-R) brief reactive psychoses among US Air Force recruits. Retrospective chart review identified six cases among 557 consecutive psychiatric admissions, the majority of which (464 patients) were treated for adjustment disorder. The strict training regime with deprivation of privacy and constant tough discipline served as precipitating stressors. All six cases presented with mixed paranoid-catatonic symptomatology and recovered within days after removing them from training. No follow-up data were available.

Clinical presentation

The reactive psychoses cannot be fully characterized by their symptoms since virtually the whole range of psychiatric symptomatology may appear, even if transiently (Birnbaum 1928; Faergeman 1963; McCabe 1975). Individual symptoms are changeable, they emerge, fade and fuse ('chameleonic, capricious and shifting' in Faergeman's wording) but they also show cultural variability. Pandurangi and Kapur (1980) found that their Indian patients presented with more histrionic behaviour, excitement and sleep disturbances and less confusion, irritability and depression than their Scandinavian counterparts. The diagnosis, therefore, depends less on certain well-circumscribed symptom-clusters than the totality of the clinical picture. There are, however, still no better guidelines than Jaspers' principles—that is, the establishment of the comprehensible relationship between trauma and the content and course of psychosis. Recent multicentre realibility studies (Dahl *et al.* 1992; Hansen *et al.* 1992) and persuasively written case reports and small series (e.g. Harry & Favazza 1984; Steiner 1991; Beighley *et al.* 1992) attest to the presence and recognizability of the classical concept of reactive psychoses.

Further issues pertaining to the diagnosis of reactive psychoses are discussed in sections on predisposing factors and precipitating events.

Follow-up studies and diagnostic stability

Follow-up studies have been conducted almost exclusively in Scandinavia and have yielded inconclusive results. Jauch and Carpenter (1988a) pointed out methodological flaws in the reported series which included lack of control groups, lack of blind assessment and failure to establish the inter-rater reliability of the diagnoses. All investigations drew their case material from hospital archives. Hospital diagnoses made by several clinicians over a long period of time are notoriously unreliable. In view of the inclination of Scandinavian psychiatrists to preferentially diagnose reactive psychoses in first-onset cases (Faergeman 1963; Odegaard 1968; Jorgensen 1985), it is not surprising that an excess of other psychoses was found at follow-up examinations. Due to restrictions in space only some of the oft-cited studies will be mentioned here. (For details, readers should consult Jauch and Carpenter's 1988a paper.)

Faergeman (1963) conducted a 14- to 19-year follow-up of 170 cases diagnosed as having reactive psychoses by Wimmer between 1924 and 1926. Faergeman managed to interview 98 of the original 170 patients, confirming the diagnosis in only 48. The least stable was the paranoid group, with a mere 24% diagnostic stability, while the emotional syndromes (53%) and disturbances of consciousness (57%) fared better, schizophrenia accounting for the majority of those reclassified at follow-up. Those with confirmed reactive psychosis had a favorable clinical outcome, with 70% recovering without relapse. In terms of social prognosis, however, the picture was bleaker, with only 60% regaining full functioning. Faergeman's inconclusive results caused Slater (1964) to doubt the usefulness of the whole concept of reactive psychoses, which has had a long-lasting effect in Anglo-Saxon psychiatry.

Retterstol (1966, 1970) conducted two long-term follow-up investigations (5–18 and 22–39 years) of the same group of consecutively admitted patients with paranoid, including reactive paranoid, psychoses. Those with reactive psychoses recovered symptomatologically in 81% of cases and 79% were able to support themselves (Retterstol & Opjordsmoen 1994). In about 12% of the cases the diagnosis of reactive paranoid psychosis had to be changed to schizophrenia. At the same time, 15% of cases with schizophrenia were rediagnosed at follow-up to have reactive paranoid psychosis.

Large-scale investigations were carried out at Gaustad Hospital, Norway during the 1950s and 1960s (e.g. Holmboe & Astrup 1957; Astrup *et al.* 1959, 1962; Noreik *et al.* 1967; Noreik 1970; Refsum & Astrup 1980, 1982). Outcome in the reactive psychoses was poorest in the paranoid subtype, better in the emotional syndromes and best in the confusional reactive psychoses. Acute onset, good premorbid personality and precipitation by somatic disease or prolonged sexual conflicts were factors positively correlated with better prognosis whereas subaverage level of intelligence predicted poor prognosis. Outcome was independent of the age of onset and the mode of treatment (Astrup *et al.* 1959). An extended follow-up of nearly the same cohort of patients revealed a somewhat more pessimistic picture. 'Schizophrenic deterioration and defects' were found in 57% and 36% of cases with a hospital diagnosis of reactive psychoses at 5- to 17-year and 15- to 27-year follow-up respectively while the corresponding figures for schizophrenia were 64% and 54% (Noreik *et al.* 1967).

A 14-year follow-up chart review of 220 first-admission reactive psychoses to a Danish institution was performed by Andersen and Laerum (1980) revealing that 50% of patients thought to have affective reactive psychosis at first admission turned out to be schizophrenic or manic-depressive at follow-up with paranoid reactive psychoses often developing into typical schizophrenia (Holmboe & Astrup 1957).

In his methodologically well-designed study, McCabe (1975) followed up his 40 prospectively ascertained reactive psychotic patients for an average of 18 months. Only one patient's diagnosis had to be changed to manic-depressive illness. Sixteen (40%) patients had to be re-admitted; the risk for re-admission was significantly higher for those with psychiatric history prior to their index admission.

A comprehensive assessment at 8- to 12-year follow-up of 41 patients diagnosed with reactive paranoid psychosis in a Danish hospital also showed significant instability of this diagnosis, with 15 (37%) patients developing definite and probable schizophrenic psychosis and a further four (10%) affective psychosis (Jorgensen 1985). Using the nationwide Danish Psychiatric Register, Jorgensen and Mortensen (1988) found that after 2 years following the first episode, when re-admitted, only 50% of reactive psychotic patients were still regarded as suffering from reactive psychoses. A nationwide survey of diagnostic practices from Norway and Denmark conducted in 1979 came to a similar conclusion (Dahl 1987). In Norway reactive psychoses took up 52% of all first-admission psychoses, falling to 25% at re-admission while, at the same time, schizophrenia rose from 18% to 51%. Danish statistics showed similar trends: the percentage of reactive psychoses decreased from 43% to 16% when that of schizophrenia increased from 7% to 34% by the time of re-admission (Dahl 1987).

The rather discouraging results of follow-up investigations led some authors (e.g. Retterstol 1987; Jorgensen & Mortensen 1990) to question the usefulness of the diagnosis of reactive psychoses as it is used currently. Narrowing the scope of reactive psychoses coupled with the introduction of operationalized criteria have been suggested to improve the reliability and validity of diagnosis (Retterstol 1987). To date, two sets of operationalized criteria have been developed, both for reactive paranoid psychoses (Opjordsmoen 1987; Jorgensen & Jensen 1988). Concurring with Jauch and Carpenter's (1988b) opinion, we feel that loose diagnostic practices, and not necessarily conceptual faults, stand behind the lack of diagnostic stability. A recent study finding reasonable multicentre and international inter-rater reliability in Nordic countries for reactive psychoses seems to support this view (Hansen *et al.* 1992).

The only study reported outside Scandinavia followed up 30 Indian patients with reactive psychoses for 6 months (Pandurangi & Kapur 1980). In 67% of the sample, the diagnosis of reactive psychosis was confirmed, while in 20% and 10% they were changed to affective psychosis and schizo-phrenia respectively.

Predisposing factors

A stressful event or life situation is the *sine qua non* for reactive psychoses but in a sizeable proportion of cases itself is not sufficient to elicit a psychotic reaction. Particularly, German authors (e.g. Jaspers 1913; Birnbaum 1928) regarded predisposition as essential to the genesis of reactive psychiatric dis-turbances questioning the possibility of reactive (psychogenic) psychosis ever occurring in a psychologically normal and balanced individual (Villinger 1920). Birnbaum (1928) asserted that constitution determines the experi-ence, content and the form of the reaction. Predisposition includes a host of somatic and personality factors. According to most early German authors, reactive psychoses may also accompany pre-existing major psychiatric disor-ders such as depression or schizophrenia (Jaspers 1913; Birnbaum 1928). Bleuler (1911/1950) listed 'Abnormal reactions of the sick psyche to emo-tionally charged experiences' (p. 206) among the acute syndromes seen in the course of schizophrenia. These abnormal reactions included Ganser's syn-drome and hysteriform twilight state which is 'then essentially the reaction of a mildly schizophrenic personality to a psychic trauma; an external event seems to be the main determinant' (Bleuler 1911/1950, p. 220).

The predisposing factors include the following.

PREMORBID PERSONALITY

Since the early descriptions there has been consensus that in the majority of cases there is a pre-existing vulnerability of the personality (Astrup *et al.* 1959; Faergeman 1963; Retterstol 1966; Noreik 1970; Stromgren 1974). There have been a wide variety of personality traits observed—for example, 'sensitive' (in Kretschmer's (1918) sense), 'neurotic' and asocial (Refsum & Astrup 1980). In contrast to these clinical impressions, McCabe (1975) sys-tematically assessed personality traits in 36 of his 40 cases and compared them with the results from their siblings. Shyness, oversensitivity, lability of affect, lack of self-confidence, and hypochondriacal and anxious traits were observed most often. Shyness and oversensitivity were found in probands significantly more frequently than in their siblings. Pandurangi and Kapur (1980) applied Cattells's 16 personality factor questionnaire (16 P-F) to their 30 reactive psychotic patients. They found abnormal levels of sensitivity, emotional instability, insecurity, timidity, tension and excitability. In a companion study, Kapur and Pandurangi (1979) compared the above-mentioned 30 reactive psychotic patients with 30 patients with non-reactive acute psychosis. Except for tension and excitability, in all the factors listed above reactive psychotic subjects had a significantly higher score than their non-reactive counterparts.

Chavan and Kulhara (1988) used the WHO's standardized test of personality assessment in their study of 22 reactive psychotic patients and a matched control group. Surprisingly, patients and controls did not differ in terms of shyness, oversensitivity, anxiety and hypochondriasis. However, reactive psychosis patients were found to be significantly more suspicious and cyclothymic.

Among modern classifications, DSM-III-R (APA 1987) mentioned that borderline personality disorder was frequently associated with brief reactive psychosis. DSM-IV (APA 1994) acknowledges further personality disorders (paranoid, histrionic, narcissistic, schizotypal and borderline) as predisposing factors for 'Brief Psychotic Disorder'. ICD-10 (WHO 1992) does not specify predisposing conditions for 'Acute and Transient Psychotic Disorders'.

ORGANIC COMPONENTS IN REACTIVE PSYCHOSES

According to European diagnostic traditions, pre-existing organic impairment was regarded as a predisposing factor and its presence did not exclude the diagnosis of reactive psychosis (Jaspers 1913; Birnbaum 1928; Stromgren 1974). In Wimmer's series followed up by Faergeman (1963), 47 of 115 cases had identifiable cerebral pathology (alcoholism, head trauma, mental retardation). Less specific organic predisposing factors included menopause, infection, sleep deprivation, physical exhaustion, surgery (Birnbaum 1928; Faergeman 1963; Stromgren 1974; Weiss & Rhoads 1979). Oftentimes the boundaries between 'organic' and 'reactive (psychogen)' causation are blurred (Astrup *et al.* 1959; Frey 1968). Recently devised operationalized criteria for reactive delusional psychosis (Opjordsmoen 1987; Jorgensen & Jensen 1988) regard organic pathology as exclusion criterion, but they are not specific enough and unnecessarily prevent clinicians from diagnosing reactive psychoses. In line with the psychopathological traditions defining part of the reactive conditions as superimposed syndromes, if it cannot be proven that manifest brain pathology or medical conditions induced and/or maintained the reactive psychosis, they should be treated as predisposing and pathoplastic factors. A simple example might clarify this reasoning. A confusional state immediately following a head trauma would not qualify as reactive psychosis even if the content was understandable within the context of the patient's personality and past and current life events. However, the organic personality disorder subsequent to the head trauma, a chronic condition, by lessening the affective-emotional and intellectual integrity and, consequently, the tolerance of the individual, would be a predisposing factor to reactive psychosis.

Occasionally head injury or other disturbance of consciousness may 'release' a reactive psychosis.

Case No. 4.3

A man in his 60s was involved in a road traffic accident in which he received a head injury sufficient to produce unconsciousness for several minutes but with no localizing neurological features and no discernible brain damage. On regaining consciousness he was initially excitable and fearful then in casualty became mute and immobile. He remained apparently stuporous for the next 48 hours then began intermittently weeping and calling for help in a state of obvious terror. He occasionally appeared to be responding to visual and auditory hallucinations. He improved with benzodiazepine sedation, gradually recovering over the next week. He had 40 years earlier been a navigator in a type of fighter bomber known as a Mosquito which had been hit by enemy fire and as these planes were wont to do had literally disintegrated. He had somehow activated his parachute and not only survived but been rescued. He had no memory for several weeks after the incident but had apparently been in a state of emotional paralysis. The head injury seemed to have produced a recapitulation of his reactive psychosis.

The precipitating events

The whole concept of reactive psychoses hinges on the presence of a stressful situation preceding the outbreak of psychosis without which the psychosis would not have occurred (Jaspers 1913; Stromgren 1974). The situation is either so powerful that would shake the very foundation of the existence of any human being, or a very specific one which strikes an individual who is, for a number of psychological and somatic reasons, vulnerable at the time to that particular event. Sensitizing previous experiences, though dormant for decades in some cases, are postulated to contribute to the underlying vulnerability and they may surface in the content of the psychosis. Maier (1912) put forward the concept of catathymia (*Katathymie*) in an attempt to explain individual, seemingly idiosyncratic, psychic vulnerability. Catathymia is the effect of a powerful and mostly subconscious affect-laden idea (*Vorstellungkomplex*), or ideas, on psychic phenomena. The content of such an idea is a desire, a wish or an ambivalent striving originating from early traumatic experience(s) that can be triggered later by specific traumatic experiences similar to, or reminding of, the original one(s). Faergeman (1963) calls catathymia a 'kind of psychic allergy', whereby a 'seemingly insignificant event will precipitate a large amount of excitation, that is, anxiety, only understandable to the observer who has knowledge of the catathymic hypersensitivity'. Thus, catathymia bridges the concepts of 'inner-psychic conflict' and 'psychic trauma' constituting the essence of psychogenesis (Faergeman 1963, p. 15). Catathymia undoubtedly brings with it a strong subjective component into the analysis of the pathogenesis of reactive psychoses paving the way for speculative psychodynamic explanations.

Pathogenic situations could be divided into acute and chronic groups, although the boundaries are not sharp between them and in any individual case they may combine with each other. Most stressful situations are complex events including more than one traumatic occurrence. Acute situations comprise interpersonal (sexual, familial, religious) conflicts, loss of loved ones or social prestige, power or wealth. Loss of freedom during social crises (e.g. war, prison, labour and concentration camps) are particularly multiplex sources of trauma (inanition, persecution, isolation, constant uncertainty and threat to life, physical and psychological torture). Natural disasters (e.g. earthquake, major accidents, floods) have similarly manifold effects. Among the chronic traumatizing situations, the classical examples are the isolation due to deafness (Kraepelin 1915), language (Allers 1920), and immigration (Frost 1938).

Judging the immediacy of the precipitating/causative event(s) in relation to the psychosis is always problematic and somewhat arbitrary. Some modern authors (e.g. Munoz *et al.* 1987) accept a very brief period, 1 week, between trauma and psychosis, others (e.g. Jorgensen & Jensen 1988) are more generous, allowing 3 months. Classical writers (e.g. Jaspers 1913;

Faergeman 1963) focused on the context in which the precipitating events unfolded and were less concerned with the exact time-frame.

The diagnosis of the reactive psychosis in most cases is not possible without the empathic and accurate rendition of the patient's 'psychological' biography (Jaspers 1948/1963). For the very same reasons, the simple cataloguing of life events by employing questionnaires does not give sufficient information without the background of a well-digested biography (McCabe 1975; Stromgren 1986). Jaspers' (1913) two masterly reconstructed case histories — 30 densely printed pages each — exemplify this empathic understanding. Boundless curiosity, empathic immersion in the patient's life and his or her current experiences and diligent investigative enquiry form the cornerstone of the diagnosis of reactive psychosis. However, it usually takes several hours of personally conducted interviews to reach the insight necessary to understand the intricate web of past and recent experiences, predisposing factors and psychopathology. Modern clinicians can rarely afford this luxury. The fundamental changes in clinical practice since Jaspers' time including, for instance, the introduction of multidisciplinary team work, the widespread use of questionnaires and rating scales employed by mental health professionals other than psychiatrists, would partly explain why (brief) reactive psychosis is seldom considered in clinical practice. In addition, the layout of multiaxial diagnostic schemes (e.g. DSM-III and its successors) listing clinical picture, personality characteristics, stressful life events separately fragments assessment and creates an environment in which dynamics and interactions are reduced to the impoverished notion of comorbidities.

Epidemiology

There are no entirely reliable data on the prevalence and incidence of reactive psychoses. National registries in Scandanavia suggest reactive psychoses occur in between 13% and 30% of all patients admitted (Dahl 1986). In Denmark, between 1970 and 1988 there were 21 615 first admission patients with reactive psychoses while the corresponding figures for manic-depressive and schizophrenic psychoses were only 18 293 and 3 825 respectively (Jorgensen & Mortensen 1992). On the basis of national statistics, Stromgren (1974) estimated a life-time expectancy of 1% for reactive psychoses with a risk period of 15–55 years of age while Faergeman's (1963) estimation was 0.3%. Using ICD-8, Canadian statistics available for the years 1969 and 1973 showed a very different picture (Allodi 1982). In 1969, reactive psychoses made up 8.3% of all first admissions for psychoses and 2.7% of all first admissions to Canadian psychiatric institutions. There were no significant changes 4 years later.

Demographic data

Due to varying diagnostic practices and lack of rigorous methodology, the following findings are more approximations than hard data. In most unselected hospital series of reactive psychoses women predominate with a ratio of 2–3 to 1 (Astrup *et al.* 1959; Faergeman 1963; Andersen & Laerum 1980; Refsum & Astrup 1980; Stromgren 1988). Age of onset peaks in the third to the fifth decade of life (Faergeman 1963; McCabe 1975; Andersen & Laerum 1980), though reactive psychosis may occur in the elderly (Raphaelsen & Stromgren 1956; Anderson & Laerum 1980; Jorgensen & Munk-Jorgensen 1985) and have been reported in children and adolescents (Warren & Cameron 1950).

Mortality

It has been long established that major psychiatric disorders increase mortality (Alstrom 1942). Although the lethality (death during an episode) of reactive psychoses is minimal (Astrup *et al.* 1959; Faergeman 1963), there is compelling evidence that reactive psychoses are associated with a mortality rate significantly higher than in the general population (Alstrom 1942; Astrup *et al.* 1959; Anderson & Laerum 1980; Jorgensen & Mortensen 1990). Based on the accurate nationwide Danish mental health and mortality statistics, Jorgensen and Mortensen (1990) found that the relative risk of mortality from reactive psychoses exceeded not only that of the general population but also those of schizophrenia and manic-depressive psychosis. Examination of the causes of death revealed that patients with reactive psychoses had an excess mortality in all major causes of death, particularly in suicide where the mortality rate was about 15 times higher than in the general population (Jorgensen & Mortensen 1992). An excess of suicide during follow-up was also found by other investigators (Astrup *et al.* 1959; Retterstol 1970; Andersen & Laerum 1980).

Biological studies

With the exception of clinical-genetic investigations, there is a conspicuous absence of biological studies although some authorities have postulated a somatic predisposition as a necessary, if not sufficient prerequisite for reactive psychoses (e.g. Jaspers 1913; Birnbaum 1928; Faergeman 1963; Stromgren 1974). In the light of the complexity of the hypothesized pathogenesis of reactive psychoses, the paucity of biological investigations is quite understandable.

Clinical-genetic investigations

No major study has been published in this area since the mid-1970s so recent methodological advances made in psychiatric genetics have not been utilized. Studies have suggested higher rates of schizophrenia and bipolar disorders in the relatives of those with reactive psychosis (Astrup *et al.* 1962; Faergeman 1963; McCabe 1975).

In McCabe's (1975) family study, while there was a sharp distinction between reactive psychoses and schizophrenia, the delimitation of reactive psychoses from manic-depressive illness was uncertain. McCabe (1975) brought together all the twin pairs from the literature where either or both of the twins had reactive psychosis. Of the 21 monozygotic twins, four were concordant for reactive psychoses in contrast to one of the 32 dizygotic twins of the same sex. The method of collapsing data from different investigations is questionable so no conclusion can be drawn from these figures.

All in all, family and twin studies have contributed modestly to the validation of reactive psychosis as a distinct entity. These inconclusive findings do not allow any firm conclusion about the role of genetic factors in the pathogenesis of reactive psychoses.

Treatment

It is somewhat paradoxical that while opinions concerning the diagnostic criteria and the very nature of reactive psychoses vary considerably, there is general agreement about their management. In the first few days symptomatic treatment with antipsychotic and/or antidepressant drugs, preferably in low doses, or even electroconvulsive therapy (ECT), is usually unavoidable (Sturup *et al.* 1942; Stromgren 1986; Stevens 1987; Beighley *et al.* 1992; Modestin & Bachmann 1992; McGlashan & Krystal 1995). Amytal sodium (Steiner 1991) and benzodiazepines (Salam & Pillai 1987) are particularly useful in reactive stupor. Having diagnostic uncertainties, as it frequently happens when facing an acute psychosis, few clinicians would share the view that patients 'may profit from experiencing spontaneous recovery and appreciating the relationship between their psychotic reaction and the precipitating stress' (Tamminga & Carpenter 1982). The increased risk of suicide in reactive psychoses (Jorgensen & Mortensen 1992) also necessitates pharmacological intervention. Attention should be paid to predisposing somatic factors such as fever, infections, malnutrition, etc. Biological treatment should be followed by individual and family psychotherapy aiming at the exploration and interpretation of the underlying conflicts helping the patient understand and 'work through' his or her problems (Stromgren 1974, 1986; McGlashan & Krystal 1995).

These general guidelines drawing on the notion that reactive psychoses are brief, self-limiting psychotic episodes, are based on clinical experience rather than well-designed clinical trials. As a consequence, they have to be applied flexibly, on an individual basis. For instance, drug treatment is not always necessary; in an earlier series 46% of the patients with reactive psychoses did not need any somatic treatment (Astrup *et al.* 1959). Drug treatment might consist of a single dose of antipsychotic or anxiolytic or may last for several days or weeks, particularly in paranoid reactive psychosis.

Maintenance medication is rarely necessary (Tamminga & Carpenter 1982; Stromgren 1986); however, it should be considered for cases where the stressful situation and the patient's vulnerability persists, the reactive psychosis was exceptionally long and severe, the patient has no insight and/or is not amenable to psychotherapy or secondary anxiety and depressive features remain as the aftereffect of the psychosis (McGlashan & Krystal 1995). Eventually, with the lack of randomized, double-blind clinical trials, prudent treatment still depends on the clinician's wisdom, i.e. the ability to analyse and integrate several biological, personality and psychosocial factors into a coherent and meaningful picture and predict the short- and long-term outcome of the particular patient.

References

Allers, R. (1920) Uber psychogene Storungen in sprachfremder Umgebung (der Verfolgunswahn der sprachlich Isolierten). *Zeitschrift fur die gesamte Neurologie und Psychiatrie* 60, 281–289.

Allodi, F. (1982) Acute paranoid reaction (bouffee delirante) in Canada. *Canadian Journal of Psychiatry* 27, 366–373.

Alstrom, C.H. (1942) *Mortality in Mental Hospitals with Especial Regard to Tuberculosis*. Munksgaard, Copenhagen.

American Psychiatric Association (1980) *Diagnostic and Statistical Manual of Mental Disorders*, 3rd edn (DSM-III). American Psychiatric Association, Washington, D.C.

American Psychiatric Association (1987) *Diagnostic and Statistical Manual of Mental Disorders*, 3rd edn revised (DSM-III-R). American Psychiatric Association, Washington, D.C.

American Psychiatric Association (1994) *Diagnostic and Statistical Manual of Mental Disorders*, 4th edn (DSM-IV). American Psychiatric Association, Washington, D.C.

Andersen, J. & Laerum, H. (1980) Psychogenic psychoses. *Acta Psychiatrica Scandinavica* 62, 332–342.

Arentsen, K. (1968) Reactive psychoses. *Acta Psychiatrica Scandinavica* 44 (Suppl. 203), 5–8.

Astrup, C., Fossum, A. & Holmboe, R. (1959) A follow-up study of 270 patients with acute affective psychoses. *Acta Psychiatrica et Neurologica Scandinavica* 34 (Suppl. 135), 1–135.

Astrup, C., Fossum, A. & Holmboe, R. (1962) *Prognosis in Functional Psychoses: Clinical, Social and Genetic Aspects*. C.C. Thomas, Springfield, Ill.

Baetz, E. (1901) Uber Emotionslahmung. *Allgemeine Zeitschrift für Psychiatrie* 58, 717–721.

Beighley, P.S., Brown, G.R. & Thompson, J.W. (1992) DSM-III-R brief reactive psychosis among air force recruits. *Journal of Clinical Psychiatry* 53, 283–288.

Birnbaum, K. (1928) Die psychoreactiven (psychogenen) Symptomenbildungen. In: *Handbuch der Geisteskrankenheiten* (ed. O. Bumke), Vol. 2, pp. 92–133. Springer, Berlin.

Bleuler, E. (1911/1950) *Dementia Praecox or the Group of Schizophrenias* (trans. J. Zinkin). International Universities Press, New York.

Bonhoeffer, K. (1911) Wie weit kommen psychogene Krankheitzustande und Krankheitsprozesse vor, die nich der Hysterie zuzurechnen sind? *Allgemeine Zeitschrift für Psychiatrie* 68, 371–386.

Bunse, P. (1918) Die reaktiven Dammerzustande und verwandte Storungen und ihre Bedeutung als Kriegspsychosen. *Zeitschrift für die gesamte Neurologie und Psychiatrie* 40, 237–282.

Cavenar, J.O., Sullivan, J.L. & Maltbie, A.A. (1979) A clinical note on hysterical psychosis. *American Journal of Psychiatry* 136, 830–832.

Chavan, B.S. & Kulhara, P. (1988) A clinical study of reactive psychosis. *Acta Psychiatrica Scandinavica* 78, 712–715.

Cooper, J.E. (1994) Relationship between chapter V(F) of the ICD-10 and national psychiatric classifications. In: *Psychiatric Diagnosis: A World Perspective* (eds J.E. Mezzich, Y. Honda & M.C. Kastrup), pp. 158–164. Springer-Verlag, New York, Berlin.

Dahl, A.A. (1986) The DSM-III classification of the functional psychoses and the Norwegian tradition. *Acta Psychiatrica Scandinavica* 73 (Suppl. 328), 45–53.

Dahl, A.A. (1987) Problems concerning the concept of reactive psychoses. *Psychopathology* **20**, 79–86.

Dahl, A.A., Cloninger, R.C., Guze, S.B. & Retterstol, N. (1992) Convergence of American and Scandinavian diagnoses of functional psychoses. *Comprehensive Psychiatry* **33**, 13–16.

Degkwitz, R. (1985) Die psychogenen Psychosen. Eine Ubersicht über die klinischen Bilder, die Genese, Prognose und Therapie. *Fortschritte der Neurologie und Psychatrie* **53**, 22–28.

Edgerton, J.E. & Campbell, R.J. (1994) *American Psychiatric Glossary*, 7th edn. American Psychiatric Association, Washington, D.C.

Eitinger, L. (1959) The incidence of mental disease among refugees in Norway. *Journal of Mental Science* **105**, 326–338.

Faergeman, P.M. (1963) *Psychogenic Psychoses*. Butterworths, London.

Frey, T.S. (1968) On reactive psychosis. *Acta Psychiatrica Scandinavica* **44** (Suppl. 203), 1–4.

Friedmann, C.T.H. (1982) The so-called hysteropsychoses. Latah, windogo and pibloktoq. In: *Extraordinary Disorders of Human Behavior* (eds C.T.H. Friedmann & R.A. Faguet), pp. 215–228. Plenum Press, New York.

Frost, I. (1938) Home-sickness and immigrant psychoses. *Journal of Mental Science* **84**, 801–847.

Guldberg, C.A., Dahl, A.A., Bertelsen, A. *et al.* (1996) The Reactivity of Psychosis Rating Form (RPRF): background, development and psychometrics. *Acta Psychiatrica Scandinavica* **93**, 113–118.

Hansen, H., Dahl, A.A., Bertelsen, A. *et al.* (1992) The Nordic concept of reactive psychosis: A multicenter reliability study. *Acta Psychiatrica Scandinavica* **86**, 55–59.

Harry, B. & Favazza A.R. (1984) Brief reactive psychosis in a deaf man. *American Journal of Psychiatry* **141**, 898–899.

Hirsch, S.R. & Hollender, M.H. (1969) Hysterical psychosis: Clarification of the concept. *American Journal of Psychiatry* **125**, 909–915.

Holmboe, R. & Astrup, C. (1957) A follow-up study of 255 patients with acute schizophrenia and schizophreniform psychoses. *Acta Psychiatrica et Neurologica Scandinavica* **32** (Suppl. 115), pp. 1–148.

Hollender, M.H. & Hirsch, S.R. (1964) Hysterical psychosis. *American Journal of Psychiatry* **120**, 1066–1074.

Jaspers, K. (1913) Kausale und 'verstandliche' Zusammenhange zwischen Schicksal und Psychose bei der Dementia praecox (Schizophrenie). *Zeitschrift für die gesamte Neurologie und Psychiatrie* **14**, 158–263.

Jaspers, K. (1948/1963) *General Psychopathology* (trans. J. Hoenig & M.W. Hamilton). Manchester University Press, Manchester.

Jauch, D.A. & Carpenter, W.T. (1988a) Reactive psychosis I: Does the pre-DSM-III concept define a third psychosis? *Journal of Nervous and Mental Disease* **176**, 72–81.

Jauch, D.A. & Carpenter, W.T. (1988b) Reactive psychosis II: Does DSM-III-R define a third psychosis? *Journal of Nervous and Mental Disease* **176**, 82–86.

Jorgensen, P. (1985) Long-term course of acute reactive paranoid psychosis: A follow-up study. *Acta Psychiatrica Scandinavica* **71**, 30–37.

Jorgensen, P. (1986) Delusional psychosis. *Acta Psychiatrica Scandinavica* **74**, 18–23.

Jorgensen, P. & Munk-Jorgensen, P. (1985) Paranoid psychosis in the elderly. *Acta Psychiatrica Scandinavica* **72**, 358–363.

Jorgensen, P. & Jensen, J. (1988) An attempt to operationalize reactive delusional psychosis. *Acta Psychiatrica Scandinavica* **78**, 627–631.

Jorgensen P. & Mortensen, P.B. (1988) Admission pattern and diagnostic stability of patients with functional psychoses in Denmark during a two-year observation period. *Acta Psychiatrica Scandinavica* **78**, 361–365.

Jorgensen, P. & Mortensen, P.B. (1990) Reactive psychosis and mortality. *Acta Psychiatrica Scandinavica* **81**, 277–279.

Jorgensen, P. & Mortensen, P.B. (1992) Cause of death in reactive psychosis. *Acta Psychiatrica Scandinavica* **85**, 351–353.

Kapur, R.L. & Pandurangi, A.K. (1979) A comparative study of reactive psychosis and acute psychosis without precipitating stress. *British Journal of Psychiatry* **135**, 544–550.

Kasanin, J. (1933) The acute schizoaffective psychoses. *American Journal of Psychiatry* **13**, 97–126.

Kendler, K.S., Spitzer, R.L. & Williams, J.B.W. (1989) Psychotic disorders in DSM-III-R. *American Journal of Psychiatry* **146**, 953–962.

Kleist, K. (1918) Schreckpsychosen. *Allgemeine Zeitschrift für Psychiatrie* **74**, 432–510.

Kleist, K. (1921) Autochtone Degenerationspsychosen. *Zeitschrift für die gesamte Neurologie und Psychiatrie* **69**, 1–11.

Kraepelin, E. (1915) *Psychiatrie: Ein Lehrbuch für Studierende und Arzte,* Vol. 4, Teil 3, 8th edn, pp. 1441–1448. Johann Ambrosius Barth, Leipzig.

Kretschmer, E. (1918) *Der sensitive Beziehungswahn.* Springer, Berlin.

Krieger, M.J. & Zussman, M. (1981) The importance of cultural factors in a brief reactive psychosis. *Journal of Clinical Psychiatry* **42**, 248–249.

Labhardt, F. (1963) *Die schizophrenie-ahnlichen Emotionspsychosen.* Springer-Verlag, Berlin.

Langness, L.L. (1967) Hysterical psychosis: The cross-cultural evidence. *American Journal of Psychiatry* **124**, 143–152.

Langfeldt, G. (1939) *The Schizophreniform States.* Munksgaard, Copenhagen.

Langfeldt, G. (1982) Definition of 'Schizophreniform Psychoses'. *American Journal of Psychiatry* **139**, 703.

Leonhard, K. (1957) *Aufteilung der endogenen Psychosen.* Akademie Verlag, Berlin.

Levine, R.E. & Gaw, A.C. (1995) Culture-bound syndromes. *The Psychiatric Clinics of North America* **18**, 523–536.

Lewin, J. (1917) Uber Situationspsychosen. *Archiv für Psychiatrie und Nervenkrankheiten* **58**, 533–598.

Lewis, A. (1972) 'Psychogenic': A word and its mutations. *Psychological Medicine* **2**, 209–215.

Maier, H.W. (1912) Uber katathyme Wahnbildung und Paranoia. *Zeitschrift für die gesamte Neurologie und Psychiatrie* **13**, 555–610.

McGlashan, T.H. & Krystal, J.H. (1995) Schizophrenia-related disorders and dual diagnosis. In: *Treatments of Psychiatric Disorders*, Vol. 1 (ed. G.O. Gabbard), 2nd edn, pp. 1039–1074. American Psychiatric Press, Washington, D.C.

McCabe, M.S. (1975) Reactive psychosis: A clinical and genetic investigation. *Acta Psychiatrica Scandinavica* **54** (Suppl. 259), 1–133.

Menuck, M., Legault, S., Schmidt, P. *et al.* (1989) The nosologic status of the remitting atypical psychoses. *Comprehensive Psychiatry*, **30**, 53–73.

Mentzos, S. (1973) Zur Psychodynamik der sogenannten "hysterischen" Psychosen. *Nervenarzt* **44**, 285–291.

Modestin, J. & Bachmann, K.M. (1992) Is the diagnosis of hysterical psychosis justified? Clinical study of hysterical psychosis, reactive/psychogenic psychosis and schizophrenia. *Comprehensive Psychiatry* **33**, 17–24.

Munoz, R.A., Amado, H. & Hyatt, S. (1987) Brief reactive psychosis. *Journal of Clinical Psychiatry* **48**, 324–327.

Noreik, K., Astrup, C., Dalgard, O.S. & Holmboe, R. (1967) A prolonged follow-up of acute schizophrenic and schizophreniform psychoses. *Acta Psychiatrica Scandinavica* **43**, 432–443.

Noreik, K. (1970) *Follow-up and Classification of Functional Psychoses with Special Reference to Reactive Psychoses*. Universitetsforlaget, Oslo.

Odegaard, O. (1968) Reactive psychoses. *Acta Psychiatrica Scandinavica* **44** (Suppl. 203), 23–26.

Okasha, A., Seif El Dawla, A. Khalil, A.H. & Saad, A. (1993) Presentation of acute psychosis in an Egyptian sample: A transcultural comparison. *Comprehensive Psychiatry* **34**, 4–9.

Opjordsmoen, S. (1987) Toward an operationalization of reactive paranoid psychoses (reactive delusional disorder). *Psychopathology* **20**, 72–78.

Pandurangi, A.K. & Kapur, R.L. (1980) Reactive psychosis. *Acta Psychiatrica Scandinavica* **61**, 89–95.

Pichot, P. (1982) The diagnosis and classification of mental disorders in French-speaking countries: Background, current views and comparison with other nomenclatures. *Psychological Medicine* **12**, 475–492.

Pichot, P. (1986) The concept of 'bouffee delirante' with special reference to the Scandinavian concept of reactive psychosis. *Psychopathology* **19**, 35–43.

Pierloot, R.A. & Ngoma, M. (1988) Hysterical manifestations in Africa and Europe. *British Journal of Psychiatry* **152**, 112–115.

Pull, C.B. (1995) Atypical psychotic disorders. In: *Schizophrenia* (eds S.R. Hirsch & D.R. Weinberger), pp. 58–72. Blackwell Science, Oxford.

Pull, C.B., Pull, M.C. & Pichot, P. (1987) Des criteres empiriques français pour les psychoses. III. Algorhytmes et arbre de decision. *Encephale* **13**, 59–66.

Raphaelsen, O.J. & Stromgren, E. (1956) Ten years' geriatrics in a Danish psychiatric hospital. *Acta Psychiatrica et Neurologica Scandinavica* **31** (Suppl. 106), 103–110.

Refsum, H.E. & Astrup, C. (1980) Reactive depression: A follow-up. *Neuropsychobiology* **6**, 79–90.

Refsum, H.E. & Astrup, C. (1982) Hysteric reactive psychoses: A follow-up. *Neuropsychobiology* **8**, 172–181.

Remington, G., Menuck, M., Schmidt, P., Legault, S. (1990) The remitting atypical psychoses: Clinical and nosologic considerations. *Canadian Journal of Psychiatry* **35**, 36–40.

Retterstol, N. (1966) *Paranoid and Paranoiac Psychoses.* C.C. Thomas, Springfield, Ill.

Retterstol, N. (1970) *Prognosis in Paranoid Psychoses.* Universitetsforlaget, Oslo.

Retterstol, N. (1987) Present state of reactive psychoses in Scandinavia. *Psychopathology* **20**, 68–71.

Retterstol, N. & Dahl, A.A. (1983) Scandinavian perspectives on DSM-III. In: *International Perspectives on DSM-III* (eds R.L. Spitzer, J.B.W. Williams & A.E. Skodol), pp. 217–234. American Psychiatric Press, Washington, D.C.

Retterstol, N. & Opjordsmoen, S. (1994) Differences in diagnosis and long-term outcome between monosymptomatic and other delusional disorders. *Psychopathology* **27**, 240–246.

Rudin, E. (1901) Uber die klinischen Formen der Gefangnispsychosen. *Allgemeine Zeitschrift für Psychiatrie* **58**, 447–462.

Ruiz, P. & Gomez, E.A. (1984) Cultural factors in the symptomatology of transient psychosis. In: *Transient Psychosis: Diagnosis, Management and Evaluation* (eds J. Tupin, U. Halbreich & J.J. Pena), pp. 31–42. Brunner/Mazel, New York.

Salam, S.A. & Pillai, A.K. (1987) Lorazepam for psychogenic catatonia. *American Journal of Psychiatry* **144**, 1082–1083.

Schioldann-Nielsen, J. (1993) August Wimmer: On possession states. Classic Text No. 15. *History of Psychiatry* **4**, 413–419.

Schneider, K. (1927) Die abnormen seelischen Reaktionen. In: *Handbuch der Psychiatrie,* Spezieller Teil, 7. Abteilung II. Teil, 1. Halfte (ed. G. Aschaffenburg), pp. 1–43. Deuticke, Leipzig-Wien.

Slater, E. (1964) Special syndromes and treatments. *British Journal of Psychiatry* **110**, 114–118.

Sommer, R. (1894) *Diagnostik der Geisteskrankheiten.* Urban & Schwarzenberg, Vienna.

Steiner, W. (1991) The use of amytal in psychogenic psychosis. *Canadian Journal of Psychiatry* **36**, 54–56.

Stephens, J.H., Shaffer, J.W. & Carpenter, W.T. (1982) Reactive psychoses. *Journal of Nervous and Mental Disease* **170**, 657–663.

Stevens, J. (1987) Brief psychoses: Do they contribute to the good prognosis and equal prevalence of schizophrenia in developing countries? *British Journal of Psychiatry* **151**, 393–396.

Stromgren, E. (1974) Psychogenic psychoses. In: *Themes and Variations in European Psychiatry* (eds S.R. Hirsch & M. Shepherd), pp. 102–125. J.J. Wright and Sons, Bristol.

Stromgren, E. (1983) The strengths and weaknesses of DSM-III. In: *International Perspective on DSM-III* (eds R.L. Spitzer, J.B.W. Williams & A.E. Skodol), pp. 69–77. American Psychiatric Press, Washington, D.C.

Stromgren, E. (1986) Reactive (psychogenic) psychoses and their relations to schizoaffective psychoses. In: *Schizoaffective Psychoses* (eds A. Marneros & M.T. Tsuang), pp. 260–271. Springer-Verlag, Berlin.

Stromgren, E. (1988) Psychiatric admissions of the elderly. *Acta Psychiatria Scandinavica* 78 (Suppl. 345), 56–60.

Stromgren, E. (1994) Scandinavian contributions to psychiatric nosology. In: *Psychiatric Diagnosis: A World Perspective* (eds J.E. Mezzich, Y. Honda & M.C. Kastrup), pp. 33–38. Springer-Verlag, New York, Berlin.

Sturup, G.K., Smith, J.C. & Hahnemann, V. (1942) Report on results of convulsion therapy. *Acta Psychiatrica et Neurologica* 17, 237–261.

Susser, E., Fennig, S., Jandorf, L., Amador, X. & Bromet, E. (1995a) Epidemiology, diagnosis and course of brief psychoses. *American Journal of Psychiatry* 152, 1743–1748.

Susser, E., Varma, V.K., Malhotra, S., Conover, S. & Amador, X.F. (1995b) Delineation of acute and transient psychotic disorders in a developing country setting. *British Journal of Psychiatry* 167, 216–219.

Tamminga, C.A. & Carpenter, W.T. (1982) The DSM-III diagnosis of schizophrenia-like illness and the clinical pharmacology of psychosis. *Journal of Nervous and Mental Diseases* 170, 744–750.

Villinger, W. (1920) Gibt es psychogenen nicht-hysterische Psychosen auf normalpsychologischer Grundlage? *Zeitschrift für die gesamte Neurologie und Psychiatrie* 57, 174–195.

Warren, W. & Cameron, K. (1950) Reactive psychosis in adolescents. *Journal of Mental Science* 96, 448–457.

Weiss, J.R. & Rhoads, J.M. (1979) Brief reactive psychosis: A psychodynamic interpretation. *Journal of Clinical Psychiatry* 40, 440–443.

Wig, N.N. (1983) DSM-III: A perspective from the third world. In: *International Perspectives on DSM-III* (eds R.L. Spitzer, J.B.W. Williams & A.E. Skodol), pp. 79–89. American Psychiatric Press, Washington, D.C.

Wig, N.N. (1990) The third-world perspective on psychiatric diagnosis and classification. In: *Sources and Traditions of Classification in Psychiatry* (eds N. Sartorius, A. Jablensky, D.A. Regier, J.D. Burke & R.M.A. Hirschfeld), pp. 181–210. Hogrefe & Huber Publishers, Toronto.

Wimmer, A. (1916) Psykogene Sindssygdomsformer. In: *St. Hans Hospital 1816–1916, Jubilee Publication*, pp. 85–216. Gad, Copenhagen.

Wimmer, A. (1924/1993) On possession states (trans. J. Schioldann-Nielsen). *History of Psychiatry* 4, 420–440.

World Health Organization (1967) *International Statistical Classification of Diseases*, 8th revision (ICD-8). World Health Organization, Geneva.

World Health Organization (1978) *Mental Disorders: Glossary and Guide to Their Classification in Accordance with the Ninth Revision of the International Classification of Diseases* (ICD-9). World Health Organization, Geneva.

World Health Organization (1992) *The ICD-10 Classification of Mental and Behavioural Disorders. Clinical Descriptions and Diagnostic Guidelines*. World Health Organization, Geneva.

Yap, P.M. (1967) Classification of the culture-bound reactive syndromes. *Australian and New Zealand Journal of Psychiatry* 1, 172–179.

CHAPTER 5

Paraphrenia

ALISTAIR MUNRO

Introduction

Paraphrenia was first described by Kraepelin (1919) early in the present century as a functional psychotic illness separate from both paranoia and schizophrenia. As the definition of schizophrenia subsequently widened, paraphrenia suffered a similar fate to paranoia, and most cases were probably diagnosed thereafter as paranoid schizophrenia or, more recently, as schizoaffective disorder. Paranoia has re-emerged, renamed delusional disorder (American Psychiatric Association (APA) 1994), and is again widely accepted as a diagnosis in its own right. Paraphrenia still remains in the wings, at present excluded from the major diagnostic classificatory systems.

The aim of this chapter is to show that paraphrenia is, at the least, a separate subcategory of illness, whose diagnosis is of some practical value. It is noteworthy that psychiatrists are increasingly unwilling to diagnose schizophrenia when markedly atypical features are present, but, as will be shown, there is often no satisfactory alternative category for such atypical cases (also see Chapter 14). It is proposed that some of these patients do fit well within the diagnosis of paraphrenia, particularly when its description is updated to match the needs of present-day practice.

Diagnostic difficulties

In most psychiatric illnesses we are still dependent on history-taking and careful observations, but very little technology, in order to make a diagnosis. Exciting research trends are demonstrating increasingly subtle brain abnormalities and are linking these to mental symptoms, but application of such methods to the clinical field is still disappointingly slow.

Appearances in psychiatric illnesses can be influenced by many things, including the acuity or chronicity of the disorder, the underlying personality of the patient, the presence of complicating features (such as alcohol abuse), the age or sex of the patient and so on. In the past, when there were virtually no effective treatments available, the clinician could observe the unimpeded evolution of a disorder over a long period, which often provided a confirmation of diagnosis as well as an indication of prognosis. Whatever perplexing form a psychiatric condition assumed when it was first observed, there was usually ample time to watch it declare its true colours with the passage of time.

In psychiatry we now have a variety of powerful treatments which we can apply to illnesses whose parameters are still only vaguely comprehended. As soon as we give a treatment, the appearance and course of the illness are modified, whether or not benefit accrues. Nowadays, it is rarely possible to observe the true natural history of a disorder, except in non-compliant patients. It is wonderful to possess these modern treatments, but they have taken away the opportunity to watch the evolution of the psychiatric disorder and have left us dependent on a 'snap-shot' approach to diagnosis. When technology eventually catches up this problem will decrease, but at present the psychiatrist is often discomfited at having to apply very specific treatments to what are, at best, provisional diagnoses.

Another confounding factor in psychiatric diagnosis lies with the personal belief system of the psychiatrist. We are only beginning to develop widely acceptable definitions of the illnesses we deal with, and a standardized terminology to describe them. One of the most striking examples of diagnostic confusion in this century was the apparent finding that schizophrenia was twice as common in the US as in the UK. It took a rigorous study (Gurland *et al.* 1970) to demonstrate that this discrepancy was apparent, not real, that a difference in philosophies and in diagnostic habits was resulting in gross overdiagnosis of schizophrenia in the US.

Schizophrenia is so obviously an overall term for a variety of superficially similar illnesses that, for many years, it has been customary to refer to 'the schizophrenias' (Harris & Jeste 1988). We are increasingly confirming that the category is heterogeneous, yet, in clinical work, we continue to diagnose schizophrenia as though it were an entity, though accepting poorly validated clinical subtypes such as the paranoid, the disorganized, etc. Often we turn a blind eye to the differential responses of individual patients to identical treatments which, in many instances, must reflect differing underlying pathologies.

Certainly we try to diagnose schizophrenia much more carefully than we did before: but we could still look much more critically at our diagnostic practices towards the schizophrenia spectrum of disorders. The future for schizophrenia will not be a magic bullet: instead it will be a process of identifying more and more subgroups with specific features and treatment responses and removing these till nothing is left. An attempt will be made here to commend paraphrenia as one of these subgroups and to suggest its separation from schizophrenia.

Paraphrenia: demonstrably different from schizophrenia?

A possible criterion in delineating subgroups would be to describe 'good outcome' and 'poor outcome' cases. In the atherapeutic past, most cases of schizophrenia-like illness had a bad prognosis but modern treatment has profoundly changed this situation. At this very time we are watching as some cases of schizophrenia with a previously bad prognosis show marked improvements with the atypical neuroleptics.

For many years, psychiatrists have reported on cases similar to schizophrenia, but with less florid symptoms and a less drastic prognosis. At present, the clinician is forced to diagnose these as 'atypical psychosis', 'psychotic disorder NOS (not otherwise specified)' or, increasingly, 'schizoaffective disorder', none of which is a satisfactory resort, since each of them necessarily lumps disparate conditions together. One of these disparate conditions is paraphrenia, no longer recognized in the DSM or ICD series, although it potentially has considerable clinical validity.

In Chapter 3, paranoia (now delusional disorder) is considered in detail and its tortuous history and eventual rehabilitation described. The delineation of that disorder was also largely the work of Emil Kraepelin (1919) who carefully distinguished paranoia from dementia praecox (which Bleuler (1950) later renamed schizophrenia). In 1909, Kraepelin introduced a further diagnostic entity, that of paraphrenia (a term originally coined by Kahlbaum (1863)), and included this in a group of four paranoid illnesses as follows:

1 paranoid dementia praecox (paranoid schizophrenia);
2 paraphrenia;
3 paranoia;
4 presenile delusions of insanity.

(Presenile delusions of insanity has not survived as a viable diagnosis and it is presumed that most cases nowadays are included with paranoid schizophrenia.)

Since Kraepelin's day, paraphrenia has continued to be diagnosed, though rarely carefully defined, by some psychiatrists but the majority in modern times tend to ignore it as a separate category. Kraepelin himself described the illness as similar to paranoid schizophrenia, having fantastic delusions and hallucinations, but with relatively slight thought disorder and much better preservation of affect. Compared with schizophrenia there was less personality deterioration and little loss of volition. The behaviour of paraphrenic patients was less disturbed than that of schizophrenics and even when their delusions were severe their manner appeared relatively reasonable. Their ability to communicate and to convey affective warmth and rapport remained good.

Now that Kraepelin had described paraphrenia as an illness lying between paranoid schizophrenia and paranoia (delusional disorder), he decided that paranoia was not associated with hallucinations: henceforth in his view a paranoia-like illness with hallucinations would be regarded as paraphrenia. Modern research on paranoia/delusional disorder discounts this distinction since both disorders can have hallucinations, though they are certainly more prominent in paraphrenia and the differentiation between the two illnesses is made on other grounds (see Chapter 3).

Paraphrenia in the psychiatric literature

Kraepelin's original description of paraphrenia is clear and he makes almost as good a case for it as for paranoia. His credentials as an observer and delineator of major psychiatric disorders are of the highest, though of course we have to make allowances for the passage of time and changes in conceptualization which inevitably have modified some of his original conclusions. If such a respected authority with such an impressive track-record in nosology could recognize paraphrenia as a legitimate diagnosis, why does it command such little respect today?

A study of the literature does little to answer this question since much of it is contradictory. 'Late paraphrenia' is currently the best-documented form of the illness but even it is controversial (Holden 1987). Many discussions on paraphrenia are dogmatic and even idiosyncratic and most of the better-quality descriptions are quite old, many of them preoccupied with ideological arguments and disagreements which have now become obscure, sometimes even quaint.

Anderson and Trethowan (1973), particularly reflecting a viewpoint of German psychiatry, had no difficulty in seeing paraphrenia as a separate illness, saying that it was 'that portion of the totality of paranoid states which do not in a few years manifest the characteristic deterioration of schizophrenia nor the full characteristics of paranoia'. Arieti (1955) similarly underlined the observation that there was minimal decay of the personality although the illness itself was often progressive.

Curran and Partridge (1969) noted another important element when they said that in paraphrenia 'emotional rapport may remain strikingly good', and many clinicians see this as a key factor in diagnosis. Even today, when the treatment outcome of schizophrenia is so much better than a generation ago, it is difficult to justify diagnosing a patient with a prolonged and sustained psychosis as schizophrenic when he or she retains a great deal of appropriate affect, good emotional range and an ability to develop a reasonable rapport, even while quite ill. This affective component was underlined by Leonhard (1960) when he referred to one of his atypical psychoses as 'affect-laden paraphrenia', though he considered this still to be linked to schizophrenia. To illustrate the importance of the affective element in paraphrenia a case description is now given.

Case No. 5.1: Paraphrenia

A woman of 45 who looks considerably younger than her stated age has had at least five admissions to a psychiatric hospital. She was originally diagnosed as suffering from paranoid schizophrenia, and when she is unwell this diagnosis is reasonable. She exhibits widespread delusions, although one —a conviction that she was cheated out of the inheritance left to her by her grandmother—is especially prominent. She also has auditory hallucinations, usually not unpleasant, and has 'visions' about her future. The latter do not appear to be actual visual hallucinations. Her thinking is vague and very mannered during relapse, and at her worst, she is verbally and behaviourally retarded. Despite this, she retains warm affect and staff always comment that she is a 'likeable' patient.

Relapses are inevitably due to her stopping her medication, which usually consists of the neuroleptic haloperidol. She cannot explain adequately why she stops taking this, but it seems to be due to a resurgence of delusional thinking. When she is well and is compliant with the drug, improvement is remarkable. She gradually becomes relaxed, quite spontaneous in manner, and shows a sense of humour. Her husband reports that she is an interesting companion and her sex-drive appears normal. She has friends who have remained attached to her, despite an intermittent history of mental illness of at least 10 years' duration. Assessment in these good periods shows slight concreteness of thinking and some inflexibility in changing themes in thought and conversation, but little else of note. When she stops her medication it takes about 2 weeks for adverse effects to appear, and she is fully psychotic in 4–6 weeks.

Despite the appearances of a florid paranoid schizophrenia when she is ill, the striking retention of personality features and of appropriate affect when she is well has led to a rediagnosis of paraphrenia.

It is noteworthy that, in contrast to the detailed descriptions of the delusional content of paranoia, the literature contains little about the nature of the prominent delusions in paraphrenia, apart from sporadic, anecdotal, single-case descriptions. Sullivan (1962) thought that a logical belief that persecution was occurring was the basis for paraphrenia and Lewis (1970) appeared to be referring to paraphrenia when he mentioned erotic delusions in some middle-aged female patients. Neither of these attributions is well documented.

Black and his colleagues (1988) paraphrased features from Kraepelin's original description when they said that paraphrenia was notable for unremitting systematized delusions, hallucinations, and no progression to dementia. Kolb (1973), however, believed that the delusions in paraphrenia lacked the quasi-logical systematization seen in paranoia. (Certainly, in the present author's view, they do not have the stability or the encapsulated quality of the delusions in paranoia/delusional disorder.)

Brink and colleagues (1979) claimed that patients with paraphrenia retain reality testing except for the persistent delusion. Merskey (1980) refers to patients with 'paranoid states or psychoses' whose illness begins after the age of 35 and who do not display the general deterioration typical of schizophrenia. Lewis (1970) believed that paraphrenia was milder than schizophrenia and had a later onset, but Bleuler (1950) underlined the illness's chronic, unremitting quality, then eventually changed his mind and decided that paraphrenia was not a separate entity anyway.

Jackson (1960) stated that the diagnosis of paraphrenia was still commonly used in Britain and Black *et al.* (1988) made a similar comment. Yet, Lewis (1970) said that the diagnosis of paraphrenia was uncommon in the UK. The term still occasionally appears in North American psychiatric publications, but then it usually refers to late paraphrenia, as is the case in the UK. On the other hand, Jordan and Farmer (1989), writing from the US, lament the neglect of the category of involutional paranoid disorder, by which they seem to mean paraphrenia. In 1980, the DSM-III (APA 1980) section on

paranoid disorder was extremely unsatisfactory and, when it described paranoia, this was really a poorly described amalgam of paranoia and paraphrenia. This has been partly remedied in DSM-III-R (APA 1987) and DSM-IV,
where the description of paranoia/delusional disorder is accurate, but at the
cost that paraphrenia is completely excluded. ICD-9 (World Health Organization (WHO) 1978) retained an inaccurate definition of paraphrenia but
even this is missing from ICD-10 (WHO 1992–1993).

It seems that the main reason for the unenthusiastic attitude towards
paraphrenia goes back to when Mayer (1921) reviewed the cases of 78
patients diagnosed with paraphrenia by Kraepelin (1919), and found that
more than half of these subsequently developed schizophrenia. As with
Kolle's (1931) work on paranoia (see Chapter 3), the subsequent literature
fails to emphasize that the remaining cases remained recognizably paraphrenic. Since Mayer's (1921) report, many prominent psychiatrists have
regarded paraphrenia as, at best, a variety of paranoid schizophrenia. Fish
(1964) and Henderson and Batchelor (1962) all advocated dropping it as a
separate category, and Lewis (1970) was lukewarm about retaining it, saying
(inaccurately) that Kraepelin's paraphrenics could have been labelled 'paranoid' (presumably meaning paranoiac) if they had not had hallucinations.
The point that Lewis (1970) overlooks is that the paraphrenic cases' delusions lacked that essential encapsulated quality typical of the delusional
symptoms seen in paranoia/delusional disorder.

Leigh and colleagues (1977) simply said that paraphrenia is 'schizophrenia arising for the first time after the age of 60 years', which was a convenient
way of diagnosing first-time schizophrenia in the elderly without actually
saying so. Kraepelin's term 'dementia praecox' emphasized the 'precocious'
onset of schizophrenia, but he himself allowed that a proportion of
cases developed later in life. However, most authorities came to believe that
schizophrenia occurred for the first time no later than middle age, so
cases arising in the 60s or later, often with relatively good preservation
of personality, had to be found an alternative name, paraphrenia being one
of these.

At the present time, we are much more prepared to diagnose first-onset
schizophrenia in older patients, although some psychiatrists are still uncom-
fortable about this. The concepts of old-age schizophrenia and late paraphrenia will be discussed briefly later.

An overall impression gained from the literature is that the great majority
of psychiatrists, whether for or against paraphrenia, are unfamiliar with the
clinical details of the delusional disorders as a group, often cannot separate

them from schizophrenia, and have great difficulty distinguishing between paraphrenia and paranoia. Since Mayer's (1921) study there has been virtually no original work on paraphrenia, with the exception of investigations into late paraphrenia. When paraphrenia was excluded from DSM-III-R, the official view on this was stated by Williams (1987) as follows:

> Some argue that such a clinical picture [i.e. of paraphrenia] distinguishes a unique syndrome and should be differentiated from schizophrenia. However, the general consensus among experts in the area is that it is premature to consider such a syndrome to be a separate disorder. Therefore, until further research proves or disproves its validity, it will still be diagnosed as schizophrenia.

That was in 1987 and little has changed since. Paraphrenia remains excluded from DSM-IV and ICD-10, and who are these 'experts in the area' and who will do the 'further' research? As will be mentioned later in the chapter, the present author and two colleagues, Drs A. Ravindran and L. Yatham, have attempted to conceptualize paraphrenia in latter-day terms and are in the process of carrying out research, but we are aware of very little other expertise or research on the subject. Yet, oddly, there are psychiatrists who continue to use the term 'paraphrenia' in their everyday practice, even if unsure of its definition.

If paraphrenia exists but is being diagnosed as schizophrenia (as Williams (1987) proposes), as psychotic disorder NOS, or as schizoaffective disorder, the chances of doing useful research are minimized, since it is thereby being confused with a variety of other conditions and cannot be studied in isolation. My colleagues and I have tried to get round this problem by doing our own case-finding and we can confirm that we not infrequently see cases of paraphrenia in hospital practice. This is because we have programmed ourselves to recognize the disorder and have the benefit of a modernized description, which is detailed later.

The concept of a paranoid spectrum

For many years, there has been some acceptance of the view that paranoia and paranoid schizophrenia represent opposite ends of a continuum of psychotic disorders in which delusions play a prominent part. Figure 5.1 displays a schema showing paranoia/delusional disorder to the left, paranoid schizophrenia to the right and paraphrenia in the middle. 'Cluster A' personality disorders (DSM-IV) are tentatively linked to the 'paranoia' end of the spectrum but lie outside it. Paranoid schizophrenia is included in the con-

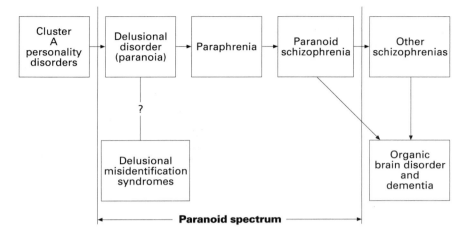

Fig. 5.1 The paranoid spectrum.

tinuum because it has features in common with delusional disorders, but other forms of schizophrenia remain outside. Dementia is also shown to the right of the spectrum since a minority of paranoid spectrum cases appear to have an underlying organic aetiology which eventually expresses itself as dementia.

It is known (Roth 1955; Jette & Winnett 1987) that a proportion of individuals with severe forms of Cluster A personality disorder develop psychotic features: when this occurs, there is some evidence that they are especially liable to develop a delusional disorder.

We know that perhaps 10% of patients with paranoia/delusional disorder or paraphrenia will show a 'shift to the right', deteriorating to schizophrenia or (especially in some older individuals) to dementia (Black *et al.* 1988). However, the great majority of cases of delusional disorder and paraphrenia remain diagnostically stable: despite this, many of them continue to be mistaken as schizophrenic or mood disorder illnesses.

Several reports have indicated that, as one moves from right to left on the spectrum, a family history of schizophrenia becomes progressively less common, suggesting that the delusional disorders are relatively unrelated to schizophrenia genetically (Munro 1982; Watt 1985). Delusional disorder itself shows no more tendency to a family history of schizophrenia than among members of the general public (Kendler 1982).

Although paranoid schizophrenia is conventionally grouped with the other clinical forms of schizophrenia, there are strong arguments for regarding it as separate and even for including it in the paranoid spectrum. Again, Kraepelin is the authority most responsible for our present-day concepts on paranoid schizophrenia, a category which has proved much less controversial than paranoia or paraphrenia. He regarded it as a subcategory of dementia praecox but, as noted above, also included it in his group of paranoid disorders. Rather than indulging in pointless argument about where paranoid schizophrenia actually lies in some hypothesized diagnostic scheme, perhaps best to acknowledge its relative separateness from either schizophrenia or delusional disorder while recognizing that it has some features in common with both of these disorders.

Paranoid schizophrenia tends to appear at a later age than the other schizophrenias and is especially characterized by delusions and well-marked auditory hallucinations. Thought disorder may be severe but there is relatively little incoherence and though behaviour may be disturbed it is usually less bizarre than in, say, disorganized schizophrenia. There is some preservation of affect and rapport but this may be masked by a prevailing mood of suspiciousness and readily aroused anger, or by attitudes of humourlessness and eccentricity. Overall, there is less tendency to degeneration than in other subtypes of schizophrenia, but considerably more so than in delusional disorder or paraphrenia.

It may be argued that paraphrenia is, at most, a subset of paranoid schizophrenia. This may be true, but, as will be shown, there are features that separate it from the latter and make it a clinically useful diagnosis in its own right. Also, there is a considerable gap in the paranoid spectrum between the constructs of delusional disorder and paranoid schizophrenia. There are cases which fall into that gap and paraphrenia appears to be a satisfactory diagnostic description for many of these.

Late paraphrenia and old-age schizophrenia

Schizophrenia may occur at an early age but the patient can live for many years, continuing to display psychotic symptoms of various sorts. This is not controversial. On the other hand, the idea that schizophrenia could appear for the first time in late middle-age or among the elderly has been the subject of very considerable argument for many years.

Nowadays there seems to be much wider acceptance that schizophrenia-like illness can occur at any age from the teens onwards (Jeste *et al.* 1988). In general, the older the age of onset, the more will the case resemble paranoid schizophrenia and the less important will be the genetic component. Unhappily, there are still arguments, often based on ideological rather than scientific grounds, as to whether late-onset cases should be regarded as truly schizophrenia or as something else (Munro 1991).

In the past decade, it has become common in the US to diagnose schizophrenia of first onset in the elderly (Templer 1989). This also happens to some extent in the UK (Grahame 1987) but arguments continue there about the differentiation between late paraphrenia and old-age schizophrenia (Almeida *et al.* 1992). It is not the intention here to join in these arguments except to remark that it seems to make little difference to treatment or ultimate outcome whether the case is called the one thing or the other. Case No. 5.2 is presented as one of paraphrenia occurring in an elderly person. Doubtless some psychiatrists would prefer to regard this as 'late' paraphrenia or even as a case of old age schizophrenia.

Case No. 5.2: *Late paraphrenia*

A lady of 83 lived alone in a house which she had inherited from her parents. Her siblings were dead, she had never married, and for the past 10 years or so she had become extremely reclusive. Prior to that she had been quiet and reserved, but well respected by neighbours. Now that her property was neglected and, on her rare appearances, she appeared unkempt and eccentric, she was regarded with some hostility. Local children would shout at her and call her a 'witch' and there had been incidents of vandalism to her house and garden. For several years, she had become increasingly convinced that she was being persecuted (which was true) but in the past 2 years she continually telephoned the local police station to say that gangs were frequently breaking into her house, that neighbours were holding noisy parties in her garden at night, that ultra-loud music was being projected into her house at all hours, and that she was being televised by the authorities inside the house (none of which were true).

Eventually, police and social services arranged for admission to the local psychogeriatric unit: the admission had to be an involuntary one. On admission, the patient was somewhat undernourished and untidy, but clean. Intellect, cognition and memory were well-preserved, but she had multiple delusions, mostly persecutory, and her thinking was scattered, with marked loosening of associations. She had auditory hallucinations and many delusional misperceptions. Her whole manner was wary and suspicious.

After approximately 2 weeks of poor cooperation, the patient finally agreed to take medication, and a low-dose neuroleptic was started. Over the next several weeks the patient gradually improved, and became calm, pleasant and compliant with her treatment regime. Although she remained reserved, affect was appropriate and she became closely attached to a small number of nurses. She also appeared comfortable in the company of two other elderly ladies who were mildly demented, and became quite maternal and caring towards them. Unfortunately, though much improved, she cannot be discharged home as she is terrified to be by herself and because she has no adequate social supports outside.

As yet, insufficient care is being taken to exclude cases of delusional disorder or paraphrenia (as opposed to late onset paraphrenia) from the overall group of schizophrenia-like disorders arising in the elderly, so this is likely to be a mixed diagnostic group in any case. Delusional disorder can arise at any age and there is evidence that this is also true of paraphrenia. It appears that no studies have been carried out to determine whether late paraphrenia is a distinct entity or whether it may be the top end of an age-continuum for paraphrenia as a whole.

A description of paraphrenia

It has been necessary to set the scene and deal with some uncertainties before moving on to the actual characterization of paraphrenia which now follows. There has been a sad lack of modern descriptions of this condition so the present author (Munro 1991) attempted to redefine paraphrenia utilizing modern terminology, a DSM-style format and the limited data which are available. This exercise was undertaken in the belief that this is a potentially useful diagnostic entity, and to inform psychiatrists of its existence and its features, thereby providing a framework for future research. With Drs Ravindran and Yatham, and using the undernoted criteria, a case-finding study has been carried out whose results are now being analysed, and we plan to submit these findings for publication shortly. We can say with reasonable confidence that we systematically recognized cases of paraphrenia in two separate in-patient psychiatric settings, and our impressions inform the following description of the illness.

PROPOSED DIAGNOSTIC CRITERIA FOR PARAPHRENIA

Paraphrenia is a distinct delusional disorder which has to have been present for at least 6 months and is characterized by the following.

1   Preoccupation with one or more semi-systematized delusions, often accompanied by auditory hallucinations. These delusions are not encapsulated from the rest of the personality.

2   The affect remaining notably well preserved and relatively appropriate. Even when severely disturbed the patient shows an ability for rapport with others and considerable affective warmth that is not typical of any form of schizophrenia.

3   None of the following: intellectual deterioration, visual hallucinations, incoherence, marked loosening of associations, flat or grossly inappropriate affect, grossly disorganized behaviour.

4   Understandability of disturbed behaviour as being related to the content of the patient's delusions and hallucinations.

5   The absence of significant organic brain disorder, and at most, only partial agreement with Criterion A for schizophrenia in DSM-IV.

ASSOCIATED FEATURES

In general, the personality is better retained than in schizophrenia and patients remain relatively higher-functioning (especially if they accept treatment). They may be able to hide their delusional beliefs and behave outwardly in a relatively normal way, at least for a time. However, distress and agitation are almost invariably present, partly because some degree of insight is often retained. As the delusions grow stronger and judgement deteriorates, irrational behaviour becomes more obvious. The patient may accuse others of intimidation, make complaints to the authorities, or sometimes show aggression to imagined persecutors. At first, their apparent justifications for such actions may be fairly convincing.

AGE OF ONSET

Traditionally it is believed that the illness begins predominantly in middle or old age, even appearing for the first time in extreme old age. In fact, the author and his colleagues have found apparently typical cases among individuals as young as their 20s.

COURSE AND PROGNOSIS

Once established, it is a chronic illness, ameliorated but not cured by treatment. It tends to cause the patient to become withdrawn and isolated, which exacerbates the social and behavioural deterioration, thereby causing further symptoms. Unfortunately, a proportion of patients, prompted by their delusional beliefs, are non-compliant with treatment, which prolongs the acute phase, sometimes indefinitely. Not uncommonly, a pattern asserts itself of improvement in hospital followed by relapse in the community due to failure to take medication. In older patients who eventually become permanently institutionalized and whose treatment can be more closely supervised, improvement seems to be well maintained unless, for example, dementia supervenes. Because no population figures for the frequency of paraphrenia are available and because no research on the entity has been carried out for such a long time, we have no idea of the relative commonness of compliance vs. non-compliance in a treated population, but non-compliance does seem to occur with more than random frequency.

FREQUENCY OF PARAPHRENIA

The frequency of paraphrenia is unknown but Fenton and colleagues (1988) possibly threw an unintentional though significant sidelight on paraphrenia when studying a series of patients who had been diagnosed as suffering from schizophrenia, using both DSM-III and DSM-III-R criteria. They found that approximately 10% of those who were diagnosed as schizophrenic utilizing DSM-III had to be excluded from the diagnosis when the stricter DSM-III-R criteria were applied. They noted that many of the excluded cases had symptoms of a delusional (paranoid) type, but had to be labelled as atypical psychoses because their delusions lacked the encapsulated quality of DSM-III-R delusional disorder.

By inference, it seems possible that many of the excluded cases could be seen as lying on the continuum between delusional disorder and paranoid schizophrenia, that is in the position said to be occupied by paraphrenia (Munro 1989). If that is so, then the frequency of paraphrenia in an inpatient psychiatric population could be provisionally estimated as being about one-tenth that of schizophrenia.

Kendler *et al.* (1982) found that patients with delusional disorders (not restricted to the DSM-III-R definition which had not then been devised) made up between 1% and 4% of psychiatric admissions and between 2% and 7% of functional psychoses. If approximately one half of the functional disorders was schizophrenic, this would suggest a frequency of between 4 and 14 paranoid disorders per 100 schizophrenics. Since paranoia/delusional disorder cases more often escape hospital admission, the majority of these 'paranoid disorders' is likely to be paraphrenic, giving a figure roughly similar to that found by Fenton *et al.* (1988).

A possible additional source of paraphrenia cases is the increasing number of patients rather loosely diagnosed nowadays as 'schizoaffective'. Certainly, some of this author's clinical colleagues appear to be using that diagnosis to describe a schizophrenia-like illness with well-retained affect.

RISK FACTORS

Predisposing factors that are generally mentioned include abnormal pre-morbid personality features, especially those characteristic of DSM-IV Cluster A personality disorders (Kendler 1982), and peripheral sensory defects, especially deafness but, to a lesser extent, visual loss (Munro 1991). Several researchers have agreed that patients with delusional-type disorders do not have a significant family history of schizophrenia, suggesting relative lack of a genetic link to schizophrenia (Kendler 1982; Munro 1982; Watt 1985).

STABILITY OF THE DIAGNOSIS

As noted, Mayer (1921) found that approximately half of Kraepelin's patients with a diagnosis of paraphrenia eventually deteriorated to schizo-phrenia. Black and colleagues (1988), on the other hand, state that 80–90% of patients with delusional disorders (probably a mixture of paraphrenia and paranoia) remain diagnostically stable, and that their demographic characteristics differ markedly from patients with schizophrenia or a major mood disorder. As ever, it is difficult to know where the apparent statistics derive from, because of the lack of published research in the last three-quarters of a century, but one's impression is that only a relatively small pro-portion of carefully diagnosed paraphrenic patients deteriorate to another disorder.

It should be emphasized that, until 40 years ago, all chronic schizophrenia-like psychoses tended to follow a deteriorative course, because of the lack of available treatments and the effects of long-term institutionalization. The end-state was not dissimilar whatever the original diagnosis. Nowadays, with treatment that is at least partly effective, that degree of degeneration is much less frequent, and good-outcome end-states are distinguishable from those with bad-outcome. Clinical experience suggests, but cannot yet confirm, that individuals with paraphrenia are considerably more likely to be in the good prognosis group as compared with core schizophrenics.

TREATMENT

Paraphrenia appears to respond to most of the standard neuroleptic drugs, and no one medication is known to be more specifically efficacious than others. But it must again be stressed that there are no scientific data on this. Behavioural therapy may reduce the degree of preoccupation with the delusions shown by the patient (Kingdon *et al.* 1994). Psychotherapy may be a useful part of the rehabilitative process in recovering treated patients but has not been shown to be of any value as a first-line treatment.

TREATMENT OUTCOME

When the patient is collaborative with medication, the clinical outcome is frequently satisfactory. The patient becomes less anxious and agitated, is considerably less preoccupied with delusional thinking and with hallucinations, and is less likely to exhibit disturbed behaviour. As the illness improves, it is noticeable that affective warmth, appropriate mood responses and good rapport in interpersonal situations becomes increasingly prominent. This, in particular, distinguishes the paraphrenic patient from the paranoid schizophrenic, whose underlying personality is commonly stiff and humourless.

Unfortunately, in the non-compliant patient this degree of improvement is only glimpsed before relapse occurs and prognosis is likely to be as bad as in schizophrenia if lack of cooperation continues. In the older patient, even though the clinical outcome is reasonably good with treatment, social outcome may be less satisfactory. Although the paraphrenic is relatively more sociable than other schizophrenics, the effects of a chronic psychiatric illness, increasing age-related problems, and relative difficulties with interpersonal relationships may make rehabilitation in the community less satisfactory and the possibility of prolonged institutional care more likely.

Conclusions

Schizophrenia — the schizophrenias — is a clustering of several disorders. A hundred years ago, Kraepelin's methodical approach to classification prompted him to recognize the similarities that appeared to link the various clinical subtypes and to describe the category of dementia praecox, subsequently named schizophrenia by E. Bleuler. This important step led to the distinction of this extremely important illness category from others such as mood disorders and dementia. At the time, dementia praecox was regarded as being almost invariably a degenerative disorder and there were no treatments available. It was more important to have the diagnosis in order to distinguish schizophrenia from other illnesses with possibly more optimistic prognoses than with any view to improving the schizophrenic patient himself.

In these circumstances, fine distinctions between clinical subtypes, based on phenomenology and course of the illness, might seem superfluous. Yet Kraepelin was a meticulous observer and he did make distinctions. He clearly separated the paranoid or delusional illnesses from dementia praecox, within schizophrenia he delineated the paranoid subtype from the others and within the delusional disorders he distinguished between paranoia and paraphrenia. Because he had no treatments for these conditions he could see all of them unaffected either in severity or in their course of evolution: we, on the other hand, rarely see untreated cases of any psychiatric disorder and are faced with appearances and a natural history that could mean almost anything, especially at the beginning of an illness.

Many of Kraepelin's observations remain valid today, and indeed form the bases for modern diagnosis and classification of the psychotic illnesses. His views on schizophrenia and mood disorders are widely accepted, and his long-neglected conceptualization of paranoia is now vindicated in DSM-IV. Was he simply wrong with paraphrenia or are there any other reasons for its disappearance from present-day diagnostic systems? Certainly, this writer's experience suggests that he was not misguided and that paraphrenia is a viable diagnosis.

Why then has it disappeared from any official classification system? My thesis is that it has not, but is simply being called a number of other things. The Fenton *et al.* (1988) study mentioned above confirms what we already know, namely that by widening the definition of schizophrenia, cases which do not really meet the criteria for that disorder can be diagnosed as schizophrenic. I would suggest that this happens with many paraphrenics who are simply labelled as 'paranoid schizophrenics' or as 'schizoaffective' cases, or are placed in some non-specific category.

Recently, with the resurgence of paranoia as delusional disorder in DSM-III-R, DSM-IV and ICD-10, one has noticed some confusion in diagnostic

practice with cases which are probably paraphrenic being diagnosed as delusional disorder because they are clearly not schizophrenic and clearly do
belong somewhere on the paranoid spectrum.

As noted previously, if the psychiatrist is aware that his case is similar to
schizophrenia but it does not completely fit into that category, and if it is not
DSM-IV/ICD-10 delusional disorder, he or she may be forced to use a non-
descript, 'atypical' diagnosis to emphasize that the patient is not schizophrenic. This usually results in heterogeneous groupings which make
research difficult. As also mentioned earlier in the chapter, there seems
to be an increasing trend towards diagnosing schizoaffective disorder,
and some of these cases are almost certainly paraphrenics who have
schizophrenic symptoms but good preservation of affective response and
warm rapport.

In the long run, does any of this matter? It seems apparent that the
treatment for paraphrenia is much the same as that for paranoid schizophrenia and there is no doubt that the two disorders have a close resemblance.
Why then separate paraphrenia if it only represents some kind of splinter
group?

There are two possible answers to that, the first being that a diagnosis of
paraphrenia may carry an implication of better prognosis than occurs in any
kind of schizophrenia, provided the patient can be persuaded to comply with
treatment. Thus, the informed psychiatrist can make his diagnosis of paraphrenia, prognosticate appropriately, and design a strategy to obtain
maximum cooperation from the patient. Secondly, if paraphrenia exists, it is
essential that we apply modern criteria to its diagnosis in order to assemble
uniform case-series and carry out worthwhile research.

Schizophrenia was a diagnostic black hole in the mid-20th century and
both paranoia and paraphrenia got sucked into it. Paranoia has re-emerged
as delusional disorder and has been revalidated as a description of verifiable
illness. Paraphrenia, because it resembles schizophrenia rather more closely,
is having difficulty in re-establishing itself as a separate entity, but there is no
doubt that there is an increasing dissatisfaction with the current situation
which insists on dismissing a functional psychosis as 'atypical' if it fails to
comply fully with the diagnostic criteria for schizophrenia. Surely we need to
investigate these so-called atypical cases to discover whether they are actually typical of something other than schizophrenia.

When the present writer started in psychiatry in the mid-1950s, some
cases of temporal lobe epilepsy, some severe obsessive-compulsive disorders,
and all cases of paranoia were regarded as aberrant forms of schizophrenia.

More accurate perception has allowed these illnesses to be studied in isolation and for them to be treated more specifically. At the same time their departure from the inflated category of schizophrenia has permitted the concept of that disorder to be refined somewhat. Paraphrenia has a fair pedigree and seems a reasonable candidate to take part in this process of identification as a separate disorder, with benefit to its sufferers and with further reduction of the confusion that is schizophrenia. It is hoped that this chapter has made a good case for supporting such an outcome.

References

Almeida, O.P., Howard, R., Förstl, H. & Levy, R. (1992) Late paraphrenia: A review. *International Journal of Geriatric Psychiatry* 7, 543–548.

American Psychiatric Association (1980) *Diagnostic and Statistical Manual of Mental Disorders*, 3rd edn (DSM-III). American Psychiatric Association, Washington, D.C.

American Psychiatric Association (1987) *Diagnostic and Statistical Manual of Mental Disorders*, 3rd edn, revised (DSM-III-R). American Psychiatric Association, Washington, D.C.

American Psychiatric Association (1994) *Diagnostic and Statistical Manual of Mental Disorders*, 4th edn (DSM-IV). American Psychiatric Association, Washington, D.C.

Anderson, E.W. & Trethowan, W.H. (1973) *Psychiatry*, 3rd edn. Baillière Tindall, London.

Arieti, S. (1955) *Interpretation of Schizophrenia*. Brunner Mazel Publishers, New York.

Black, D.W., Yates, W.R. & Andreasen, N.C. (1988) Delusional (paranoid) disorders. In: *Textbook of Psychiatry* (eds J.A.Talbott, R.E. Hales & S.C. Yudofsky), pp. 391–396. American Psychiatric Press, Washington, D.C.

Bleuler, E. (1950) *Dementia Praecox or the Group of Schizophrenias* (transl. J. Zinkin). International Universities Press, New York.

Brink, T.L., Capri, D., Deneeve, V. *et al.* (1979) Hypochondriasis and paranoia: Similar delusional systems in an institutionalized geriatric population. *Journal of Nervous and Mental Disorders* 167, 224–228.

Curran, D. & Partridge, M. (1969) *Psychological Medicine*, 6th edn. Livingstone, Edinburgh.

Fenton, W.S., McGlashan, T.H. & Heinssen, R.K. (1988) A comparison of DSM-III and DSM-III-R schizophrenia. *American Journal of Psychiatry* 145, 1446–1449.

Fish, F.J. (1964) *An Outline of Psychiatry*. John Wright & Sons, Bristol.

Grahame, P.S. (1987) Late paraphrenia or the paraphrenias. *British Journal of Psychiatry* 151, 268–269.

Gurland, B.J., Fleiss, J.L., Cooper, J.E., Sharpe, L., Kendell, R.E. & Roberts, P. (1970) Cross-national study of diagnosis of mental disorders, hospital diagnoses and hospital patients in New York and London. *Comprehensive Psychiatry* 11, 18–25.

Harris, M.J. & Jeste, D.V. (1988) Late-onset schizophrenia: An overview. *Schizophrenia Bulletin* 14, 39–55.

Henderson, D. & Batchelor, I.R. (1962) *Henderson and Gillespie's Textbook of Psychiatry*, 9th edn. Oxford University Press, London.

Holden, N.L. (1987) Late paraphrenia or the paraphrenias? A descriptive study with a 10-year follow-up. *British Journal of Psychiatry* **150**, 635–639.

Jackson, D.D. (1960) *The Etiology of Schizophrenia*. Basic Books, New York.

Jeste, D., Harris, M.J. & Pearlson, G.D. *et al.* (1988) Late-onset schizophrenia, studying clinical validity. *Psychiatric Clinics of North America* **11**, 1–13.

Jette, C.C.B. & Winnett, R.L. (1987) Late-onset paranoid disorder. *American Journal of Orthopsychiatry* **57**, 485–494.

Jordan, H.W. & Farmer, M.W. (1989) Involutional paranoid disorder: A forgotten syndrome. *Journal of National Medical Association* **81**, 950–952.

Kahlbaum, K. (1863) *Die Gruppirung der Psychischen Krankheiten*. Kafemann, Danzig.

Kendler, K.S. (1982) Demography of paranoid psychosis (delusional disorder). *Archives of General Psychiatry* **39**, 890–902.

Kendler, K.S., Gruenberg, A.M. & Strauss, J.S. (1982) An independent analysis of the Copenhagen sample of the Danish adoption study of schizophrenia. III. The relationship between paranoid psychosis (delusional disorder) and the schizophrenia spectrum disorders. *Archives of General Psychiatry* **39**, 985–987.

Kingdon, D., Turkington, D. & John, C. (1994) Cognitive behaviour therapy of schizophrenia. *British Journal of Psychiatry* **164**, 581–587.

Kolb, L.C. (1973) *Modern Clinical Psychiatry*, 8th edn. W.B. Saunders, Philadelphia, Penn.

Kolle, K. (1931) *Die Primäre Verücktheit, Psychopathologische, Klinische und Genealogische Untersuchungen*. Thieme, Leipzig.

Kraepelin, E. (1919) *Dementia Praecox and Paraphrenia* (transl. R.M. Barclay; from the 8th edn of E. Kraepelin (1909–13) *Clinical Psychiatry: A Textbook for Students and Physicians*). Livingstone, Edinburgh.

Leigh, D., Pare, C.M.B. & Marks, J.A. (1977) *Concise Encyclopedia of Psychiatry*. M.T.P. Press, Lancaster.

Leonhard, K. (1960) Die Atypischen Psychosen und Kleists Lehre von den Endogenen Psychosen. In: *Psychiatrie der Gegenwart*, Vol. 2 (eds H. Gruhle, E. Neele & H. Schwab). Springer, Berlin.

Lewis, A. (1970) Paranoia and paranoid: A historical perspective. *Psychological Medicine* **1**, 2–12.

Mayer, W. (1921) On paraphrenic psychoses. *Zentralblatt für die Gesamte Neurologie und Psychiatrie* **71**, 187–206.

Merskey, H. (1980) *Psychiatric Illness*, 3rd edn. Baillière Tindall, London.

Munro, A. (1982) *Delusional Hypochondriasis*. Clarke Institute of Psychiatry Monograph No. 5, Toronto.

Munro, A. (1989) Classification of patients not meeting DSM-III-R criteria for schizophrenia (letter). *American Journal of Psychiatry* **146**, 816–817.

Munro, A. (1991) A plea for paraphrenia. *Canadian Journal of Psychiatry* **36**, 667–672.

Roth, M. (1955) The natural history of mental disorder in old age. *Journal of Mental Science* **101**, 281–301.

Sullivan, H.S. (1962) *Schizophrenia as a Human Process*. W.W. Norton & Co., New York.

Templer, D.I. (1989) A comment on late-onset schizophrenia. *Schizophrenia Bulletin* 15, 173–175.

Watt, J.A.G. (1985) The relationship of paranoid states to schizophrenia. *American Journal of Psychiatry* 145, 1456–1458.

Williams, J.B.W. (1987) Psychotic and mood disorders. *Hospital Community Psychiatry* 38, 13–14.

World Health Organization (1978) *International Statistical Classification of Diseases*, 9th revision (ICD-9). World Health Organization, Geneva.

World Health Organization (1992–1993) *The ICD-10 Classification of Mental and Behavioural Disorders*. World Health Organization, Geneva.

CHAPTER 6

Factitious Disorders

DINESH BHUGRA

Introduction

Factitious disorders cover a multitude and complex range of symptoms which can mimic most illnesses under the sun. Perhaps the more obvious of all these cases are those with symptoms consistent with the diagnosis of Munchausen's syndrome.

Pathological factitious illness has been conceptualized as a pyramid of physical and behavioural patterns in which the base of the pyramid represents an exaggeration of physical symptoms or feigned illness behaviour that may allow the patient to abdicate responsibility, deny failure and to look around for and encourage caring responses from family, medical and social networks (Phillips *et al.* 1983). Folks and Freeman (1985) suggest that of the pyramidal hierarchy, Munchausen's syndrome is the most extreme type characterized by simulation of disease, pathological lying, frequent wanderings, especially in men of lower class, associated with long periods of behavioural and social maladjustment (also see Pallis & Bamji 1979). On the other hand, women of higher social class who may be well educated, intelligent and employed in a medically related field may too present with factitious disorders (Reich & Gottfried 1983).

These disorders fall within a large and heretofore undefined grey zone between hysteria and clear-cut malingering; at the same time, they occupy an interesting but diagnostically perplexing interface between medicine and psychiatry (Hyler & Spitzer 1978).

Various terms used to describe factitious disorders have included Munchausen's syndrome, polysurgical addiction, hospital addiction, desire to be ill, self-induced illness, self-induced injury, self-mutilation, artefactual illness, dermatitis interfacta, feigned illness, hospital hoboes, feigned bereavement, peregrinating patients, hospital vagrants, hospital fraud, Ahasuerus' syndrome, Van Gogh syndrome, pathomime, and apothecary attraction syndrome. The number of synonyms for factitious disorders suggests multiple pathology as well as diagnostic confusion. Such complexity also leads to ambivalence among the teams looking after such patients.

In this chapter, I aim to cover current perspectives on diagnosis and clinical management including managing self-destructive behaviour (for management of repeated deliberate self-harm see Chapter 10).

Historical concepts

Self-injurious behaviour for the purposes of gaining attention is not a recent phenomenon. Veith (1965) has suggested that even though self-inflicted diseases had been recognized in biblical times, in the Middle Ages, the 'hysterics' were seen as being able to induce haemoptysis by placing leeches in their mouths or skin lesions following excoriation. In 1843, Gavin proposed that 'one may feign the symptoms of a disease, without any disease existing or else one may excite a state of real but temporary disease in order to have it taken for a more chronic or permanent disease' (p. 9). He suggested that there were four types—feigned or purely fictitious (which could be pretended or simulated), exaggerated diseases, factitious or wholly produced with the patient's concurrence and aggravated. These were often seen in soldiers, seamen, prisoners, conscripts, revengeful members of the lower classes who preferred idleness to industry, imitators, sycophants, fanatics and slaves, and their main purpose was to obtain discharge. He cites Marshall in 1816 who noticed that knowledge and experiences greater than generally believed, along with an acquaintance with anatomy, physiology and pathology, was especially required to decide upon the health and general efficiency of recruits. In simulating an illness, Gavin (1843) argues that an impostor finds it difficult to give a consistent account of the origin and progress of his alleged disability.

With interest in hysteria increasing dramatically in the late 19th century, interest in factitious disorders appeared to wane (Hyler & Sussman 1981). Even though Meninger (1934) described polysurgical addiction in case reports, Asher (1951) was the first clinician to use the term Munchausen's syndrome following the adventures of Baron Munchausen already fictionalized by Raspe (1948). Like the baron, such patients travel from hospital to hospital reciting tall tales about their illnesses. Wingate (1951) suggested abandoning the term on grounds that the real baron was too wise and would not have countenanced any abdominal surgery and proposed

Ahasuerus' syndrome instead, appealing to the wandering Jew of the Old Testament, thereby emphasizing the constant suffering, the lack of permanent residences, the multiple aliases and the apparent immortality of these patients.

The physical varieties of factitious disorder as defined by Asher (1951) were: acute abdominal type, haemorrhagic type and the neurological type. Although Schechter (1973) suggested that this was ipsepathogenesis recognizing the patient's active participation (psychic or physical) in the disease is crucial and no doubt the choice of symptoms will be linked with the underlying factors.

Definitions

Although very many types of syndromes have been identified, it is conceded that presenting symptomatology is limited only by the individual's medical knowledge, sophistication, imagination and daring, as Hyler and Sussman (1981) remind us.

Psychiatric Munchausen's syndrome has been described (Bhugra 1988). The essential features of this variety will include pseudologia fantastica — often the patient will feign bereavement and give a very dramatic account of whole family being wiped out in a road traffic accident or similar incident — although these stories are often very difficult to corroborate. Carney (1980) has suggested that the evidence of deliberate deception is often very obvious. He differentiated between wanderers and non-wanderers and proposed that the former be called (true) Munchausen and the latter (hospital) addicts. He stressed that the wanderers were more likely to be male, unemployed, aggressive and low achievers and generally less stable. Cheng and Hummel (1978) proposed that Munchausen's syndrome was a psychiatric condition and should be seen and managed as such. Barker (1962) reported that in his series of Munchausen, patients were more likely to be aggressive, restless, attention-seeking and difficult individuals to establish rapport with because of their glib, evasive, uninformative or facile responses. However, Bursten (1965) suggested three criteria for the diagnosis of Munchausen's syndrome: dramatic presentation of one or more complaints, pseudologia fantastica and wandering.

Bhugra (1988) proposed that the following factors need to be taken into account while making a diagnosis.

1   Definitive features:
    (a)   evidence of 'falsified' symptoms — whether they are psychiatric or physical or both;

(b) other evidence of falsehood, for example lying, using aliases;

(c) difficulties in forming relationships.

2 Pointers towards diagnosis:

(a) history of alcohol abuse;

(b) masochistic tendencies;

(c) disturbed sexual functioning;

(d) history of criminal behaviour;

(e) multiple admissions without specific reasons;

(f) extensive knowledge of symptoms and working of hospitals — possible nursing or medical backgrounds.

To these, the absence of visitors can be added as a possible sign.

Hyler and Sussman (1981) suggest pseudologia fantastica, wandering and evidence of prior treatment, medical sophistication and disruptive hospitalization, demands for medication and absence of visitors as key factors.

Diagnostic features

According to DSM-IV (American Psychiatric Association (APA) 1994), the essential feature of factitious disorder is the intentional production of physical or psychological signs or symptoms. The presentation may include fabrication of subjective complaints (e.g. complaints of acute abdominal pain in the absence of any such pain), self-inflicted conditions (e.g. the production of abscesses by injecting saliva into the skin), exaggeration or exacerbation of pre-existing general medical conditions (e.g. feigning of *grand mal* seizure with previous history of epilepsy) or any combination or variation of these. The motivation is to assume the sick role and external incentives are absent (Table 6.1).

Table 6.1 Diagnostic criteria for factitious disorder.

A Intentional production or feigning of physical or psychological signs or symptoms

B The motivation for the behaviour is to assume the sick role

C External incentives for the behaviour (such as economic gains, avoiding legal responsibility, or improving physical well-being, as in malingering, are absent

Types

300.16 With predominantly psychological signs and symptoms

300.19 With predominantly physical signs and symptoms

300.19 With combined psychological and physical signs and symptoms

According to DSM-IV criteria, the disorder is of three further subtypes—predominant psychological signs or symptoms, predominant physical signs or symptoms, and a combination of the two.

Associated features may well include approximate answers and use of psychoactive substances to mimic symptoms which may then present with an unusual clinical picture. Substance misuse comorbidity is not unknown in this group. Furthermore, multiple admissions for surgical investigations will lead to multiple surgical interventions.

In the International Classification of Diseases, 10th revision (ICD-10; World Health Organization (WHO) 1992), factitious disorder is subsumed under the category of personality disorder in which the individual, in the absence of a confirmed physical or mental disorder, disease or disability, feigns symptoms *repeatedly* and *consistently* (author's emphasis). Individuals with this pattern of behaviour usually show signs of a number of other marked abnormalities of personality and relationships.

Factitious disorder must be differentiated from malingering, which is defined as the intentional production or feigning of either physical or psychological symptoms or disabilities, motivated by external stresses or incentives. The commonest external motives for malingering include evading criminal prosecution, obtaining drugs, avoiding military conscription or dangerous military duties, and attempting to obtain sickness benefits or improvement in living conditions such as housing. In malingering the goal may be apparent especially if symptoms 'disappear' if challenged or goal obtained.

Commonly presenting features of chronic factitious illness include bizarre demeanour or behaviour which is demanding, dramatic, evasive, medically sophisticated, unruly or self-harming. In addition to the three categories described by Asher (1951) and mentioned earlier in this chapter, there have been other features like fraudulent fever (Petersdorf & Bennet 1957; Thompson *et al.* 1964; Rumans & Vosti 1978; Aduan *et al.* 1979), haemoptysis (Feinisilver *et al.* 1983; O'Shea *et al.* 1984), proteinuria (Mitas 1985), torsion dystonia (Batshaw *et al.* 1985), multiple abscesses (Tunbridge 1969), feculent urine (Reich *et al.* 1977), cessation of menstruation (D'Souza *et al.* 1977), open wounds (Ciak *et al.* 1981), self-mutilation (Ireland *et al.* 1967), haematuria (Kerr *et al.* 1980), and pulmonary manifestations (Roethe *et al.* 1981). Even pseudo-Munchausen's syndrome has been reported (Gurwith & Lingston 1980). The Munchausen patients have not lagged behind the advancing technologies and have modified their symptoms accordingly. Repeated cardioversion (Tizes 1977) and even electronic Munchausen's syndrome have been reported (Mitchell & Frank 1982). A Munchausen family (Ireland *et al.* 1967) as well as a *folie à deux* involving a mother–daughter dyad with Munchausen's syndrome (Janofsky 1986) have been reported.

Munchausen by proxy

First described by Meadow (1977), Munchausen by proxy is exemplified usually by mothers who systematically fabricate information about their children's health or intentionally make their children gravely ill. The children usually require extensive medical investigation which may be invasive and dangerous. As with Munchausen (in the adult), these patients will seemingly stop at nothing to gain access to doctors and the inner circle or care in hospitals. They may seek public recognition of or public adulation for their devoted and dedicated caretaking of a sick child. The term was coined to highlight the similarities in that Munchausen by proxy uses children as a proxy or substitute for the adult's own body. Unfortunately, the similarity in the two terms has led to a degree of confusion and has been misunderstood as a variation of the adult disorder (Schreier & Libow 1993). It is clear that for every published case, there are many more that are dealt with less publicly. Although this phenomenon is more common in mothers than fathers, fathers may well play a passive colluding part in this form of abuse of their children.

SUBTYPES

Schreier and Libow (1993) suggest that initially they thought of three categories of fabrication: help-seekers (excluded from the Munchausen-by-proxy syndrome because they (the parents) were seeking help for a burdened parent) and two primary categories: doctor addicts and active inducers. They then went on to suggest that because of clear differences between mothers of infants and mothers of older children in terms of personal style, along with presentation to the health-care system, a distinction between 'mild' and 'severe' forms of Munchausen-by-proxy syndrome certainly carries significance for the child's physical well-being and is also likely to define the child's psychological risk as well.

Munchausen-by-proxy syndrome remains a qualitatively different phenomenon. The overanxious parent does not want her child to be ill and shows relief (even if only temporarily) when reassured that her child is well.

On the other hand, a Munchausen-by-proxy syndrome parent has a tremendous degree of difficulty in acknowledging any personal problems but instead focuses on the child's medical problems. They may tell falsehoods about their own backgrounds, medical histories and life experiences. Their affect may well reflect a surprising and inappropriate level of satisfaction with their child's problems (Schreier & Libow 1993). Such mothers may appear insatiably needy and continue to demand, ostensibly on their child's behalf, but in reality on their own.

The common usage of the terms 'Munchausen's syndrome' and 'Munchausen by proxy' leads to an element of confusion in the clinical arena. Furthermore, it would appear that a significant minority of mothers engaged in a 'by proxy' behaviour themselves may manifest the adult Munchausen's syndrome either before, parallel with or after the child's factitious illness. Rosenberg (1987) estimates that between a tenth and a quarter of such mothers suffer from Munchausen's syndrome.

Also known as Polle's syndrome or Meadow's syndrome, these mothers often have a history of previous nurse or medical training and a history of fabricating symptoms or signs relating to themselves. Warner and Hathaway (1984) reported on a series of 17 cases presenting with allergic manifestations and observed that the mothers were well educated, middle class and articulate, with a preponderance of marital problems and a pathological attachment to their children. These mothers may have detailed knowledge of the medical and hospital systems either through their training or prolonged admissions for their own factitious illnesses. It has been suggested that these children usually do not suffer from any other form of abuse.

Meadow (1982) has proposed various warning signs which include persistent or recurring illness that cannot be explained, investigations resulting in signs at variance with the child's health, symptoms and signs that make the specialist state that they have never seen such a case, symptoms and signs do not occur in the absence of the parent, overly attentive mother (who refuses to leave the hospital), treatments that are not tolerated, a very rare disorder, a mother who is not especially worried, and clinical symptoms that do not respond as expected to appropriate and careful administration of medication.

Epidemiology

The prevalence of Munchausen's syndrome is widely disputed. It is likely that many cases get reported several times over thereby artificially inflating the numbers. Blackwell (1968) reported on a patient with 178 documented hospitalizations along with numerous visits to the Accident and Emergency departments. Similarly, Maur *et al.* (1973) observed that one of their cases had had 423 documented admissions by the age of 52. These multiple admissions and medical and surgical treatments may well lead to genuine iatrogenic problems leading to further admissions but do not give the true incidence or prevalence. Pope *et al.* (1982) reported that fabrication of symptomatology by adults on an in-patient unit accounted for 6.4% of admissions.

Bhugra (1988) reported that in 1 year, of 775 admissions under the age of 65 to a psychiatric hospital, four clear cases of Munchausen's were identified. This is likely to be an underestimate because admissions to general medical/surgical wards were not included. True incidence is even more difficult to identify simply because the precipitating and predisposing factors may well lead to help-seeking elsewhere in the health-care system. Although O'Shea *et al.* (1984) have argued that free health-care encourages this kind of behaviour, cases have been reported from various health-care systems.

Psychopathology

Patients with factitious disorders are different in one important aspect from others presenting with functional somatic symptoms in that even though a pathophysiologic process is present, it is not necessarily objective and the disease process is produced by the patients themselves, as opposed to being the expression of an autonomous pathophysiologic process (Stinnet 1987).

Folks and Freeman (1985) suggest that predominant personality types are antisocial, histrionic and narcissistic. Bhugra (1988) proposed that factitious disorders were a form of generalized chaos syndrome that patients suffered from and predominant personality traits may lead to presentation with certain characteristics, be they sexual dysfunction or eating disorders.

Psychiatric symptoms may well replace medical or surgical presentations. Pathognomonic signs include factitious bereavement or grief including the absence of expected dysphoric affect, thoughts of self-harm and urgent demands for hospitalization. Underlying motivations can be multiple and vary according to individuals. Such individuals may be looking for control or may be looking for being controlled. Physical or sexual abuse may play a part in the genesis of such disorders. Such individuals may place special value on the secrecy of their transitional object (see Feldman & Ford 1994).

The perceived control over one's symptoms has been seen as an important factor in the production of factitious illnesses. Predisposing factors may include a history of physical illness or disability or a history of prolonged or serious physical illness in the family, anger against the medical establishment, employment in medical or paramedical field, significant relationships with a physician in the past or in the family, and parental influence (Hyler & Sussman 1981). These factors are very likely to have a role in aetiology of factitious disorders.

Psychiatric/psychological features

Clinicians attempting a psychodynamic understanding of factitious disorders must take into account developmental factors, personal history, ongoing life stresses and the relationship of these stresses within the context of the medical settings (Carney 1980). The relationship between factitious disorders and borderline personality disorders and history of immature behaviour with limited parental control in childhood all contribute towards a pattern of broken homes, foster placements or institutional placements with subsequent delinquency, conduct disorders and behavioural disturbances. Such patterns are very likely to lead to behaviours which will compensate for developmental traumas and secondary escape from stressful life situations.

Differential diagnosis

Following diagnoses must be considered when dealing with cases of factitious disorders or Munchausen's syndrome. Given sufficient time and background history, it should be possible to pinpoint motivation even if the patient is unaware of the forces responsible for presentation of certain symptoms. For diagnosing factitious disorders (excluding feigned psychosis, for which see below) the following conditions should be considered.

1 *Genuine physical illness*. It may sometimes be very difficult to differentiate between genuine physical illness and factitious disorders, especially if factitious disorders may have led to injections of feculent material thereby producing genuine fever and associated symptoms. Until the factitious nature of the illness and its aetiology is recognized, treatment measures may well not prove to be adequate.

2 *Malingering*. Malingering differs from factitious disorder in that under-

lying secondary gain may be evident. In addition, such gain is easily under-standable in the context of the individual's personality.

3   *Somatization*. Sometimes it may be difficult to differentiate between som-atization and factitious disorders in that in both conditions physical symp-toms appear to be a result of underlying psychological distress. However, in somatoform disorders, the patient does not produce the symptoms voluntar-ily. They may also not be very familiar with medical terminology or hospital procedures. In conversion or dissociation disorders, the individual cannot control the production of the symptoms. In hypochondriasis, on the other hand, the patient believes that he or she is ill and has a disease and is worried about it, whereas in factitious disorders, the worry is limited and not as pronounced.

4   *Substance abuse*. Substance abusers, though dependent upon change, do not seek multiple hospitalizations.

Psychiatric Munchausen's syndrome may show antisocial behaviour, character neurosis, brain damage, and primitive pre-super ego self-aggression (Ireland *et al.* 1967). Justus *et al.* (1980) propose that as the patient is re-enacting the trauma of his childhood in the relationships with hospital staff, it is more than likely that their ties are false and may show marked hostility and anger towards their carers after presenting with feigned psychosis. Three out of four cases reported by Bhugra (1988) appeared to have learning dis-ability. Factitious psychosis is seen as a last ditch effort to prevent further dis-integration to a genuine psychosis and Berney (1973) observed that four out of five cases went on to develop schizophrenia. Underlying borderline person-ality was seen as a key factor. O'Shea (1982), using 16 P-F Inventory (16 per-sonality factor of Cattell) and MMPI (Minnesota Multiphasic Personality Inventory), highlighted that patients were troubled by checking, slowness, repetition and doubting. In addition, typical traits of hypochondriasis, depression, hysteria, psychopathic deviation, paranoia and psychasthenia were noted. As these patients can vary their symptoms with tremendous medical sophistication, use aliases and have no visitors (Maue 1986), the atti-tude of hospital staff will have a very important role in reaching a satisfactory diagnosis and setting up appropriate management in place.

Management

GENERAL

Chapman (1957) emphasized that the patients with factitious disorders or

Munchausen's syndrome have a remarkable threshold for tolerating procedures at the time of admission but this tolerance disappears very rapidly after that and invariably they become uncooperative after a few days in hospital. Reed (1978) urged that all initial efforts should therefore be directed towards stopping these patients discharging themselves. The first step is a tolerant, sympathetic attitude (Ireland *et al.* 1967). These authors recommend that for factitious disorders, arrangements must be made for long-term psychotherapy and supervision.

Whether these patients should be detained compulsorily under legal provision raises not only legal but ethical dilemmas as well. Different states and countries have different definitions of mental illness and justification for detention and the local interpretation of such laws must be taken into account.

The management should aim at: (i) controlling the feeling of generalized chaos as discussed above; and (ii) preventing further chaos.

For controlling the feeling of generalized chaos, the patient must be involved in identifying his or her needs and negotiating these from the onset. Hospitalization with clear indications and identified periods may allow the patient to control his or her environment, for example by getting regular attention from the staff, by participating actively in the environment on the ward and by channelling anger and hostility in an appropriate way.

The attitudes of the staff towards such patients play an important part in their management. Scully *et al.* (1984) advocated that attention to physician's counter-transference reactions may reduce premature discharge. Staff must be allowed to express their own reactions in order to develop insight into their own responses (Snowdon *et al.* 1978). With developing such strategies, pathogenesis of such a condition can be understood and more effective strategies for its management will be formulated (Scoggin 1981). Although only one case of Munchausen's syndrome has been successfully treated, this patient was willing to stay in the hospital for 3 years (Yassa 1978). Folks and Freeman (1985) suggest that successful therapy involves careful and empathic history-taking and change in therapeutic goal from cure of the simulated disease to redefining or coping with Munchausen's syndrome and the patient is allowed to keep the illness in order to maintain contact with health-care professionals. As Folk and Freeman (1985) propose, perhaps the best treatment is early recognition, as dangerous interventions can be avoided.

Suggestions for blacklisting these patients are usually more problematic in their implementation (see Wright *et al.* 1995).

LIAISON APPROACH

As Hyler and Sussman (1981) suggest that as these patients often use their peculiar empathy for the unconscious impulses of the medical staff (Ireland *et al.* 1967), the dynamics of physician behaviour will respond accordingly. The liaison psychiatrist should educate staff, safeguarding the patient and direct efforts towards obtaining adequate knowledge of developmental history and psychological testing if indicated.

Confrontation is not necessarily appropriate and building rapport, offering support and appropriate treatment can produce a degree of acceptance. For factitious disorders, family members can be involved in the process of assessment and management. If confronted with the factitious nature of the illness, the patient may admit that the factitious illness is present but refuse psychiatric intervention or may decide to cooperate with psychiatric intervention.

PSYCHOTHERAPIES

The best first step is simply to identify by means of accurate assessment and prompt diagnosis. Satisfactory outcome is rare, largely because a majority of the patients do not stick around to cooperate with treatment. In addition, psychotherapy, behaviour modifications and pharmacotherapy have been tried generally with little success. In addition, there may well be a subgroup of patients who may have underlying psychological symptoms or psychiatric syndromes which are amenable to treatment. These include affective disorders, psychotic disorders, organic disorders and personality disorders. Positive contributing factors are capability of establishing and maintaining rapport with the treating clinician and stable psychosocial support systems as evinced by long-term relationship, occupation, etc.

Treatable psychopathology such as anxiety disorder, depressive syndromes, conversion symptoms and major psychoses need to be evaluated and treated. Some patients with transient anxiety and depression may initially retain their illness behaviour but accept treatment for the anxiety and depression (Folks & Freeman 1985).

Psychodynamic psychotherapy may prove to be of limited use. Cognitive therapy or cognitive analytical therapy may well prove to be of much greater impact in long-term management of factitious disorders.

Hyler and Sussman (1981) caution the psychiatrist to be aware of patient–staff and staff–staff tensions, and even though no clear treatments are available, the psychiatrist should not end up promising too much to the staff and the patient, ending up delivering too little. The psychiatrist must have made an attempt to understand dynamics, have realistic expectations and work with the team and the patient.

References

Aduan, R., Fauci, A., Dale, D., Herzberg, J. & Wolff, S. (1979) Factitious fever and self-induced infection. *Annals of Internal Medicine* 90, 230–242.

American Psychiatric Association (1994) *Diagnostic and Statistical Manual of Mental Disorders*, 4th edn (DSM-IV). American Psychiatric Association, Washington, D.C.

Asher, R. (1951) Munchausen's syndrome. *Lancet* i, 339–341.

Barker, J.C. (1962) The syndrome of hospital addiction. *Journal of Mental Sciences* 108, 167–182.

Batshaw, M., Wachtel, R., Deckel, A. *et al.* (1985) Munchausen's syndrome simulating torsion dystonia. *New England Journal of Medicine* 312, 1437–1439.

Berney, T.P. (1973) A review of simulated illness. *South African Medical Journal* 47, 1429–1434.

Bhugra, D. (1988) Psychiatric Munchausen's syndrome: Literature review with case reports. *Acta Psychiatrica Scandinavica* 77, 497–503.

Blackwell, B. (1968) The Munchausen's syndrome. *British Journal of Hospital Medicine* 1, 98–102.

Bursten, B. (1965) On Munchausen's syndrome. *Archives of General Psychiatry* 13, 261–268.

Carney, M. (1980) Artefactual illness to attract attention. *British Journal of Psychiatry* 136, 542–547.

Chapman, J. (1957) Peregrinating problem patients: Munchausen's syndrome. *Journal of the American Medical Association* 165, 927–933.

Cheng, L. & Hummel, L. (1978) The Munchausen's syndrome as a psychiatric condition. *British Journal of Psychiatry* 133, 20–21.

Ciak, C., Frederick, W. & Glew, R. (1981) Another Munchausen's patient. *New England Journal of Medicine* 305, 289.

D'Souza, D., Bharucha, M. & Shah, M. (1977) Munchausen's syndrome. *Journal of Postgraduate Medicine* 23, 95–98.

Feinisilver, S., Raffni, T., Kornei M. *et al.* (1983) Factitious haemoptysis: The case of the red towel. *Archives of Internal Medicine* 143, 567–568.

Feldman, M.B. & Ford, C.V. (1994) *Patient or Pretender*. John Wiley, New York.

Folks, D. & Freeman, A. (1985) Munchausen's syndrome and other factitious illness. *Psychiatric Clinics of North America* 8, 263–278.

Gavin, H. (1843) *Feigned and Factitious Diseases*. J. Churchill, London.

Gurwith, M. & Lingston, C. (1980) Factitious Munchausen's syndrome. *New England Journal of Medicine* 302, 1482–1484.

Hyler, S. & Spitzer, R. (1978) Hysteria split asunder. *American Journal of Psychiatry* 135, 1500–1504.

Hyler, S. & Sussman, N. (1981) Chronic factitious diseases with physical symptoms. *Psychiatric Clinics of North America* 4, 365–377.

Ireland, P., Sapira, J. & Templeton, B. (1967) Munchausen's syndrome: Review and report of an additional case. *American Journal of Medicine* 43, 579–592.

Janofsky, J. (1986) Munchausen's syndrome in a mother and daughter: An unusual presentation of folie à deux. *Journal of Nervous and Mental Disease* 174, 268–270.

Justus, P., Kreutzinger, M. & Kirchens, C. (1980) Probing the dynamics of Munchausen's syndrome. *Annals of Internal Medicine* 93, 120–127.

Kerr, D., Wilkinson, R., Horler, A., Schapira, K. & Walls, J. (1980) Factitious haematuria and urinary tract infection. *Archives of Internal Medicine* 140, 631–633.

Maue, F.R. (1986) Functional somatic disorders. *Postgraduate Medicine* 79, 201–210.

Maur, K.V., Wasson, K. & Deford, J.W. *et al.* (1973) Munchausen's syndrome. *Southern Medical Journal* 66, 629.

Meadow, R. (1977) Munchausen's syndrome by proxy: The hinterland of child abuse. *Lancet* ii, 343–345.

Meadow, R. (1982) Munchausen's syndrome by proxy. *Archives of Disease in Childhood* 57, 92–98.

Meninger, K. (1934) Polysurgery and polysurgical addiction. *Psychoanalytical Quarterly* 3, 173–199.

Mitas, J. (1985) Exogenous protein as the cause of nephrotic range proteinuria. *American Journal of Medicine* 79, 115–118.

Mitchell, C.C. & Frank, M. (1982) Pseudobradycharia during holter monitoring: The electronic Munchausen's syndrome? *Journal of the American Medical Association* 248, 469–470.

O'Shea, B., McGinnis, A., Cahill, M. & Falvey, J. (1984) Munchausen's syndrome. *British Journal of Hospital Medicine* 31, 269–274.

O'Shea, B., McGinnis, A., Lowe, N. *et al.* (1982) Psychiatric evaluation of Munchausen's syndrome. *Irish Medical Journal* 75, 200–202.

Pallis, C. & Bamji, A. (1979) McElroy was here: Or was he? *British Medical Journal* 1, 973–975.

Petersdorf, R. & Bennet, I. (1957) Factitious fever. *Annals of Internal Medicine* 46, 1039–1042.

Phillips, M., Ward, N. & Ries, R. (1983) Factitious mourning: Painless patienthood. *American Journal of Psychiatry* 140, 420–425.

Pope, H.G., Jonas, J. & Jones, B. (1982) Factitious psychoses: Phenomenology, family history and long-term outcome of nine patients. *American Journal of Psychiatry* 139, 1480–1486.

Raspe, R. (1948) *The Singular Travels, Campaigns and Adventures of Baron Munchausen.* Cresset Press, London.

Reed, J. (1978) Compensation neurosis and Munchausen's syndrome. *British Journal of Hospital Medicine* 19, 314–321.

Reich, P. & Gottfried, L. (1983) Factitious disorders in a training hospital. *Annals of Internal Medicine* 99, 240–247.

Reich, P., Lazarus, M., Kelly, M. & Rogers, M. (1977) Factitious faeculent urine in an adolescent boy. *Journal of the American Medical Association* 238, 420–421.

Roethe, R., Fuller, P., Byrd, R., Stanford, W. & Fisk, D. (1981) Munchausen's syndrome with pulmonary manifestations. *Chest* 79, 487–488.

Rosenberg, D. (1987) Web of deceit: A literature review of Munchausen's syndrome by proxy. *Child Abuse and Neglect* 11, 547–568.

Rumans, L. & Vosti, K. (1978) Factitious and fraudulent fever. *American Journal of Medicine* 65, 745–755.

Schechter, D. (1973) Self-induced diseases and disabilities. *Lawyers Medical Journal* 1, 281–296.

Schreier, H. & Libow, J. (1993) *Hurting for Love: Munchausen by Proxy.* Guilford, New York.

Scoggin, C. (1981) Factitious illness. *Postgraduate Medicine* 74, 259–265.

Scully, R., Mark, E. & McNeely, B. (1984) Case 28–1984. *New England Journal of Medicine* 311, 108–116.

Snowdon, J., Solomons, R. & Druce, H. (1978) Feigned bereavement: Twelve cases. *British Journal of Psychiatry* 133, 15–19.

Stinnet, J.L. (1987) The functional somatic symptom. *Psychiatric Clinics of North America* 10, 19–34.

Thompson, G., Shuster, J., Williams, R. & Kaye, M. (1964) Munchausen's syndrome: A cause of pyrexia of unknown origin. *Canadian Medical Association Journal* 91, 1021–1023.

Tizes, R. (1977) The professional cardioversion patient. *Chest* 71, 434–435.

Tunbridge, W. (1969) Munchausen's syndrome. *New England Journal of Medicine* 280, 1130–1131.

Veith, I. (1965) *Hysteria: The History of a Disease.* University of Chicago Press, Chicago, Ill.

Warner, J. & Hathaway, M. (1984) Allergic forms of Meadow's syndrome. *Archives of Disease in Childhood* 59, 151–156.

Wingate, P. (1951) Munchausen's syndrome. *Lancet* i, 412–413.

World Health Organization (1992) *The ICD-10 Classification of Mental and Behavioural Disorders. Clinical Descriptions and Diagnostic Guidelines.* World Health Organization, Geneva.

Wright, B., Bhugra, D. & Booth, J. (1995) Computers, communication and confidentiality: Tales of Baron Munchausen. *Journal of Accident and Emergency Medicine* 13, 18–20.

Yassa, R. (1978) Munchausen's syndrome: A successfully treated case. *Psychosomatics* 19, 242–243.

CHAPTER 7

Disorders of Passion

PAUL E. MULLEN

Introduction

Paranoia has returned from the nosological wilderness in the form of the delusional disorders with DSM-IV (American Psychiatric Association (APA) 1994) listing a number of subtypes, including the erotomanic, the jealous, the persecutory and the somatic. This has rekindled a wider interest in delusional syndromes which present as organized extensions and elaborations of preoccupations and suspicions which, far from being bizarre, are part of the experience of most of us at some time in our lives. Suspicions of infidelity, unrequited love, the fear of rejection and ridicule, these are among the states of mind that lie at the centre of such delusional systems just as they lie at the core of much everyday distress and discomfort. The concept of paranoia fell into disrepute, at least in part, because of the difficulties separating many cases so labelled from the schizophrenias, on the one side, and the fanatical preoccupations and overvalued ideas, on the other. This chapter will begin by revisiting part of the debate on the delusional syndromes represented by de Clérambault's attempt to carve out a subcategory of disorders of passion and use this to address the clinical and nosological issues raised by the pathological extensions of such powerful human experiences as love, jealousy and indignation. This chapter is driven neither by a taste for history nor an obsession with how terminology has been used, and misused, but by a more pragmatic desire to articulate a framework which will aid the clinician's understanding of these forms of psychopathology and make subsequent management more effective.

De Clérambault and psychoses passionels

De Clérambault (1942) proposed the category 'psychoses passionels' for patients displaying either erotomania, litigious behaviour or morbid jealousy. He argued that these states are characterized by delusional systems with special characteristics of their own differing sharply from the persecutory or other paranoid delusions (Baruk 1974). De Clérambault suggested what he termed the interpretative delusions of paranoia, such as those involving persecutory delusions, were based on a feeling of suspicion in which the patient is driven to seek explanations in a world experienced as hostile and constantly changing, a world which leaves the patient fearful and largely passive. He contrasted this with those in the grips of *psychoses passionels* which have at their core an all-absorbing sense of purpose with a precise aim which leads to a constant striving and to desires which bring the patient into direct conflict with the world. The patient in the grips of a persecutory delusion may come into conflict with those around him or her and even launch attacks against supposed enemies. The distinction being advanced suggests that patients in the grip of a persecutory delusion experience themselves as the object of others' malevolence and their attacks are usually pre-emptive strikes driven by fear. The morbidly jealous or the paranoid litigant is engaged in an active battle for his or her perceived rights, not a mere warding off of a threatening world. The litigious, for example, experience themselves as proactive subjects accusing and seeking redress, whereas the persecuted tend to be reactive with their attempts to protect themselves from the plots and incursions of their tormenters. In de Clérambault's view, persecutory or grandiose forms of paranoia spread, gradually affecting the whole personality, and the delusional content is many-sided, changing and progressive, whereas in the delusions of passion there is a rapid, if not immediate, onset with the emergence of a well-formed and focused organizing principle around which the delusional system revolves. Signer (1991), in an excellent account of the development of the ideas of de Clérambault, notes that he viewed these disorders as precipitated by a shock or crisis which moved the patient from ordinary emotionality to a pathology of passion. Once initiated, these disorders were prolonged, forceful and usually ended in action. It is important to note with regard to the views of de Clérambault that though he emphasized the continuity of disorders of passion with antecedent psychic life, and the reactive elements, he remained wedded to a fundamentally organic origin. It was his followers and pupils who gave a strongly psychodynamic coloration to theories of the aetiology of disorders of passion (Lagache 1938).

Central to de Clérambault's idea is the notion of passions which involve an active striving to fulfil desires and attain ends. 'Passion' in English originally carried the implication of suffering and of something that is done to us, or happens to us. Passions overwhelm, but traditionally this is an overwhelming by outside forces foreign to one's true nature rather than a willed commitment to an aim which absorbs all of the subject's energies. This notion of being overcome by an external influence is expressed idiomatically when we say, infected by jealousy, bowled over by love, overcome by anger and blinded by rage. In French, '*passion*' carries similar implications of 'sufferance' and the involuntary but, to an even greater extent than in traditional English usage, it has connotations of being at the explosive end of the emotional spectrum. The notion of passions and their disorders as involving the wilful pursuit of desires does, however, accord with more recent conceptualizations which regard emotions as involving judgements, intentionality and motives (Solomon 1976, 1980; Gordon 1987; Greenspan 1988).

The term 'passion' itself may thus be criticized. The separation of persecutory and grandiose delusions from passionate delusions is rarely so clear-cut in clinical practice as suggested by de Clérambault. The sudden and dramatic onset is far from a universal feature of these disorders. Despite these and other caveats, the creating of a category of disorders of passion may nevertheless bring heuristic and practical benefits. De Clérambault's disorders of passion comprised the trio of morbid jealousy, erotomania and querulousness, reflecting as they do the pathologies of jealousy, love and indignation. The querulents include not just paranoid litigants but hypochondriacal claimants. There may be a case for extending the ambit of disorders of passion to include resentment, pride and destructive envy, which are among the other emotions which could be regarded as laying a basis for further examples of such conditions. A broader view of the disorders of passion will be taken than approved by de Clérambault in that this chapter will range beyond the pure, or primary, syndromes to the secondary, or symptomatic, variants (which only partly correspond to de Clérambault's associated syndromes) and will not be confined to disorders with clear-cut delusions.

Restrictions on length, and respect for the reader's tolerance, dictate that following a general introduction to the disorders of passion only one of de Clérambault's trio of *psychoses passionels* will be considered in detail. Erotomania, or pathological love, has been chosen for a more detailed account. Pathological jealousy has been described and discussed at greater depth and length than other disorders of passion (Langfeldt 1961; Shepherd 1961; Retterstøl 1967; Vaukhonen 1968; White & Mullen 1989) whereas, conversely, the various forms of pathological querulousness have, with a few notable exceptions (Kraepelin 1917; Kolle 1931; Stalstrom 1980; Astrup

1984; Rowlands 1988), attracted so little attention as to make its extended consideration problematic. Finally, erotomania has emerged in recent years as a focus of renewed interest and its detailed reconsideration may be timely.

Clinical and nosological issues

Those with disorders of passion have an overwhelming sense of entitlement and are convinced that others are abrogating their rights (Mullen *et al.* 1993). The morbidly jealous believe they are the victims of an infidelity which has deprived them of the fealty which is their due and they are driven to expose this disloyalty, reassert their control and punish the transgression. The querulent are indignant at the infringements of what they consider their self-evident rights and prerogatives and are driven by the desire for public vindication and retribution on those who would deprive them of both justice and their rightful possessions. The erotomanic, as Esquirol (1965) wrote, are 'possessed of an exaggerated and sentimental attachment to someone who in reality has little or no relation to the sufferer' and they are driven to assert the rights of their love and attempt to realize the intimate relationship which they believe has been vouchsafed them, irrespective of the expressed wishes of the object of their attentions. In all three of these states, there is an intense focus on another individual who is the object of the passion (in the querulant, this may be an organization or group). They know what they want and they know what obstructs their desires. Each in their different ways usually asserts their supposed rights with a self-absorption and self-righteousness which puts at nought the interests of the object of their concerns, and which all too often disregards the constraints on acceptable interpersonal behaviour and even the obligation to conform to the law. When frustrated, as they inevitably are, there is a risk of eruptions of vindictiveness and rage. It is perhaps for these reasons that this trio of disorders is more familiar to the forensic specialist than the general psychiatrist.

Morbid jealousy and erotomania, if not morbid querulousness, are far from uncommon disorders. In the clinical evaluation of a patient, however, they are too often either not recognized or dismissed. In part this reflects a tendency to subordinate the morbid passion to a formulation in terms of a so-called 'Axis I' diagnosis such as schizophrenia or major depression, of which the passion is a mere symptom, or as in delusional disorder to consider that the passion forms the manifest content of the disorder which merely functions to consign the patient to the correct subtype. This tendency has weighty support. Shepherd (1961) regarded morbid jealousy primarily as a symptom and similar arguments have been advanced with regard to erotomania (Hollender & Callahan 1975; Ellis & Mellsop 1985; Bowden 1990). The low profile of these disorders also derives from our tendency to overlook them because of their ambiguous status which is created by being stretched over a broad range of experience from the more extreme variants of those intense emotional states, to which we are all prone, through to clear delusional processes. In cases where delusions are absent, the attribution of pathology rests on judgements about the intensity and the facility with which the passion is evoked and the extent to which the passion seems understandable, given the actual situation and the subject's cultural and social background. Love, the sense of justice and jealousy are aspects of the human experience which naturally tend to the extreme and to be accompanied by enthusiasms. It is no easy matter to decide when a committed concern for fairness and justice translates into querulousness or where a proper pursuit of civil redress crosses the line into morbid litigiousness. These boundary issues are no less problematic in the areas of love and jealousy.

The limits of normality in jealousy, love and indignation are further complicated by the changing constructions placed on these passions in different cultures and at different historical periods within the same culture. Singer (1966) traced the changing expressions of love through European history, vividly illustrating the radical shifts that have occurred not only in what would be considered acceptable behaviour but in acceptable ways of articulating, for yourself and others, being in love. Jealousy has also been subject over time to dramatic shifts in what constitutes its acceptable expression (Stearns 1989; Mullen 1991). The changing construction of jealousy in our own culture has gradually transformed it from a socially sanctioned response to infidelity into an individual's psychological state, redolent of immaturity, possessiveness and insecurity. In, for example, agrarian societies, where personal honour is a central organizing social principle, infidelity not only publicly shames the partner but also presents a threat to the whole social power structure which, having its roots in kinship, is dependent on female fidelity for its legitimacy (Gullerot 1971; Mullen 1993). In such societies the behaviour accepted, if not actively sanctioned, from the jealous would be labelled in most modern Western societies as not only excessive but almost certainly suggestive of pathology. Similarly, there have been shifts in what constitutes legitimate grounds for jealousy, assuming any legitimacy is still credited to this unfashionable emotion. Even the way we understand our own feelings, desires and impulses evoked by a passion appears to shift with social and cultural influences. As jealousy has increasingly been banished from the acceptable into the realms of the disapproved and disordered, so love, particularly in its purely erotic manifestations, has benefited from rising prestige and from a rescuing of a wide range of sexual expressions from the disapproved and the disordered to a status where they claim, if not universal acceptance, at least a tolerance virtually impossible to gainsay. Even attempting to erect a boundary around an area of pathology in such shifting sands raises questions about the extent to which social and cultural judgements are being reified into mental disorders. Few would argue that the entry and exit of homosexuality into the lists of the mental disorders represented such processes at work. Attempts to avoid the problems of such relativism by claiming that the pathological emotion is the emotion which has its origins in a pathological process (such as schizophrenia) either shifts the focus of doubt or produces a circularity. It would, however, be an error to argue that because the boundaries of the normal are fluid and shifting that no area remains for the pathological. That love and jealousy could be not only excessive and misplaced but part of a madness seems to have been recognized almost as long as there have been categories of mental illness. Pragmatically, it is reasonable to assume there is a realm of the pathological in reference to the passions though its boundaries are neither fixed nor above challenge.

Reactive and symptomatic disorders

The disorders of passion can be broadly divided between those which emerge as a symptom complex within some underlying process, such as schizophrenia, and those which emerge as a pure or primary disorder in response to a situation which can be meaningfully related to the emergent passion.

Pathologies of passion are most frequently encountered as part of a recognizable psychiatric syndrome where they form part of the symptomatology of the underlying disorder. In theory, any condition capable of giving rise to a delusional development can generate a pathology of passion. Further obsessive-compulsive disorders can centre on fears over a partner's fidelity and in theory could drive either a morbid infatuation or a compulsive pursuit of supposed justice.

The features of a symptomatic (or secondary) disorder of passion are:
1   they owe their genesis and evolution to an underlying mental disorder which emerges prior to, or contemporaneously with, the pathology of passion;

2 the clinical features of the underlying disorder are present alongside the pathology of passion;

3 they usually resolve as the underlying disorder resolves.

A number of psychotic processes, including the schizophrenias, are associated with a delusional configuration conforming to a disorder of passion. Delusions of infidelity are, for example, reported to be a prominent feature in 14% of those with schizophrenia (Shepherd 1961). In a far more extensive study of 8134 in-patients, Soyka *et al.* (1991) reported delusions of infidelity to be found in 7.0% of organic psychosis, 6.7% of paranoid disorders and 2.5% of those with schizophrenia. These disorders are rarely problematic diagnostically, given the history and the presence in the mental state of features, unrelated to the passion, which point to the presence of an underlying psychotic process. It is with the delusional disorders (paranoia) and the paranoid personality disorders that the nosological problems begin.

A number of authorities consider that the disorders of passion do not form a discrete entity but can be found as a particular symptom complex within a wide range of mental disorders (Hollender & Callahan 1975). Similarly, at least with reference to pathological jealousy, DSM-IV (p. 635) regards it as one of the potential diagnostic features of a paranoid personality disorder and by implication a symptom. Munro (1988a, 1988b) considers delusional (paranoid) disorders, paraphrenia and paranoid schizophrenia to form a continuum which shares at least some aetiological factors and rejects delusional disorders as being in any way understandable developments of personality (also see Chapter 4). This would place delusional disorders on a par with schizophrenia and when its manifest content conforms to pathological jealousy, pathological love or pathological querulousness, these should be regarded as symptoms. If these views are accepted, all disorders of passion are symptomatic, or at the very least all that involve delusional convictions are symptomatic. Conversely, there is an alternative tradition which, though accepting that most such disorders are indeed secondary, or symptomatic, regards a subgroup (which overlaps with, but is not necessarily coextensive with, delusional (paranoid) disorders) as to be understood as emerging from an interaction between personality and a particular life situation, with or without the influence of additional mental or physical factors (Jaspers 1910, 1963; de Clérambault 1942; Retterstøl 1967; Kretschmer in Hirsch & Shepherd 1974; Retterstøl & Opjordsmoen 1991). It should be emphasized that such views do not equate with causal psychodynamic explanations as they all appeal to elements within the basic personality (or *anlagen*) which are regarded by most of these authorities as a biological given and potentially heritable.

Jaspers (1910) used morbid jealousy to illustrate the classic division of mental disorders into processes, developments and reactions. Jaspers' (1910, 1963) notion of a morbid reaction involved a response to a precipitating event in which the intensity and content of the provoking experience was sufficient to make understandable the emergence of the disorder, and in which there was a close temporal relationship between the provoking experience and the onset of the disorder. Ideally, the progress of the disorder should be linked to the evolution of the situation which precipitated it and the disorder should come to an end when the provoking cause is removed. Though such a description may make theoretical sense, it is difficult to apply to clinical realities. In practice, the passions which may emerge in ordinary, well-balanced individuals in response to infidelity, injustice or intense attraction do not become morbid, and it is only in those peculiarly sensitized by, for example, their personality or their past experiences, who are vulnerable to disorders of passion. It is only by grafting on the elements of what Jaspers (1910) calls a developmental disorder onto the idea of a reaction that a clinically coherent category emerges, at least with regard to disorders of passion. Jaspers hypothesized a developmental disorder to arise out of the interaction of the provoking situation with the individual's basic character structure (which he regarded as a product of a lifetime of interaction between the biologically given dispositions and environmental contingencies, physical, social and psychological). As in the reactive disorders, there is a provocation which, for example, in morbid jealousy would be events interpreted as implying the partner's infidelity. The progress of such disorders of passion, once set in motion, would rarely have the immediate connection to the evolution of the provoking situation suggested by Jaspers as a condition of a reactive disorder, but the disorder would be likely to be open to some modification by changes in the provoking situation. By combining and slightly modifying the Jasperian categories, a grouping of morbid reactions is produced, characterized by the following.

1   The presence at the onset of the disorder of a situation that can reasonably be related to evoking the particular passion (e.g. supposed infidelity or experienced injustice).

2   A state of affairs which renders the individual vulnerable to an extreme reaction which almost always involves a personality vulnerability or disorder (e.g. paranoid personality disorder or the sensitive self-referential personality) and which in addition may involve any of the following:

(a)   past experiences which leave the individual peculiarly vulnerable (e.g. previous desertion or infidelity);

(b)   chronic or recurrent confusion or intoxication (arising from, for example, cocaine abuse or alcoholism);

(c)   a mental disorder, most frequently depressive, which may effect both the interpretation of events and the nature of the response.

3   The response is exaggerated psychologically and often behaviourally (with respect to the norms for the individual and their culture).

4   The evolution of the morbid reaction may be influenced by factors in the provoking situation which tend to ameliorate or aggravate the evoked passion.

In practice, the personality vulnerability is the common ground from which these disorders spring. Such morbid reactions would be both a response to a situation and are usually understandable as an extension of the habitual way in which the individual elaborates and reacts to his or her lived experiences. For all their pathology, these morbid reactions usually remain part of the individual's praxis or human destiny.

Given this formulation, the kinship to an intense reaction which should be considered as within the normal range is clear. To assist in the distinction, it is necessary to provide at least a general outline of the characteristics of a normal reaction. In broad terms, jealous and amorous responses, together with reactions to perceived injustice or malfeasance, remain within normal limits if:

1   they are a response to events which can reasonably be related to evoking the particular passion (this may be difficult in love, which is notoriously indiscriminate);

2   the passion focuses on a plausible object;

3   the feelings, desires and behaviours evoked broadly remain within the limits acceptable to the individual's self-concept and within the wider cultural norms;

4   the passion has a course and evolution that can understandably relate to the provoking events and subsequent developments;

5   the subjects seek (and eventually accept) a reasonable resolution of their desires, or strive to extricate themselves from the situation if an irreconcilable conflict is generated.

Pathological reactions can give rise to delusional developments and the symptomatic forms of the pathologies of passion do not always involve delusions, as with those which arise on the basis of an obsessive-compulsive disorder. The distinction should not therefore be confused with a psychotic–non-psychotic dichotomy.

The view advanced in this chapter is that both de Clérambault's pure disorders of passion and those morbid forms of jealousy, love and querulousness which would be classified currently as delusional disorders can usefully be regarded as one group of pathological reactions.

Labels such as 'reactive' or 'endogenous', which claim an aetiological specificity and understanding with little, if any, empirical basis, have rightly come to be regarded with suspicion. The construction of the category of morbid reaction being suggested here, though essentially clinical, is contaminated by its inescapable link to postulated, but unproven, causal elements. One alternative is to attempt a purely phenomenological division which would generate delusional and non-delusional categories, further subdivided between those with accompanying disturbances of mental state, such as hallucinations or depressed mood suggestive of specific disorders, and those where the jealousy, erotomania or querulousness forms the totality of the psychopathology. This would be a tidier classification but would not offer as much guidance to the clinician on how to conceptualize and treat these conditions.

Regarding disorders of passion as symptom complexes which may be associated with organic psychoses, functional psychoses, neuroses and personality disorders is an example of a medical reductionism in which the jealousy, erotomania or querulousness becomes mere epiphenomena generated by the underlying illness or disorder. Though often justifiable on theoretical and pragmatic clinical grounds, it is dubious when a delusional disorder is presented as the generating condition, for here the totality of the discernible psychopathology may well be restricted to the pathological passion so that the morbid emotion becomes in practice a symptom of itself, or at the very least the only evidence for the condition of which it is supposed to be a symptom. This approach also tends to sever the connections between the normal emotions of love, jealousy and indignation and the morbid states to which they give shape. Such a severance is justified in those states where the symptom complex emerges from a pre-existing mental illness such as schizophrenia, though even here the personality and past experiences of the patient are often critical in determining the content of morbid preoccupations and emotions. In what we have termed 'the morbid reactions', the kinship to extreme reactions is clear and the terminology directs our attention to the specifics of the passion as well as the specifics of the individual and the context from which the passion emerged. This has clinical advantages and, in practice, even those such as Hollender and Callahan (1975) and Shepherd (1961), who advance for erotomania and morbid jealousy respectively, a universally symptomatic construction place considerable emphasis on the personalities, life experiences and immediate contexts from which the morbid passions emerge.

The category of overvalued ideas has been considered to have particular relevance to morbid jealousy, morbid querulousness and erotomania (McKenna 1984). Overvalued ideas are convictions of overriding personal significance out of all proportion to their overt content. They differ from the strongly held beliefs of the commonality in the degree of emotional investment and the central place they occupy in the mental life of the individual (Fish 1967; Mullen 1986). They are regarded as sitting on a continuum between the deeply held convictions of normal individuals and delusional beliefs. They are similar to strongly held religious and political beliefs, differing largely in their highly personalized, not to say egocentric, quality. They usually develop on the basis of a previously abnormal personality (or, occasionally, as the expression of an underlying psychotic or organic process), often in response to an experience understandably related to the content of the overvalued idea. Fish (1967) noted that in overvalued ideas the convictions directed actions to a far greater degree than in most delusions. Those with overvalued ideas often act on their beliefs determinedly and repeatedly (McKenna 1984).

The biopsychosocial conceptualization of mental disorders which receives almost universal support does theoretically allow for all mental disorders to be viewed in the context of a potentially dynamic interaction between biological, psychological and social factors. This framework allows, in theory, ample room for delusional disorders, or any other mental disorder, to be regarded as representing in an individual case the influences of a social or psychological challenge on a vulnerable individual. DSM-IV and ICD-10 (World Health Organization 1992) do not claim to offer aetiological understanding nor do they attempt to advance meaningful or causal connections between the disorders' defined and putative influences, be they biological, social or psychological. The attempt to delineate specific criteria for a particular disorder inevitably produces a discontinuous categorical system. This, it can be argued, is merely an assistance to precise communication rather than representing an endorsement of qualitatively distinct conditions. Thus, though many personality disorders can be regarded as lying at the extreme end of a continuum and differing only quantitatively from the general population, nevertheless it facilitates communication to lay down clear criteria for when a given clinical picture is to be properly labelled as representing a personality disorder. Though DSM-IV and ICD-10 are theoretically innocent of aetiological assumptions and employ a categorical system without necessarily endorsing qualitative distinctions, nevertheless they are applied in a context where notions of disease entities predominate and where interest and commitment focus on postulated physical (biological) causes for nearly all psychotic disorders, and not a few of those conditions characterized by less severe disruptions of mental state. The approach taken in this chapter has no necessary conflict with the currently employed classificatory systems, but is somewhat out of step with the 'biological' enthusiasm of the age.

This chapter will assume that what is termed the pathologies of passion are in part an extreme form of normally occurring emotions, with the reactive forms in a continuum with normal emotional experiences. A commitment to this formulation derives in part from a disquiet with the degree to which modern psychiatry is trapped within its own constructions of disease entities (both Axis I and II), and in part from a clinical experience heavily biased towards forensic practice. It is not uncommon for individuals whose stalking behaviours, domestic violence or harassing claims have raised questions about their state of mind to be referred for assessment by courts or lawyers. Such individuals often inhabit the borderlands between extreme and pathological forms of love, jealousy or indignation. This clinical experience reinforces a tendency to see disorders of passion as in continuity with normal emotional experience.

Management

In theory, the symptomatic pathologies of passion should resolve when the generating mental disorder is treated. In practice, the underlying disorder may be of a type in which attaining full remission is difficult, as with some schizophrenias. In most cases, however, sufficient response is obtainable to produce an effective resolution of the passional symptom complex. In most cases of schizophrenia, the morbid jealousy, erotomania or querulousness will abate as the active symptoms of the condition respond to treatment, or subside with time and the progress of the disorder's own natural history. Echoes of the disorder may persist, when the patient with schizophrenia is in full remission, though these muted preoccupations usually remain dormant unless directly broached and rarely produce either active distress or action. In affective disorders, a more complete resolution can be expected with treatment and the attainment of insight into the irrational or exaggerated nature of the passion is usual. The occasional manic patient will cling onto aspects of their delusional preoccupations following a return to the euthymic state, but, as with those who have had schizophrenia, such remnants of pathologies of passion rarely create distress or motivate action. In the management of affective disorders complicated by disorders of passion, it is usual to add specific anti-psychotic drugs to the treatment of the mood disorder, just as when other delusional developments emerge in depression or mania.

Disorders of passion usually create considerable interpersonal and social conflict for the sufferer. Part of effective management is whilst they are actively symptomatic, protecting them, and protecting potential victims, from the effects of their morbid preoccupations and desires. This usually involves an active engagement with the patient and their ideas which goes way beyond prescribing. Similarly, as the underlying disorder subsides, the patients will need specific assistance in reintegrating into relationships and social contexts which have often been all but destroyed by their jealousy, misplaced amorous pursuits or clamorous claims. The need for such ongoing counselling and support is particularly marked in those who have had an affective disorder, partly because their aspirations in terms of future functioning are usually greater than in those damaged by schizophrenia, and partly because they have often been particularly effective, and therefore disruptive, in pursuing their misplaced passion.

Disorders of passion, particularly morbid jealousy, may emerge as part of organic disorders ranging from thyroid dysfunction to multiple sclerosis. In some of these cases the primary pathology is irreversible but the pathology of passion will usually respond to anti-psychotic medication and appropriate psychotherapy. Occasionally, as in cases of thyroid disease, the resolution of the generating physical disorder will not automatically abolish the disorder of passion which may have acquired an autonomous existence and will require to be treated directly.

Intense suspicions of infidelity have been reported to form the content of an obsessive-compulsive disorder (Cobb & Marks 1979; Mullen 1990; Stein *et al.* 1994) and, though it is not reported, there is no reason to exclude the possibility of erotomanic and querulous preoccupation forming the content of an obsessive-compulsive disorder. In those who could be construed as obsessive in the everyday sense of that word, the quality of disorders of passion may lead to their being conceptualized as a clinical form of obsessive-compulsive disorder and, perhaps more importantly, in the case of morbid jealousy, to being subjected to therapeutic strategies developed primarily for the management of obsessive-compulsive disorder (Cobb &

Marks 1979; Bishay *et al.* 1989; Stein *et al.* 1994; Dolan & Bishay, in press). The efficacy in selected cases of cognitive behavioural approaches and of drugs known to be effective in obsessive-compulsive disorder is important when considering therapeutic options and may well need to be incorporated into our understanding of the nosology and aetiology of these conditions. The group which appears to respond best to such approaches are the delusional disorders and the intense, but non-delusional, preoccupations in which the subject retains insight into their excessive and irrational nature, even if such insight is often fluctuating and partial.

The pathological reactions usually emerge on the basis of a marked underlying disorder of personality. The characterological anomalies include excessive suspiciousness, oversensitivity, a propensity to self-reference, and in some cases the subjects exhibit either a gross narcissism (with its attendant overweening sense of entitlement) or a fragile facade of self-confidence which is easily breached to reveal the oversensitivity and suspiciousness. The immediate management of pathological jealousy, love or indignation does not require that the personality vulnerabilities be corrected, though they often intrude on therapy. The pathology of passion must be managed directly. In the case of clearly delusional preoccupations, the use of anti-psychotics is usually indicated. Pimozide has been advocated as having specific efficacy but low to moderate doses of most anti-psychotics can be employed (Mooney 1965; Munro 1984; Munro *et al.* 1985; Ungvari & Hollokoi 1993; Mullen & Pathé 1994a). Regular psychotherapy is necessary, if only to maintain compliance, for it is not easy to persuade someone that by taking a pill their amorous quest, or the illicit amorous activities of their partner, will be influenced in a positive manner. Gentle confrontation, the pointing out of the distortions which sustain the beliefs, and the reiteration of the damage being done to the patient's own interests, are an integral part of good clinical management. To employ such approaches, a relationship must be sustained with the patient over time, no easy matter with these groups.

Delusions have been proposed to result from attempts to make sense of abnormal perceptual experiences rather than representing a disorder in either reasoning or inferential thinking (Maher 1988). Though such theories may have utility in understanding some delusional developments in those with schizophrenia, where 'delusions of explanation' may arise from abnormal experiences such as hallucinations and passivity experiences, they seem difficult to apply to delusional disorders where perceptual anomalies, if any, seem to follow and serve the delusional thinking. Alternatively, those with delusions have been claimed to show anomalies in attribution, judgement and probabilistic reasoning (Garety 1991). Chadwick and Lowe (1994) suggest that what is common to delusions is an attempt to make sense of particular events, which are not restricted to perceptual disturbances, and that the deluded individual constructs the belief to explain particular experiences. This approach to delusions stresses a continuity with normal processes which lead to judgements and convictions but would appear more relevant to the delusions found in delusional disorders than those found in most examples of schizophrenia or affective psychosis. These approaches, which can broadly be termed 'cognitive theories of delusional beliefs', have generated a range of therapeutic techniques for 'persuading' patients out of their delusional convictions (Alford & Beck 1994; Chadwick & Lowe 1994). Their applicability to disorders of passion remains to be tested.

Jealousy has attracted the largest literature on treatment and management (for reviews, see White & Mullen 1989; Pines 1992; Mullen 1995) and there has been particular attention to exaggerated or pathological reactions. Techniques involving desensitization, cognitive restructuring and reframing as well as a wide range of conjoint and couples therapies have been employed (Constantine 1986; Friedman 1989; Tarrier *et al.* 1989; Crowe & Ridley 1990; White 1991; Pines 1992). These approaches broadly aim to alter the cognitions which created and sustained the jealousy. Similar treatment strategies may well have a place in the erotomanias and querulants (also see Chapter 12).

Substance abuse, particularly involving alcohol or psychostimulants such as cocaine, may be related both to the genesis of disorders of passion and to sustaining and enhancing the conditions once initiated. Control over the underlying abuse is an essential element in management. The contribution to violence of substance abuse in these disorders also needs emphasizing.

Erotomania or pathological love

DEFINITION

'Erotomania' is well established as the term for pathological forms of love. The term is unfortunate, given the implications of both the erotic and the manic, neither of which are entirely appropriate. It is also unfortunate because of the historic baggage attached to the term, in particular that acquired in de Clérambault's attempt to clarify the concept. Alternative terms have been proposed, including 'erotic paranoia' (Krafft-Ebing 1904), 'erotic self-reference delusions' (Kretschmer in Hirsch & Shepherd 1974), 'delusional loving' (Seeman 1978) and 'pathological extensions of love' (Mullen & Pathé 1994a). A term such as 'pathological love' would be the most satisfactory and would avoid the phenomenological limitations of 'delusional love' and the ideological commitment of 'pathological extensions'. For the present, we remain saddled with 'erotomania' and this term will continue to be used in this chapter.

The term 'erotomania' was employed in the 19th century to describe at least three putative disorders.

1   Love melancholies, in which a wide range of symptoms, including, but not restricted to, those we would recognize as depression, were attributed to sentimental or erotic attractions which had either been unrequited or indulged in excessively (Burton 1621; Harvey 1672, quoted in Hunter & McAlpine 1963).

2   Erotic manias (nymphomania, satyriasis), which were described vividly by Isaac Ray (1839) as 'states of the most unbridled excitement, filling the mind with a crowd of voluptuous images, and ever hurrying its victim to acts of the grossest licentiousness' (pp. 192–193). This enviable form of erotomania was also on occasion extended to incorporate those sexual behaviours we now pusillanimously refer to as 'the paraphilias' (Macpherson 1889).

3   Erotomania, which Esquirol (1965) included amongst his monomanias as a disorder characterized by an exaggerated and irrational sentimental attachment usually to someone who in reality has little or no relationship to the sufferer.

It is the latter use of the term 'erotomania' which gave rise to our current concepts as it was redescribed and modified by authorities over the next century. Krafft-Ebing (1904) wrote, 'the nucleus of the whole malady is the delusion of being distinguished and loved by a person of the opposite sex who regularly belongs to one of the higher classes of society . . . the love, as should be emphasised [is] romantic, enthusiastic, but absolutely platonic' (p. 408). Kraepelin (1921) gives the pre-eminent clinical description:

> . . . the patient perceives that a person of the other sex distinguished really or presumedly by high position is kindly disposed to him . . . an intercepted glance, a chance meeting . . . let this hidden love become certainty to the patient. . . . Very soon every chance occurrence, clothing, meetings, reading, conversation acquire for the patient a relation to his imagined adventure . . . the whole colouring of the love is visionary and romantic . . . finally the patient resolves on further steps. He promenades before the window of the adored one, sends letters . . . but [if] things take an unfavourable turn the

loved one can become the enemy and the persecutor of the patient.
(pp. 245–249)

If Kraepelin apparently could not conceive of homosexual attachments giving rise to such a disorder, his English contemporary Hart (1912) seemed to imply it was specifically a malady of aged females when he wrote 'in Old Maids' Insanity an unmarried lady of considerable age, and blameless reputation, begins to complain of the undesirable attentions to which she is subjected by some male acquaintance . . . [who, she explains] is obviously anxious to marry her and persistently follows her about' (p. 122). De Clérambault (1942), whose name has come to be attached specifically to this syndrome, added to existing descriptions an emphasis on a sudden explosive onset, and on the patients insisting that it is the object of their attentions who made the first approach, and remains the prime mover in the supposed affair. He also modified the previous literature's emphasis on the love being sentimental and platonic, recognizing that overt carnal desires and clearly sexual behaviours could form part of the clinical picture.

PREVALENCE

Pathologies of love occur in men and women, the homosexual and the heterosexual, and in a variety of cultural contexts (Lovett Doust & Christie 1978; Taylor *et al.* 1983; Dunlop 1988; Eminson *et al.* 1988; El-Assra 1989). They are regarded as a rarity, being reported in 0.3% of in-patients (Retterstøl & Opjordsmoen 1991) and make up between 3% and 10% of delusional disorders, though with higher rates among forensic patients (Rudden *et al.* 1983; Menzies *et al.* 1995). The condition was long considered to be almost exclusively a disorder of females. Only Krafft-Ebing (1904), among the classical accounts, considered it to be found more frequently among men. Taylor *et al.* (1983) were the first to point to the male preponderance when subjects were drawn from a forensic population, an observation which has been amply confirmed subsequently (Leong 1994; Mullen & Pathé 1994a; Harmon *et al.* 1995; Menzies *et al.* 1995). The gender ratio for erotomanic syndromes overall must still be considered uncertain, though in the pure (reactive) forms females almost certainly predominate. Enoch and Trethowan (1979) noted the condition is 'still so infrequently mentioned as to appear virtually unknown'. There seems little doubt that the supposed rarity of pathologies of love owes more to a failure of recognition than a paucity of cases. The emergence of stalking as a category of offence in many jurisdictions, and as a matter of public concern throughout the Western world, will almost certainly increase rates of ascertainment. The DSM-IV, despite its limitations, will assist the recognition of this syndrome.

MORBID BELIEFS IN BEING LOVED AND MORBID INFATUATIONS

Kretschmer (in Hirsch & Shepherd 1974) considered erotomania to be based on an exaggeration of those dispositions to be found in normal lovers and therefore could involve both beliefs that one was loved as well as a morbidly enhanced infatuation. This goes against the trend in the literature strongly emphasized by de Clérambault (1942) which had shifted Esquirol's (1965) 'exaggerated attention' to a claim that cases should be confined to those who believe they are loved and are either merely responding to the other's supposed advances or have made every effort to discourage the claimed interest. The focus on a false belief of being loved in defining the psychopathology appears understandable, for a claim to be loved, and to have had that love revealed by specific actions and events, is usually open to falsification, whereas the assertion that one loves another is difficult to argue with, let alone declare to be false, particularly when no accompanying claim is made that the affection is returned. In practice, however, it is not so much the falsifiability of the central belief which indicates a psychopathological process but the reasons advanced for believing either that they are loved or that their infatuation will be crowned by establishing a relationship.* The associated behaviours also alert the clinician to possible pathology. When one of our

---

* Current definitions of delusion often begin by emphasizing it is a false belief. The inadequacy of falseness as a criterion is that we are often dealing with convictions which are either unverifiable (as, for example, many instances of jealousy) or depend on perspective and balance (as in the litigant) which places the assertions in the realm of probabilities, not truth and falsehood. Clear delusions may have at their core an essentially correct evaluation of the world (as with delusional jealousy) or may depend on personalized extensions of widely accepted beliefs (that there is a God who does direct, and in various ways communicate with, his or her creations). One suspects those who advocate false beliefs as the touchstone of delusion either hold a simple correspondence notion of truth or would appeal to a pragmatism which regards true propositions as those leading to effective (good) actions or as partaking of socially and culturally shared beliefs. The objection to the truth criterion is not, however, based on philosophical quibbles but on its inadequacy. It is from Jaspers' approach, particularly his emphasis on the way the delusion emerges and the effects on the life of the patient, that a more clinically robust understanding, and recognition of delusions, is to be obtained. (Jaspers 1963)

patients declared that love had been initially revealed when the object of her affections complained one morning in the lift about the difficulties he had had with the traffic driving to work, and when she later said she had had her beliefs confirmed by his angry demand she cease writing him embarrassing and inappropriate love letters, it was hardly necessary to establish with the supposed lover that he did not harbour the loving sentiments attributed to him by the patient. The assumption of disorder depends in large part on the eccentric, if not bizarre, grounds on which the patients base their convictions of being loved, and their remarkable capacity to reinterpret even the clearest of rejections as encouragement, if not outright expressions of love. One of our patients earnestly recounted how he had approached the object of his affections in the street to declare his love and she had told him to fuck off and leave her alone. When it was suggested that this might indicate rejection, he happily explained that, on the contrary, it was another hopeful indication of their developing intimacy for, after all, fucking was part of loving. The other elements which indicate pathology are: the degree of preoccupation with the supposed lover; the tenacity with which the beliefs are upheld against objections and contrary experience; as well as the extent to which the passion disrupts the affected individual's functioning. Similarly, in a morbid infatuation the pathology is revealed less by the core belief itself and more by the all-absorbing nature of the preoccupation, the unrealistic expectations, and the outrageous behaviour which potentially damages the proclaimed object of affection and certainly damages the would-be lover.

Pathological beliefs in being loved can be characterized as involving:

1 a conviction of being loved despite the supposed lover having done nothing to encourage or sustain that belief but on the contrary having either made clear their lack of interest or remained unaware of the claimed relationship;

2 a propensity to reinterpret the words and actions of the object of their attentions to maintain the belief in their supposed romance;

3 preoccupation with the supposed love which comes to form a central part of the subject's existence.

These three essential criteria are often accompanied by:

4 a conviction that the claimed relationship will eventually be crowned by a permanent and loving union;

5 repeated attempts to approach or communicate with the supposed lover.

Pathological beliefs in being loved may be clearly delusional as when the love is revealed in some extraordinary manner (as with one of our patients, who recognized the messages of love in a television news item about Israel), are sustained by ideas of reference, and extend to effect a wide area of the patient's experience of the world (as with a patient who became convinced that the telephone and mail service were in league with the secret service to interrupt the communications of love from the object of his affections). On occasion, however, the pathological beliefs in being loved seem to conform phenomenologically more closely to overvalued ideas than frank delusions. In clinical practice, it is not uncommon to be left in some uncertainty, with the amorous ideas lying in that transitional area between the extreme emotional responses of normal individuals and clear delusional developments.

In clinical practice, the subjects' convictions that the objects of their affections love them is usually accompanied with an acknowledged reciprocal affection. It is only the occasional patient who claims to be pursued by a lover to whom they remain indifferent. In one of our cases, the patient claimed to have been plagued for many months by the unwanted attentions of a young clergyman. She believed he repeatedly drove past her house with the intention of seeing her, prowled unseen around the house at night, and constantly communicated with her via barely audible blips which could be heard from the telephone, both when the receiver was in place and when she lifted the receiver. Though initially she said she found these attentions frightening, she gradually came to realize that the behaviours were the attempts of a shy man, encumbered by an unwanted wife, to communicate his love. Her fear was replaced by concern, then by love, and she began to respond with letters and repeated phone calls declaring their now mutual affection.

In the series of 16 erotomanic cases of Mullen and Pathé (1994a) in which they attempted to distinguish between morbid beliefs in being loved and morbid infatuation, in most cases it was a mixture of being loved and loving in return which characterized the condition. The two cases who claimed initially to have been passive and unwilling recipients of the object's affections admitted to having eventually succumbed to the supposed approaches. The occasional case in which the erotomanic claims to have no reciprocal feelings for the supposed lover create no theoretical difficulties. In contrast, those cases which predominantly, or exclusively, involve a morbid infatuation do create both practical and theoretical difficulties.

The definition promulgated in DSM-IV requires that erotomania be equated with 'a delusion that another person, usually of a higher status, is in love with the individual' (p. 765). The potential implications of such exclusivity was dramatically illustrated in the trial of John Hinkley Junior, who attempted to assassinate President Reagan. Hinkley had developed an intense and preoccupying infatuation with Jodi Foster and had claimed that his desire to attract her attention lay behind the attack on the president. Evidence was given at the trial to indicate that Hinkley did not have erotomania because he at no time claimed that Jodi Foster loved him, or even currently reciprocated his interest. The consuming infatuation with Jodi Foster, which had directly led, through a tortured reasoning process, to his trying to kill the president, was not considered capable of sustaining a diagnosis of delusional disorder because Hinkley made no claim that Jodi Foster had reciprocated his affections (Low *et al.* 1986; Goldstein 1987; Meloy 1989). The question of a severe mental disorder based on a morbid infatuation, though important, was just one of the diagnostic issues in this trial where clinical experience confronted the word of DSM-III, and the word won (Stone 1984).

The nosological problem is further illustrated by the following cases.

Case No. 7.1

A 36-year-old man, when first seen, had pursued a young woman with declarations of love and offers of marriage for 8 years. He was the only child of an elderly couple. The father had been effectively absent from the home and the mother an intrusive and domineering presence. Socially isolated at school and with only one friend during adolescence, he had nevertheless completed an apprenticeship and established with the friend a thriving business. Some months prior to his first encounter with the young woman, he had gone on holiday with his friend and business partner and, though the precise events were never revealed, there appears to have been a confrontation with his sexuality and possibly the homosexual elements in their relationship. This led to a complete severance of contact with his only companion. He became preoccupied with the need to marry and to find a pure and virginal bride. He began frequenting discos and clubs. One evening he encountered a 15-year-old woman whom he immediately recognized as his 'God chosen bride'. This recognition was based on her wearing predominantly white, and an air or emanation he discerned from observing her. He asked her to dance; she accepted. He approached her a second time, but whether due to his manner or lack of terpsichoreal skill, she declined to repeat the performance. He returned to the same club the next night in the hope of seeing her but was disappointed. He eventually managed to trace her and find out where she lived.

He sent flowers and an invitation to go out. She wrote a polite refusal. He repeated the process several times and received a response from her parents that they and their daughter wished him to cease these attentions. He began following her in the street. He would stand in a park opposite her house at night. He continued to send letters. An older sister approached him and demanded he stop harassing the young woman. He continued. The family contacted the police and were informed no offence had been committed. (This was in the days prior to anti-stalking legislation.) The father and an older brother confronted him one night as he kept vigil outside their house and threatened him. The next night he returned armed with a firearm which he brandished when approached. He was arrested. On release from police custody, having received a non-custodial sentence, he returned to his pursuit of the young woman. By this time his business had collapsed. His every waking moment was occupied with pursuing or thinking about the young woman. He had exhausted his financial resources in part by buying flowers and gifts (which were repeatedly returned), in part by paying for cosmetic surgery in the belief that if his receding hairline, slightly off-centre nose and possibly overprominent ears were corrected, she would respond to his approaches. This man's dogged pursuits of the object of his affections continued for years. He was imprisoned and committed to hospital (though not treated) but this produced only interruptions in his quest. The family moved; the young woman changed her name; she married; but still he was there. When examined over these years, he insisted she would one day be his wife and that they were destined for each other but he recognized she was currently frightened of him and did not, nor ever had, borne him any affection. He believed her mind had been poisoned against him by her family, particularly by the sister who on one occasion he assaulted. He was convinced, however, that eventually she would see through these falsehoods and recognize in him her destiny.

Case No. 7.2

A man in his late 40s became infatuated with a woman of a similar age. This man was the youngest of a large family and had had a close relationship with his mother. He was apparently socially successful at school and in adolescence and in adult life had considerable success working as a salesman. He had had numerous brief heterosexual affairs. He was a heavy drinker and, in later life, a regular smoker of marijuana. He dressed immaculately and he had an expensive sports car even though in recent years he lacked the finances to support such an indulgence. On first meeting, he radiated charm with an easy and expansive manner and an engaging verbal fluency. It became obvious, however, on closer acquaintance, that he was vulnerable to even the slightest criticism and was prone to blame and accuse others for any reverse, however minor. In the 2 or 3 years prior to his meeting the object of his affections, his life had been going badly. His business had collapsed and his attempt to redress the decline through dishonest handling had resulted in a prison sentence. His substance abuse had increased. He had alienated most of his acquaintances and all of his surviving family. His boyish charm had abandoned him and he no longer had much, if any, success in finding sexual partners. The object of his affections was a reasonably senior civil servant whom he had encountered while trying to establish yet another business. Initially taken by his charm, she had gone out with him on two occasions. He claims, but she denied, they had had sexual intercourse. She had become disenchanted with him and declined further invitations. He began phoning her repeatedly at home and at work. She had her calls monitored to prevent this. He wrote numerous letters. She returned them unopened. He took to intruding on her at work. She had him barred from the building. He followed her in the street and repeatedly came to her flat. She obtained a court order restraining him from approaching her or her flat. He responded by breaking into her flat so when she returned home he had literally moved in. She called the police. He was bound over to keep the peace. He broke into her flat once more and when she attempted to call for help, he threatened and eventually struck her. He was imprisoned but on release took a taxi from the door of the prison to her flat. He was serving a third prison sentence when eventually seen by our service. He made no claim that she loved him, going only as far as stating a belief that she might have been beginning to fall for him and because she was afraid of a developing relationship had stopped seeing him. He accepted she was now terrified of him because of his acknowledged inept attempts to win back her affections. He was adamant, however, that he loved her and she was the perfect partner. He was convinced he would eventually wear down her resistance and she would give him another chance. He was certain they were destined for each other. He thought about her constantly and ruminated on potential strategies to gain her love and attention.

Cases such as these have taken on a new prominence, with the emergence of stalking as a category of criminal offending and as a constellation of behaviours of concern to mental health professionals to whom police and the courts are turning for assessment and remedies. Among those who stalk are erotomanics who are convinced the object of their attentions loves them, but equally a group have been recognized who, though they persistently pursue the object of their affections, make no strong claims to their love being reciprocated. This group have been considered by some to constitute a subgroup of erotomania termed 'borderline erotomanics' by Meloy (1989) and 'pathological infatuation' by Mullen and Pathé (1984a). Meloy (1989, and in press) refers to an 'extreme disorder of attachment' which involves repetitive and persistent preoccupations with the beloved and manifests in the pursuit of the object of attention. Though Meloy (1989) derives his concept of borderline erotomania from a coherent psychodynamic theory, the acknowledged need for postulating a new subgroup of erotomania is that DSM-III and DSM-IV specify that the central feature of erotomania is that the object of the patient's attentions is believed to love the patient. Confined by the words of the manual, a new category must be created for these cases. Mullen and Pathé (1994a, 1994b) reject the currently accepted form of words for defining erotomania and appeal to a far longer clinical and nosological tradition which does not accept the exclusive emphasis on a morbid belief in being loved. They suggest that pathologies of love (erotomania) can include pathological infatuation, which is characterized by the following:

1   an intense infatuation without necessarily any marked accompanying conviction that the affection is currently reciprocated;
2   the object of the infatuation has either done nothing to encourage the feelings or clearly rejected any continuing interest or concern;
3   the infatuation preoccupies the patient to the exclusion of other interests resulting in serious disruption of their lives;
4   the subject insists on the legitimacy and probable success of their quest.

These elements are usually accompanied by a persistent pursuit of the object of affection with gradually escalating intrusiveness which creates fear and distress in the object of these unwanted attentions.

Pathological infatuations can phenomenologically be considered delusions or overvalued ideas or even occasionally be true obsessional phenomena.

In normal individuals, periods of such infatuation may occur (particularly in adolescents) but they fade when it is clear that no favourable response is to be expected from the beloved. The teenage 'crush' lacks the conviction of eventual fulfilment (though fantasies of such fulfilment are common) and acts as a pleasurable embellishment of their life, not as a preoccupying and disruptive element. Adolescent crushes are often social experiences in which the absorbing interest in a particular figure in the teenage culture is shared with like-minded peers and pursued through groups and clubs. This is in stark contrast to the isolating nature of pathological infatuations. Even the adolescents' passion for some admired, though usually unavailable, figure in their immediate environment is usually shared with friends and becomes a matter for joint interest and enjoyment.

In most erotomanics, morbid infatuation coexists with a morbid conviction of being loved, but there can be states which are virtually exclusively either morbid beliefs in being loved or morbid infatuations.

Symptomatic erotomanias

Psychiatrists, as already noted, are usually more likely to encounter pathological love as part of wider disturbances of mental state and it has been specifically described in association with schizophrenia (Hayes & O'Shea 1985), affective disorders (Raskin & Sullivan 1974; Rudden *et al.* 1990), schizoaffective disorders (Gillett *et al.* 1990) and a range of organic psychosyndromes (Lovett Doust & Christie 1978; Drevets & Rubin 1987; Signer & Cummings 1987; Gaddall 1989). Rudden *et al.* (1990) reported 12 of their 28 cases had schizophrenia, Mullen and Pathé (1994a) reported that, of their 16 cases, seven had a primary diagnosis of schizophrenia and three of mania as part of a bipolar disorder; in the series of Menzies *et al.* (1995), of 13 cases, nine had a primary diagnosis of schizophrenia and of Gillett *et al.*'s (1990) 11 cases, three had schizophrenia and four a bipolar illness.

The symptomatic pathologies of love differ from those occurring as pathological reactions (or from those falling within the delusional disorder category), not only by being accompanied by the other disturbances of mental state specific to the generating disorder, but also by being more fickle in changing the object of their attentions over time and in tending to have more obviously carnal desires and intentions (Mullen & Pathé 1994a). In erotomanic syndromes occurring in manic states, the preoccupations usually disperse when the mania settles, but with a recurrence of the disorder, the pathology of love can recur, often fixing on a new object of attention. In the schizophrenic disorders, the pathology of love tends to fluctuate with the course of illness, again with resolution during periods of relative quiescence and a return, often with a new object, during exacerbations. One of our cases with schizophrenia had pursued six different women over a period of 10 years, convinced that they loved him. His victims were selected from health staff and, on one occasion, a young woman he saw in the street.

Erotomanic symptoms associated with the schizophrenias may be associated with a greater frequency of sexual attacks on the object of their attentions (Mullen & Pathé 1994b). The risks of assaultative behaviour in general and sexual violence in particular was not, however, reported by Menzies *et al.* (1995) to be significantly associated with a primary diagnosis of schizophrenia.

A typical example of a symptomatic erotomania arising as part of a schizophrenic disorder is illustrated by the following case.

Case No. 7.3

Mr AF was the eldest of a family of three children. His father was a successful professional man with whom AF had a close relationship. His mother had her first episode of schizophrenia when AF was 10 years old. She subsequently remained on regular medication, though was not readmitted. AF was apparently a normal, reasonably sociable child until his mid-teens. Academically, he had always been poor and fell well below the attainments of his two siblings. On leaving school AF began an apprenticeship but in his late teens became increasingly withdrawn and erratic in his work attendance. He was first admitted at the age of 20 following an outburst of aggression at home. At that time he was reported as having an odd mechanical gait with posturing and occasional echopraxia. Subsequently, he was reported to be hallucinated and have a number of poorly systematized delusions. AF had a series of admissions over the next 6 years with the picture becoming increasingly that of a withdrawn, hallucinated individual with a number of persecutory preoccupations. He was assaultative towards relatives and staff on a number of occasions.

The first erotic fixation was reported some 7 years after his initial presentation. He apparently began to write love letters to a nurse. He followed her constantly. On discharge he repeatedly appeared at the nurse's home and followed her in the street. He made a number of attempts to embrace her. The nurse appears to have been sufficiently discomforted by this to change her place of employment. Two years later he attempted to embrace another nurse and subsequently exposed himself to her. He was again reported as stalking this nurse and following her. An attempt to rehabilitate him in the community was brought to an abrupt end when he attempted to rape a 14-year-old schoolgirl. It transpired that he had been following this young girl for some weeks and had made a number of approaches to her. Her family had contacted both mental health services and the police to try and have him stopped. When charged, he claimed that the young woman was in love with him. He said that she had been giving him signs and signals to encourage him. She also spoke to him at night and had had messages placed in television programmes declaring her love. Prior to the actual assault, he claimed that she enticed him both by the colour of the clothes she was wearing and by movements of her hand.

There were four further episodes recorded in the next 10 years when this man became fixated on female members of staff. On all occasions, he believed that they were in love with him and sexually desired him. He interpreted their clothes, their gestures and any statement they made as declarations of sexual interest. He made at least two further indecent assaults on the objects of his affection. On each of these four occasions he claimed that in fact the nurses were the 14-year-old schoolgirl that he had previously assaulted. He said that it was her in disguise, or using a different name, coming back to renew their relationship. The only attempt to discharge this man during the previous 10 years had been rapidly terminated when he had pursued a young woman in the street, calling her by the name of the schoolgirl and making indecent suggestions. This occurred at a time when the other positive symptoms of his long-standing schizophrenic illness appeared to be in full remission. He remains in a secure psychiatric unit on regular medication.

REACTIVE (PURE) EROTOMANIAS

The central feature of the reactive or pure pathologies of love is that they are discrete entities unaccompanied by features of other disorders. Their emergence is usually understandably related to the patients' previous personality and to their current personal and social situation. A provoking event can often plausibly by related to the onset. This precipitating event has been suggested to involve a 'narcissistic wound' or loss (usually of a supportive relationship) (Hollender & Callahan 1975; Enoch & Trethowan 1979; Evans *et al.* 1982). Pure pathologies of love often appear to emerge from a context of emptiness to fill a vacuum in the patients' lives. Taylor *et al.* (1983) noted all their cases to have led lonely and solitary existences with no sexual partners for many years prior to the emergence of the delusion. Segal (1989) pointed to certain common themes in the lives of these patients which included socially empty lives, a lack of sexual contact and low socioeconomic status. Mullen and Pathé (1994a) noted that all their five cases of pure erotomania were, at the time the disorder emerged, facing a life which appeared to them bleak, unrewarding and bereft of intimacy. The eroto-manic fixation can be postulated to provide at least a semblance of an intimate relationship and a route to the engagement of the loving and erotic affections of the patients. Scheler (1954) in his classic study of the phenomenology of love suggested that we do not love someone because they give us pleasure but we experience joy through loving. The act of love, even if unrequited, is itself still accompanied by a feeling of great happiness. For those whose life is empty of intimacy, the rewards of even a pathological love may be considerable.

The premorbid personalities in pure cases of erotomania have variously been described as shy and awkward (Krafft-Ebing 1904), hypersensitive and self-referential (Kretschmer in Hirsch & Shepherd 1974), proud and rebellious (de Clérambault 1942), narcissistic (Enoch & Trethowan 1979; Meloy 1989), schizoid (Munro *et al.* 1985), lacking in confidence, suspicious and socially avoidant (Retterstøl & Opjordsmoen 1991) and, finally, timid and withdrawn (Seeman 1978). The features common to these various formulations is of a socially inept individual isolated from others, be it by sensitivity, suspiciousness or assumed superiority (Mullen & Pathé 1994a). These patients tend to be described as living socially empty lives, often working in menial occupations and being, or feeling themselves to be, unattractive (de Clérambault 1942; Hollender & Callahan 1975; Enoch & Trethowan 1979; Segal 1989). The desire for a relationship in many cases is balanced by a fear of rejection or a fear of the realities of intimacy, both sexual and emotional. The following case history illustrates a pure or reactive pathology of love.

Case No. 7.4

LT, a female aged 47, was the youngest of four children. LT's father was disabled as a result of a work injury and her mother was the dominant figure. LT was described as shy and isolated both at school and as a teenager. On leaving school she obtained a job as an accounts clerk which she had retained until a year prior to admission.

Her husband was her first and only boyfriend. They married when she was 22 and he was 30 years of age. He was always the dominant figure in the relationship, making all of the decisions and controlling the money. His views always prevailed, giving her no opportunity even to ventilate her own opinion or feelings.

LT was always painfully shy and self-conscious. She reported frequently feeling that people looked at her and laughed at her behind her back. At work she was occasionally overwhelmed by suspicions that others were ganging up on her and talking about her. She said she always put these fears back in control by using logic because 'I know it's not real'. She avoided social contacts outside of the family. She was a well-organized individual but had no obsessional or phobic symptoms.

Four years prior to admission she had come 'to realize' that a senior partner in the firm for which she worked entertained romantic feelings about her. She had always admired him and considered him a gentle and concerned individual. Her preoccupations with this man increased markedly after the sudden death of a younger brother who had been the person with whom she had had the closest relationship. The love crystallized out following an incident when the object of her affections spoke to her one morning about the weather and the prospects for the upcoming ski season. It was this, she claimed, that made her realize he reciprocated her affection. She said, 'I knew this meant he had strong feelings for me, because usually I am completely ignored. No one chats to me. They think I'm not intelligent enough.' Over the next few months she felt that he expressed his love in a variety of roundabout ways; clothes that he wore, the way he nodded a greeting, and the occasional exchanged good morning. It was not, she said, so much what he said but the tone of voice and the way he said it. She became interested in her appearance for the first time in many years, took up aerobics, lost 10 kg and began dyeing her hair.

The object of her attentions, in a victim impact statement, said he had been aware for some years that she was infatuated with him, but this was entirely one-sided and had never been encouraged. He tried to ignore it but it became, in the last 3 years, increasingly intrusive. She would follow him, turn up unexpectedly, stand next to his car after work awaiting his departure, write notes to him and phone him both at work and at home. He arranged for her to be made redundant to prevent continuing harassment at work.

Eight months prior to the admission, whilst trailing the object of her affections, LT observed him meeting and having a drink with a senior secretary from the firm's office. Over the next week she tailed both this lady and the object of her affections. She became convinced that he was having an affair with this woman. She found herself troubled by intrusive images of her would-be lover in the arms of this other woman. She became increasingly distressed and angry. She made a number of accusatory phone calls to both the object of her affections, his wife and the secretary she supposed to have stolen his affections from her. At one point she attempted to throw herself in front of his car. She caused a major incident at his place of work by accusing him in front of a number of colleagues of having an affair and having deserted her. At this time she began to develop signs of depression with sleep disturbance, loss of appetite, self-denigratory ruminations and suicidal thoughts. Immediately prior to her admission she confronted the object of her affections with a rifle she had taken from her husband's gun cupboard. He claims she pointed it at him and threatened him; she denies actually directing the gun at him. The gun was discharged but the circumstances are in dispute. She left to return home; where she attempted to stab herself through the heart and in fact succeeded in inflicting a serious chest wound.

On admission, she acknowledged she was still preoccupied by thoughts of her supposed lover. She believed that there would still be a reconciliation between them because he remained in love with her and she returned his affection. She acknowledged that she was still plagued by jealousy and that vivid images would intrude into her consciousness of him having intercourse with her supposed rival. She claimed no longer to be actively suicidal because she recognized that eventually this hiccup in their relationship would be sorted out and they would have a future together.

This lady was commenced on both antidepressants and 6 mg of pimozide and, over the subsequent 4 weeks, the intensity of her preoccupations with this supposed beloved gradually decreased. She came to recognize that the relationship was now over and there was no future, given what had occurred. She still retained the belief that he had returned her affections, though she would accept that she may have been over-hopeful in her expectations for the relationship. She remains on medication.

Mullen and Pathé (1994a) noted that in all the pure syndromes in their series the premorbid personality was marked by exquisite self-consciousness with a tendency to refer the actions and utterances of others to themselves, usually endowing them with a denigratory or malevolent colouring. It is not difficult to extrapolate from such a tendency to the development of a pathology of love, given that all that may be required to set such a development in motion is seeing the actions and utterances of one particular person not as malevolent but as loving. These character traits may also provide some rationale for why apparently intelligent and not unattractive people are so handicapped in social and erotic relationships that they are driven into fantasy and delusion to satisfy their needs of intimacy.

The view advanced here of the pure or reactive forms of pathologies of passion being an extension of normal emotional reactions leaves problems over the boundary between the pathological and the morbid. The boundary issues are particularly acute in instances where there has been some form of real relationship, however fleeting, between the individual and the object of their affections (see Case No. 7.1). That the feelings were reciprocal at some stage makes it difficult subsequently to designate the love pathological. The other area of potential confusion is where unrequited love is pursued with such misplaced enthusiasm that it gives the mistaken impression of pathology. The following case exemplifies this latter quandary.

Case No. 7.5

Ms K was a 27-year-old of borderline intelligence from a stable middle-class background. She had worked as an office cleaner. She was shy and self-conscious, having little social life. Following a Christmas party she had intercourse with an office worker in his 30s who was married with children. They were both intoxicated at the time. This was her first sexual experience. She approached him subsequently but he, apparently embarrassed by the connection, rejected her with increasingly brutal directness.

Ms K believed that the man must care for her and that his actions indicated that he loved her. She was distressed and confused by his subsequent behaviour and, having no basis for comparison, decided he could not mean what he said. Over the next 4 months she approached him repeatedly, she telephoned him frequently, she turned up at his home and followed him to his golf club. She understood he was trying to put her off but could not accept that he had no feelings for her. Following one particularly direct and abusive rejection, she became angry and vandalized his car. She still kept pestering him, hoping to reawaken his interest. He took out a restraining order. She was enraged and went to his house and in front of his wife and children accused him of destroying her life. She refused to leave. The police were called and she was committed to hospital.

The behaviour of this young woman resembles that of someone with erotomania. All her hopes and fantasies about the future became dependent on the supposed love. She was totally preoccupied with this man to the extent of neglecting her work and herself. She certainly made repeated and sustained attempts to approach the supposed lover despite increasingly insistent rejections. She did not, however, reinterpret the man's words and actions to maintain the belief in his love but simply found herself incapable of crediting his change of heart. When she finally accepted the relationship was over, she moved to anger and distress. Her behaviour was based on a misinterpretation, fostered by naivety and sustained by a desperate hope, and though she behaved like someone with a pathological infatuation, she did not think like such an individual.

THE OBJECT OF AFFECTION

De Clérambault (1942), following Kraepelin (1921), considered that the erotomanic fixed their attentions on individuals of higher social status. This was given even greater emphasis by Segal (1989), who contrasts the physically unattractive erotomanic employed in some menial occupation with the attractive, high-status, intelligent(!) object of their affections. The popular attention given to the erotomanic followers of the rich and famous has reinforced this stereotype.

Part of normal love is endowing the beloved with attractive attributes, and it would be a poor suitor who could divine no claim to excellence in the object of their affections. The love of the erotomanic, being little constrained by practicalities or even plausibility, is free to fix on almost anyone, so their desire for excellence need not be mitigated by pragmatic considerations about likely success. In our experience, however, the objects of pathological love are almost as variable in their personal and professional attributes as are the objects of normal love. Erotomanic individuals fix their attentions on those they find attractive and with whom they have a real or supposed contact. The famous who intrude themselves, via television and videos, into our homes, often creating a pseudo-intimacy, clearly become targets more frequently than most. Objects of attention are often chosen from among individuals encountered in the work environment, either through employment relationships or by being a customer or client of the service offered by the future victim (Harmon *et al.* 1995; Meloy in press). At high risk are professionals, particularly health professionals, whose work not only brings them in contact with vulnerable people but often does so in a context of being helpful and concerned. In our experience, male erotomanics, like their non-disordered brothers, most often bestow their affections largely by virtue of the perceived physical attractiveness of the object of affection. Anyone can become the object of the disordered affections of the erotomanic and though the high-risk groups do have high status, they do not account for all victims. Similarly, although erotomanics are drawn from the lonely, socially incompetent and disordered, they are in our experience far from universally physically unattractive and some have attained high social status. (There is a medical practitioner, an academic and a lawyer among the erotomanic stalkers known to our clinic.)

STALKING AND OTHER FORMS OF VIOLENCE

Erotomania has long been known to be associated with stalking behaviours and to have the potential to lead to overt aggression. Esquirol (1965) reported a case who both attempted to lift the skirts of the actress he stalked and assaulted the husband he believed stood between him and his beloved. Morrison wrote in 1848, 'erotomania sometimes prompts those labouring under it to destroy themselves or others, for although in general tranquil and respectful, the patient sometimes becomes irritable, passionate and jealous' (quoted in Enoch & Trethowan 1979). De Clérambault (1942) believed that although erotomania began in pride, love and hope, it all too easily degenerated into resentment and anger.

Stalking behaviours are an almost inevitable accompaniment of erotomanic disorders. The core features of stalking are repeated attempts to establish contact and/or otherwise communicate with the object of the stalker's attention. This can involve following, maintaining surveillance over the object of attention's place of work or residence and approaches. Repeated attempts to communicate, be it by telephone, letter or electronic mail, are also common. In addition, following rebuffs the erotomanic may become enraged, make threats, interfere with the victim's property or try and cause disruption to the victim's life (by such things as ordering goods on their behalf or making vexatious complaints). Overt sexual approaches and attacks may also occur (Mullen & Pathé 1994b; Menzies *et al.* 1995).

Taylor *et al.* (1983) described four male erotomanics who as a result of their disorder acted violently. Zona *et al.* (1993) reported on the stalking behaviours in a group of 74 of what they termed 'obsessional followers', of whom seven fulfilled their criteria for erotomania. Meloy and Gothard (1995), looking at a similarly constituted group of 20 obsessional followers, noted frequent threats and an incidence of 25% for physically assaulting the victim. Leong (1994) reports five cases of erotomania referred for psychiatric assessment by the courts, all of whom had stalked the object of their affections; in addition, two had made threats, one had broken into the house of his victim and one into their car. The series of 48 subjects referred for assessment following charges of harassment reported by Harmon *et al.* (1995) contained six women diagnosed as delusional disorder erotomanic type and five men they regarded as having many of the symptoms of erotomania. They also had 10 cases of schizophrenia, several of which may have met our criteria for a symptomatic pathology of love. In their 'amorous group', 12 of 18 made threats and seven were assaultative. In the study of Mullen and Pathé (1994b), the cases were also drawn from a forensic population and, perhaps not surprisingly, showed high levels of threatening and assaultive behaviour. Menzies *et al.* (1995) also drew their cases of erotomania in part from a forensic population and again found significant levels of antisocial behaviour related to erotomanic delusions. These latter two studies almost certainly overestimate the risk of physical assault in erotomanic patients, but it should be emphasized that the impact of being stalked can be devastating even when no overt physical violence is involved. The victims of the extended and dedicated pursuit of erotomanic patients are often seriously traumatized. The repeated intrusions from telephone calls, letters, approaches and following create a state of constant apprehension, if not frank fear. Many victims curtail their social lives, change or abandon their employment, change residence and even change country in an effort to escape the unwanted attentions. A significant proportion of victims suffer post-traumatic stress symptoms and the development of significant depressive disorders is common after prolonged harassment (M. Pathé & P.E. Mullen, in preparation).

Erotomanics can resort to overt violence against the object of their affections, motivated by rage at rejection or jealousy. Occasionally, the assault may be an inadvertent by-product of the patient's clumsy attempts to approach the object of their attention (Mullen & Pathé 1994b). Those believed to impede access to the beloved may also fall victim to the violence of an erotomanic. Taylor *et al.* (1983) and Menzies *et al.* (1995) found the violence to be directed most frequently at someone other than the object of the patient's affections but in the series of Mullen and Pathé (1994b) and Harmon *et al.* (1995), the supposed beloved was the usual victim.

MANAGEMENT AND PROGNOSIS

The general approach to the management of symptomatic and reactive (pure) disorders of passion has already been discussed. In the symptomatic erotomanic syndromes, the treatment relevant to the generating disorder is provided, augmented where appropriate with anti-psychotic agents and psychotherapeutic interventions directed at the pathology of love. In the reactive (pure) syndromes, the mainstay of management is anti-psychotics in low to moderate dosage (e.g. pimozide, 2–6 mg per day) combined with counselling and support which both confronts the cognitive distortions sustaining the erotomanic fixation and hopes to move the patient to a more effective engagement with other people. This is often a protracted and frustrating process with slow progress and frequent reverses, but real therapeutic gains are usually possible if the patient remains engaged in treatment.

The literature in general does not indicate a good response to treatment even in the symptomatic conditions. Gillett *et al.* (1990) suggest a poor response in their four cases, with a primary diagnosis of schizophrenia and, even more surprisingly, a refractory erotomania in a case of mania which persisted despite effective treatment of the mood disorder. Segal (1989), on the basis of a literature review and his own experience, noted the extreme persistence of the erotic delusions with, at best, some remnant of the delusion remaining in all except the rare case. These gloomy prognostications are reiterated by Leong (1994), who goes so far as to suggest courts and social policy makers 'should not place much emphasis on psychiatry and other mental health disciplines in diminishing the erotomanic delusion' (p. 384) and seems to imply that criminal and civil sanctions may be more appropriate. One of the few long-term follow-up studies suggests a somewhat less grim outlook with favourable outcomes in two cases, relatively favourable in one and poor or uncertain in three (Retterstøl & Opjordsmoen 1991). Claims for the efficacy of pimozide or other antipsychotics in the pure (reactive) syndromes have been made (Munro *et al.* 1985; Stein 1986).

An abiding problem with managing these cases is the almost total lack of motivation for treatment. Those caught up in pathological love do not see themselves as ill but blessed with a romance whose only blemish is the tardiness of response in the beloved or the interference of third parties (often including the would-be therapist). The benefits for these disorders for the patient should not be forgotten, for they provide some solace for their loneliness, some support for their damaged self-esteem and some purpose to their otherwise empty existences. As Segal (1989) pointed out, 'erotomania, if kept under control, is not an altogether negative phenomenon, since it may provide solace for a few lonely souls, who might otherwise spend their lives in unrelieved isolation and solitude' (p. 1265), though one might question whether if unrequited love is 'kept under control', it qualifies as an erotomania.

A somewhat more optimistic picture was painted by Mullen and Pathé (1994a), who considered the general therapeutic pessimism about eroto-manic syndromes to be misplaced. Their experience was that the response to treatment in the symptomatic disorders reflected the nature and severity of the underlying disorder, with their three cases secondary to manic illnesses making a complete recovery but those with intractable schizophrenia disorders often continuing to harbour erotomanic delusions, though usually in a less florid and preoccupying form. The pure or reactive pathologies of love had a variable outcome, although four out of five either made a full recovery or showed marked amelioration of symptoms with low doses of anti-psychotics and supportive psychotherapy. They emphasized the need to persist with treatment in the pure syndromes over many months before improvement can be expected.

An element worthy of emphasis in the management is improving the social supports and networks of patients with pathologies of love. Though in our experience it is rarely possible to assist these patients to find and maintain intimate relationships, it has in some been possible to engage them in social activities and contacts which provide considerable support. If their lives remain bereft of human contact, let alone intimacy, it will be difficult to induce them to abandon the only semblance of a relationship they possess.

The widely held pessimism about the effective management of eroto-manic syndromes is a self-fulfilling prophesy made prior to any substantial trials of treatment. It is particularly unfortunate at a moment when mental health professionals are likely to be increasingly asked for opinions by the courts about the appropriate disposal of stalkers driven by erotomanic pre-occupations. It is probable that only effective treatment is capable of freeing the victim from pursuit and the patient from an all-encompassing preoccupa-tion. We are failing both our patients and their victims by not using the man-agement approaches already available and working on developing more effective therapeutic interventions.

Conclusion

The disorders of passion cut across existing psychiatric classifications. They take their origin in normal mental processes and their definition in deviance from those normal emotional experiences. In the symptomatic form, they can be brought into an easy correspondence with the dominant psychiatric systems of classification and thought, but if the pure or reactive construction is allowed, they begin to conflict with a strong tendency in psychiatry which would prefer, particularly when confronted with psychotic phenomena, to think in terms of the discontinuities of qualitative differences and the process of disease. Contemporary psychiatrists rarely have a problem, with so-called personality disorders being on the extreme end of a continuum which includes the normal, nor do they baulk at anxiety and mood disorders being generated by reactions to various forms of stress and trauma. In psychotic disorders, there is currently a general acceptance that the timing of the emergence of active symptoms and elements in course and evolution of the disorder can be influenced by social and psychological factors but the notion of delusional developments arising on the basis of an interaction between personality, past experience and current realities is, however, foreign to current thinking and the psychogenic psychosis (see Chapter 4) have all but been consigned to limbo. The clinical realities of the disorders of passion particularly in their pure and reactive form can provide a gentle challenge to such orthodoxy.

References

Alford, B.A. & Beck, A.T. (1994) Cognitive therapy of delusional beliefs. *Behavioural Research and Therapy* 32, 369–380.

American Psychiatric Association (1994) *Diagnostic and Statistical Manual of Mental Disorders*, 4th edn. (DSM-IV). American Psychiatric Association, Washington, D.C.

Astrup, C. (1984) Querulent paranoia: A follow-up. *Neuropsychobiology* 11, 149–154.

Baruk, H. (1974) Delusions of passion. In: *Themes and Variations in European Psychiatry* (eds M. Shepherd & S.R. Hirsch), pp. 375–384. Wright, Bristol.

Bishay, N., Petersen, N. & Tarrier, N. (1989) An uncontrolled study of cognitive therapy for morbid jealousy. *British Journal of Psychiatry* 154, 386–389.

Bowden, P. (1990) De Clérambault syndrome. In: *Principles and Practice of Forensic Psychiatry* (eds R. Bluglass & P. Bowden), pp. 821–822. Churchill Livingstone, London.

Burton, R. (1621) *The Anatomy of Melancholy*. [Numerous reprints and editions.]

Chadwick, P.D.J. & Lowe, C.F. (1994) A cognitive approach to measuring and modifying delusions. *Behavioural Research and Therapy* 32, 353–367.

Cobb, J.P. & Marks, I.M. (1979) Morbid jealousy featuring as obsessional compulsive neurosis: Treatment of behavioural psychotherapy. *British Journal of Psychiatry* 134, 301–305.

Constantine, L.L. (1986) Jealousy and extramarital sexual relations. In: *Clinical Handbook of Marital Therapy* (eds N.S. Jacobson & A.S. Gurman). The Guilford Press, New York.

Crowe, M.J. & Ridley, J. (eds) (1990) *Therapy with Couples*. Basil Blackwell, Oxford.

De Clérambault, C.G. (1942) Les psychoses passionelles. In: *Oeuvres Psychiatriques*, pp. 315–322. Presses Universitaires, Paris.

Dolan, M. & Bishay, N. (in press) The effectiveness of cognitive therapy in the treatment of non psychotic morbid jealousy. *British Journal of Psychiatry*.

Drevets, W.C. & Rubin, E.H. (1987) Erotomania and senile dementia of Alzheimer type. *British Journal of Psychiatry* **151**, 400–402.

Dunlop, J.L. (1988) Does erotomania exist between women? *British Journal of Psychiatry* **153**, 830–833.

El-Assra, A. (1989) Erotomania in a Saudi woman. *British Journal of Psychiatry* **155**, 553–555.

Ellis, P. & Mellsop, G. (1985) De Clérambault's syndrome: A nosological entity? *British Journal of Psychiatry* **146**, 90–95.

Eminson, S., Gillett, T. & Hassanyeh, F. (1988) Homosexual erotomania. *British Journal of Psychiatry* **154**, 128–129.

Enoch, M.D. & Trethowan, W.H. (eds) (1979) *Uncommon Psychiatric Syndromes*. John Wright, Bristol.

Esquirol, J.E.D. (ed.) (1965) *Mental Maladies: A Treatise on Insanity* (trans. R. de Saussure). Hafner Publishing Co., New York.

Evans, D.L., Jechel, L.L. & Slott, N.E. (1982) Erotomania: A variant of pathological mourning. *Bulletin of the Menninger Clinic* **46**, 507–520.

Fish, F. (ed.) (1967) *Clinical Psychopathology*. Wright, Bristol.

Friedman, S. (1989) Strategic reframing in a case of delusional jealousy. *Journal of Strategic and Systematic Therapy* **8**, 1–4.

Gaddall, Y.Y. (1989) De Clérambault's syndrome (erotomania) in organic delusional syndrome. *British Journal of Psychiatry* **154**, 714–716.

Garety, P.A. (1991) Reasoning and delusions. *British Journal of Psychiatry* **159**, 14–18.

Gillett, T., Eminson, S.R. & Hassanyeh, F. (1990) Primary and secondary erotomania: Clinical characteristics and follow up. *Acta Psychiatrica Scandinavica* **82**, 65–69.

Goldstein, R.L. (1987) More forensic romances: De Clerambault's syndrome in men. *Bulletin of American Academy Psychiatry Law* **15**, 267–274.

Gordon, R.M. (ed.) (1987) *The Structure of Emotions*. Cambridge University Press, Cambridge.

Greenspan, P.S. (ed.) (1988) *Emotions and Reasons*. Routledge, New York.

Gullerot, E. (1971) In: *Women, Society and Change*, pp. 19–28. McGraw Hill, New York.

Harmon, R.B., Rosner, R. & Owens, H. (1995) Obsessional harrassment and erotomania in a criminal court population. *Journal of Forensic Sciences* **40**, 188–196.

Hart, B. (ed.) (1912) *The Psychology of Insanity*. Cambridge University Press, Cambridge.

Hayes, M. & O'Shea, B. (1985) Erotomania in Schneider positive schizophrenia. *British Journal of Psychiatry* **146**, 661–663.

Hirsch, S.R. & Shepherd, M. (eds) (1974) *Themes and Variations in European Psychiatry*. Wright, Bristol.

Hollender, M.H. & Callahan, A.S. (1975) Erotomania or de Clérambault's syndrome. *Archives of General Psychiatry* **32**, 1574–1576.

Hunter, R. & Macalpine, I. (1963) *Three Hundred Years of Psychiatry, 1535–1860*, pp. 196–197. Oxford University Press, Oxford.

Jaspers, K. (1910) *Eifersuchtswahn*. Heidelberg.

Jaspers, K. (1963) *General Psychopathology*, 7th edn (trans. J. Hoenig & M.W. Hamilton). Manchester University Press, Manchester.

Kolle, K. (1931) Über querulanten. *Archiv für Psychiatrie und Nervenkrankheiten* **95**, 24–100.

Kraepelin, E. (1917) *Lectures on Clinical Psychiatry* (trans. T. Johnstone). Macmillan, London.

Kraepelin, E. (1921) *Manic Depressive Insanity and Paranoia* (trans. M. Barclay). E.S. Livingstone, Edinburgh.

Krafft-Ebing, R. von (1904) *Text Book of Insanity* (trans. C.G. Chaddock). F.A. Davis, Philadelphia.

Lagache, D. (1938) Erotomanie et jalousie. *Journal de Psychologie Normale et Pathologique* Avril–Juin, 127–160.

Langfeldt, G. (1961) The erotic jealousy syndrome: A clinical study. *Acta Psychiatrica Scandinavica* **36** (Suppl. 151), 7–68.

Leong, G.B. (1994) De Clerambault syndrome (erotomania) in the criminal justice system: Another look at this recurring problem. *Journal of Forensic Sciences* **39**, 378–385.

Lovett Doust, J.W. & Christie, E.H. (1978) The pathology of love: Some clinical variants of de Clérambault's syndrome. *Social Science and Medicine* **12**, 99–106.

Low, P.W., Jeffries, J.C. & Bonnie, R.J. (eds) (1986) *The Trial of John W. Hinckley, Jr: A Case Study in the Insanity Defence*. Foundation Press, Mineola, N.Y.

Macpherson, J. (ed.) (1889) *An Introduction to the Study of Insanity*. Macmillan, London.

Maher, B.A. (1988) Anomalous experience and delusional thinking: The logic of explanation. In: *Delusional Beliefs* (eds T.F. Oltmanns & B.A. Maher), pp. 15–33. Wiley, New York.

McKenna, P.J. (1984) Disorders with overvalued ideas. *British Journal of Psychiatry* **143**, 579–585.

Meloy, R.J. (1989) Unrequited love and the wish to kill. *Bulletin of the Menninger Clinic* **53**, 477–492.

Meloy, J.R. (in press) A clinical investigation of the obsessional follower. In: *Explorations in Criminal Psychopathology* (ed. L. Schlesinger). C.C. Thomas, Springfield, Ill.

Meloy, J.R. & Gothard, S. (1995) Demographic and clinical comparison of obsessional followers and offenders with mental disorders. *American Journal of Psychiatry* **152**, pp. 258–263.

Menzies, R.P.D., Fedoroff, J.P., Green, C.M. & Isaacson, K. (1995) Prediction of dangerous behaviour in male erotomanics. *British Journal of Psychiatry* **166**, 529–536.

Mooney, H.B. (1965) Pathologic jealousy and psychochemotherapy. *British Journal of Psychiatry* **111**, 1023–1042.

Mullen, P.E. (1986) The mental state and states of mind. In: *Essentials of Postgraduate Psychiatry*, pp. 3–36. Academic Press, London.

Mullen, P.E. (1990) Morbid jealousy and the delusion of infidelity. In: *Principles and Practice of Forensic Psychiatry* (eds R. Bluglass & P. Bowden), pp. 823–834. Churchill Livingstone, London.

Mullen, P.E. (1991) Jealousy: The pathology of passion. *British Journal of Psychiatry* **158**, 593–601.

Mullen, P.E. (1993) The crime of passion and the changing cultural construction of jealousy. *Criminal Behaviour and Mental Health* **3**, 1–11.

Mullen, P.E. (1995) The clinical management of jealousy. *Directions in Psychiatry* **15**, 1–8.

Mullen, P.E. & Pathé, M. (1994a) The pathological extensions of love. *British Journal of Psychiatry* **165**, 614–623.

Mullen, P.E. & Pathé, M. (1994b) Stalking and the pathologies of love. *Australian and New Zealand Journal of Psychiatry* **28**, 469–477.

Mullen, P.E., Taylor, P.J. & Wessely, S. (1993) Psychosis, violence and crime. In: *Forensic Psychiatry: Clinical, Legal and Ethical Issues* (eds J. Gunn & P. Taylor). Butterworth Heinemann, Oxford.

Munro, A. (1984) Excellent response of pathological jealousy to pimozide. *Canadian Medical Association Journal* **131**, 852–853.

Munro, A. (1988a) Delusional (paranoid) disorders: Etiologic and taxonomic considerations. I. The possible significance of organic brain factors in etiology of delusional disorders. *Canadian Journal of Psychiatry* **33**, 171–174.

Munro, A. (1988b) Delusional (paranoid) disorders: Etiologic and taxonomic considerations. II. A possible relationship between delusional and affective disorders. *Canadian Journal of Psychiatry* **33**, 175–178.

Munro, A., Obrien, J.V. & Ross, D. (1985) Two cases of 'pure' or 'primary' erotomania successfully treated with pimozide. *Canadian Journal of Psychiatry* **30**, 619–621.

Pines, A.M. (ed.) (1992) *Romantic Jealousy: Understanding and Conquering the Shadow of Love*. St Martin's Press, New York.

Raskin, D.E. & Sullivan, K.E. (1974) Erotomania. *American Journal of Psychiatry* **131**, 1033–1035.

Ray, I. (ed.) (1839) *Medical Jurisprudence of Insanity*. Charles C. Little & J. Brown, Boston.

Retterstøl, N. (1967) Jealousy: Paranoic psychosis. *Acta Psychiatrica Scandinavica* **34**, 75–107.

Retterstøl, N. & Opjordsmoen, S. (1991) Erotic self reference psychosis in old maids: A long term follow up. *Psychopathology* **24**, 388–397.

Rowlands, M.W.D. (1988) Psychiatric and legal aspects of persistent litigation. *British Journal of Psychiatry* **153**, 317–323.

Rudden, M., Sweeney, J. & Frances, A. (1983) A comparison of delusional disorders in women and men. *American Journal of Psychiatry* **140**, 1575–1578.

Rudden, M., Sweeney, J. & Frances, A. (1990) Diagnosis and clinical course of erotomanic and other delusional patients. *American Journal of Psychiatry* **147**, 625–628.

Scheler, M. (1954) *The Nature of Sympathy* (trans. P. Heath). Routledge & Kegan Paul, London.

Seeman, M.V. (1978) Delusional loving. *Archives of General Psychiatry* **35**, 1265–1267.

Segal, J. (1989) Erotomania revisited: From Kraepelin to DSMIII-R. *American Journal of Psychiatry* **146**, 1261–1266.

Shepherd, M. (1961) Morbid jealousy: Some clinical and social aspects of a psychiatric symptom. *Journal of Mental Science* **107**, 607–753.

Signer, S.F. (1991) De Clerambault's concept of erotomania and its place in his thought. *History of Psychiatry* **2**, 409–417.

Signer, S.F. & Cummings, J.L. (1987) De Clérambault's syndrome in organic affective disorder. *British Journal of Psychiatry* 151, 404–407.

Singer, I. (ed.) (1966) *The Nature of Love*, Vol. 1. *Plato to Luther*. Random House, New York.

Solomon, R.C. (ed.) (1976) *The Passions*. Anchor Press, New York.

Solomon, R.C. (1980) Emotions and choice. In: *Explaining Emotions* (ed. A.O. Rorty). University of California Press, Berkeley, Calif.

Soyka, M., Naber, G. & Völcher, A. (1991) Prevalence of delusional jealousy in different psychiatric disorders. *British Journal of Psychiatry* 158, 549–553.

Stalstrom, O.H. (1980) Querulous paranoia: Diagnosis and dissent. *Australian and New Zealand Journal of Psychiatry* 14, 145–150.

Stearns, P.N. (ed.) (1989) *Jealousy: The Evolution of an Emotion in American History*. New York University Press, New York.

Stein, D.J., Hollander, E. & Josephson, S.C. (1994) Serotonin Reuptake Blockers for the treatment of obsessive jealousy. *Journal of Clinical Psychiatry* 55, 30–33.

Stein, M.B. (1986) Two cases of 'pure' or 'primary' erotomania successfully treated with pimozide. *Canadian Journal of Psychiatry* 31, 289–290.

Stone, A.A. (ed.) (1984) *Law, Psychiatry and Morality*. American Psychiatric Press, Washington, D.C.

Tarrier, N., Beckett, R., Harwood, S. & Ahmed, Y. (1989) Comparison of a morbidly jealous and a normal female population on the Eysenck Personality Questionnaire (EPQ). *Personality and Individual Difference* 10, 1327–1328.

Taylor, P., Mahendra, B. & Gunn, J. (1983) Erotomania in males. *Psychological Medicine* 13, 645–650.

Ungvari, G.S. & Hollokoi, R.I.M. (1993) Successful treatment of litigious paranoia with pimozide. *Canadian Journal of Psychiatry* 38, 4–8.

Vaukhonen, K. (1968) On the pathogenesis of morbid jealousy. *Acta Psychiatrica Scandinavica* 202 (Suppl. 202).

White, G.L. (1991) Self, relationship, friends and family: Some applications of systems theory to romantic jealousy. In: *The Psychology of Jealousy and Envy* (ed. P. Salovey). Guilford Press, New York.

White, G.L. & Mullen, P.E. (eds) (1989) *Jealousy: Theory Research and Clinical Strategies*. Guilford Press, New York.

World Health Organization (1992) *The ICD-10 Classification of Mental and Behavioural Disorders. Clinical Descriptions and Diagnostic Guidelines*. World Health Organization, Geneva.

Zona, M.A., Kaushal, K.S. & Lane, J. (1993) A comparative study of erotomania and obsessional subjects in a forensic sample. *Journal of Forensic Sciences* 38, 894–903.

CHAPTER 8

Folie à Deux

THOMAS A. HUGHES AND
ANDREW C.P. SIMS

Introduction

It is of the essence of a delusion that it is an individual or idiosyncratic idea,
notion or belief; it is not shared by other people even from that person's cultural or religious group; and it is not amenable to reason. It is therefore
highly exceptional and hence noteworthy when two or more people share
the same delusion. *Folie à deux* implies insanity, expressed as shared delusional notions, affecting two or more people in close association with each
other. Synonyms are therefore 'shared insanity', 'communicated insanity',
'contagious insanity', 'infectious insanity', 'psychosis of association',
'induced psychosis' and 'multiple insanity' (Enoch & Trethowan 1991). In
some of those involved, *folie à deux* may be the only psychiatric disorder
present. In others the syndrome may be present with a number of other psychiatric disorders.

The syndrome is frequently seen as arising first in one patient and
being acquired by a second patient. There are many terms to distinguish
those first and second involved: 'primary agent and passive agent', 'inductor
and inductee', 'primary and secondary case', 'inducer and acceptor',
'inducer and recipient', 'principal and associate'. There is confusion
in the literature over the meaning of these terms. The former should
refer to the person who first develops the delusional belief, who may or
may not be the dominant partner in the relationship. 'Primary patient
and secondary patient' have been proposed as the simplest and clearest
(Munro 1986) when discussing the subtype *folie imposée* (see later). In
relation to the other subtypes, the distinction is less relevant (also see
Chapter 3).

The syndrome has been reported frequently to involve children, but in
this account the involvement of children is not dwelt upon at length. There

are particular difficulties in differentiating the important but distinct response of normal children to the beliefs of a psychotic parent from the particular phenomenon of *folie à deux*.

History

The condition may have been noted first by William Harvey in 1651 when he described a case of pseudocyesis:

> A noble lady who had borne more than ten children, and in whom the catamenia never disappeared except as the result of impregnation. Afterwards, however, being married to a second husband, she considered herself pregnant, forming her judgement not only from the symptoms on which she usually relied, but also from the movements of the child, which were frequently felt both by herself and her sister, who occupied the same bed with her. No arguments of mine could divest her of this belief. The symptoms depended on flatulence and fat.' (Hunter & MacAlpine 1963)

A clearer description was given by Sir Kenelm Digby in 1658:

> A very melancholy woman . . . while she continued in that mood, she thought herself possessed, and did strange things . . . and all this happened, because of the deep resentment she had for the death of her Husband: She had attending her four or five young Gentlewomen, whereof some were her Kinswomen, and others served her as Chambermaids. All these came to be possessed as she was, and did prodigious actions. These young Maids were separated from her . . . they came to be all cured by their absence; and this Lady was also cured afterwards by a Physician.' (Hunter & MacAlpine 1963)

The French term *'folie à deux'*, which means 'insanity of two', was first used by Lasègue and Falret in a preliminary communication to the Societé Médico-Psychologique in 1873 (Enoch & Trethowan 1991), and in a subsequent paper (Lasègue & Falret 1877). It had been alluded to by others such as Berlyn; Ideler, who spoke of the 'infectiousness of insanity'; Hoffbauer, who wrote 'about psychic infection'; and Wollenberg, who described instances of familial mental 'infection' (Gralnick 1942). Baillarger used the term *'folie communiquée'* in 1860 to describe two members of the same family admitted to hospital on the same day suffering from similar delusions (Enoch & Trethowan 1991). The condition was subsequently divided into four subgroups. Lasègue and Falret delineated only the group later termed '*folie imposée*'; *folie simultanée* was first described by Regis in 1880; *folie communiquée* by Marandon de Montyel in 1881; and *folie induite* by Lehmann in 1885 (Gralnick 1942).

Gralnick (1942) claimed to have reviewed all the cases reported in the English language literature from 1879 until 1942, a total of 103. Other reviews in the English language since this time are those of Rioux (1963); McNiel *et al.* (1972), which was concerned with subjects aged 65 and over; Soni and Rockley (1974); and Mentjox *et al.* (1993), who reviewed the case reports between 1974 and 1991, reporting on 76 case descriptions, with a total of 107 recipients.

Diagnostic criteria

Gralnick (1942) referred to *folie à deux* as 'the psychosis of association' and defined it as 'the transference of delusional ideas and/or abnormal behaviour from one person to one or more others who have been in close association with the primary affected patient'. One would, however, take exception to 'abnormal behaviour being transferred from one person to another', as it broadens the concept to such an extent that it is no longer useful. Fortunately, jumping off a bridge to one's doom is an uncommon experience; it would not be appropriate to describe every occasion where such behaviour is reported in the newspaper and imitated by another person as *folie à deux*. The transference of abnormal behaviour should only be taken to imply *folie à deux* when the associate is acting on shared abnormal beliefs, or is clearly behaving in such a way as to indicate acceptance of abnormal beliefs without these being formally elicited.

Dewhurst and Todd (1956) list the following as prerequisite for the diagnosis: definite evidence that the partners have been intimately associated; a high degree of similarity in the content of the delusions of those involved, though the nature of the psychosis may differ; and unequivocal evidence that the partners share, support and accept each other's delusions. Others have also observed that in some cases the content of the delusions may not be identical in those involved, because of the elaboration of the delusions by the associate.

Classification of clinical subtypes

Several attempts have been made to classify subtypes of *folie à deux*. The most often cited is that of Gralnick (1942).

1 *Folie imposée* (imposed psychosis), in which the delusions of a psychotic person are transferred to a non-psychotic ('mentally sound') one. Those involved must be intimately associated and free from outside influences. The recipient, who is 'intellectually and morally weaker', offers little resistance to the delusional ideas and does not elaborate them himself. The condition of the recipient 'tends' to resolve very soon after separation.

2 *Folie simultanée* (simultaneous psychosis), in which identical psychoses characterized by depression and persecutory ideas appear simultaneously in two people, both of whom have a predisposition to psychosis. A long and intimate association is necessary, and the two are of similar intellect. The psychosis usually appears directly after an 'accidental' (non-specific precipitating) cause, usually of a depressive nature.

3 *Folie communiquée* (communicated psychosis), in which delusions are transmitted only after a long period of resistance. It is not essential that those involved should present the same psychosis. After acceptance of the delusions, they are maintained by the associate even after separation and continue to develop independently of the principal.

4 *Folie induite* (induced psychosis), in which new delusions are added to those of a (psychotic) patient, under the influence of another (psychotic) patient.

Gralnick (1942) reviewed the literature and reported on the relative frequency of these subtypes when this could be decided: *folie imposée*, 64%; *folie simultanée*, 6%; *folie communiquée*, 25%; and *folie induite*, 5%. However, Mentjox *et al.* (1993) found 21% of cases probably suffered *folie induite*. The difference in reported relative frequency may reflect changes in diagnostic practice or publication bias rather than a real change in incidence. Sims *et al.* (1977) have described a single case where these four phenomena are all present.

Criticisms of clinical subtypes

That Gralnick could identify the various subtypes from the literature could be interpreted as support for the validity of his system of classification. However, even he doubted the existence of *folie simultanée*. Also, though the subtypes were identified in over 90% of cases, the subtype was often offered by Gralnick rather than those who reported the case and Gralnick conceded such assumptions were not neccessarily correct.

Dewhurst and Todd (1956) criticized the theoretical validity and usefulness of this classification. They view the stability of the delusion in the secondary case as an artefact associated with duration of the psychosis; as the duration of the psychosis increases, so does the stability of the delusions, and a diagnosis of *folie imposée* becomes one of *folie communiquée*. In an extension of this view, Sacks (1988) regards *folie imposée* and *folie communiquée* as opposite ends of a continuum (see later). Dewhurst and Todd (1956) view *folie induite* as redundant, merely complicating the classification system, and consider that such cases are better classified under the other subtypes because the same mechanisms are involved whether the secondary subject is psychotic or not.

If the subject who first developed the delusion cannot be identified, subtyping becomes less useful, and *folie simultanée* or *folie induite* may be decided by default. Soni and Rockley (1974) consider that there have only been a few cases reported where it has not been possible to distinguish the principal from the associate. Dewhurst and Todd (1956) take a different view and share Gralnick's scepticism about the existence of *folie simultanée*, as it is likely that one partner develops the delusion first, however short the time interval between the onset in the partners. The diagnosis is only reached because a clear history of the onset of the beliefs was not obtained. Most other writers, including Gralnick (1942) and Mentjox *et al.* (1993) agree it is often difficult to tell who has influenced whom, and emphasize the reciprocal nature of this process. *Folie simultanée* has been reported to be more frequent in the elderly, occurring in almost half of published cases reviewed by McNiel *et al.* (1972). It is suggested that in the elderly the syndrome is associated with particularly marked interdependent relationships. Therefore, there may be special difficulties in determining the primary case in this group, and the over-representation of this subtype may partly be explained by the difficulties in obtaining an adequate history of the evolution of the syndrome.

Mentjox *et al.* (1993) argue that in many cases the type can only be specified *post hoc*. This applies particularly to *folie imposée* and *folie communiquée* because in the acute situation the effect of separation is not yet known. Munro (1986) regards only the division into *folie imposée* and *folie simultanée* as useful, because the management of each is quite different, *folie communiquée* and *folie induite* being variations of *folie simultanée*.

Although it is reasonable clinical practice to designate the situation where a delusional notion is shared by two or more closely associated people 'folie à deux', another psychiatric disorder will be present in at least one of those involved. The distinction into subtypes is only useful inasmuch as it comments upon the diagnosis of the associate, whether or not that person suffers from a psychiatric illness, and hence the need for treatment. Psychopathology should be the servant and not the master of clinical needs for diagnosis and management.

Classification in ICD-10 and DSM-IV

The classification of *folie à deux* is shown in Table 8.1.

In the *International Classification of Diseases* (ICD-10; World Health Organization (WHO) 1992), *folie à deux* is classified under 'Schizophrenia, schizotypal and delusional disorders' as 'Induced delusional disorder', although it is recognized that the illness in the dominant person is not invariably schizophrenia. The similarity between the diagnostic guidelines in ICD-10 and the criteria proposed by Dewhurst and Todd (1956) are apparent. The system includes a description of the main clinical features and allows a degree of flexibility in clinical diagnosis; diagnostic guidelines rather than strict criteria are given, so that a diagnosis can be reached with varying degrees of confidence. Though the guidelines use the term 'delusion' in relation to the associate, this is qualified by adding that only one person suffers from a genuine psychotic disorder.

Table 8.1 Diagnostic criteria in ICD-10 and DSM-IV.

ICD-10: Induced delusional disorder (F.24)
A   Two or more people share the same delusion or delusional system and support one another in this belief
B   They have an unusually close relationship
C   There is temporal or other contextual evidence that the delusion was induced in the passive member(s) of the pair or group by contact with the active member

DSM-IV: Shared psychotic disorder (297.3)
A   A delusion develops in an individual in the context of a close relationship with another person(s), who has an already-established delusion
B   The delusion is similar in content to that of the person who already has the established delusion
C   The disturbance is not better accounted for by another psychotic disorder (e.g. schizophrenia) or a mood disorder with psychotic features and is not due to the direct physiological effects of a substance (e.g. a drug of abuse, a medication) or a general medical condition

ICD-10, *The International Classification of Diseases* (World Health Organization 1992); DSM-IV, *Diagnostic and Statistical Manual of Mental Disorders* (American Psychiatric Association 1994).

There are a number of shortcomings particular to this system. First, the clarity of the description of the syndrome is not helped by the use of the term 'dominant' to describe the primary patient, nor in the statement that the secondary patient is usually subservient. This serves only to cloud the separate considerations of who first develops the abnormal belief, and who is dominant in the relationship. Secondly, it is inaccurate to state that only one person suffers from a genuine psychotic disorder; in *folie communiquée* more than one may do so. Thirdly, the absence of a clear primary partner in many cases may mean the third diagnostic guideline is difficult to apply in a clinical situation.

In the *Diagnostic and Statistical Manual of Mental Disorders* (DSM-IV; American Psychiatric Association (APA) 1994), *folie à deux* is classified under 'Schizophrenia and Other Psychotic Disorders', as 'Shared Psychotic Disorder'. It is recognized that the primary case may not necessarily suffer schizophrenia, though this is usual, but may be suffering from illnesses such as delusional disorder or an affective disorder. The manual states that for the purposes of this disorder, the term 'psychotic' is equivalent to 'delusional', abandoning the previously over-restrictive specification that the delusions must be persecutory in content (APA 1987).

A problem particular to this classification is that the diagnostic criteria specify that a delusion develops in the associate, though in many cases encountered by clinicians, the beliefs of the associate are not held with full delusional intensity, and would be better described as an overvalued idea, a delusion-like idea or a misinterpretation (Sims 1995). If the criteria are applied rigorously, many such cases will be difficult to classify.

Folie simultanée is specifically excluded in ICD-10, and appears to be excluded in DSM-IV by Criterion A, which may be appropriate in those situations where two patients have independent psychoses, even if some of their delusions are shared (Munro 1987). This should not simply mean that cases where it cannot be decided that either patient is the primary are considered to be *folie simultánee* and classified elsewhere.

Both systems share a number of problems. Both ICD-10 and DSM-IV state that the delusions in the secondary patient usually disappear if the relationship with the primary patient is interrupted. This is questionable, as will be seen later. DSM-IV goes further, stating that if the delusions in the secondary patient do not disappear, then another diagnosis is probably appropriate. Finally, hallucinations are said to be unusual in the secondary patient in ICD-10, and this is also implied in DSM-IV. This is questionable, particularly in cases other than *folie imposée*, as will be shown later. Thus, both ICD-10 and DSM-IV specify a narrow group with a good prognosis, and in which the associate is likely to recover after separation without additional treatment. This may have limited relevance to clinical practice.

In both systems, the clinician is permitted to record more than one diagnosis, so that both *folie à deux* and any underlying or associated condition may be recorded. This should be done so that examination of close associates is not overlooked in future presentations.

Associated conditions

Folie à deux has been reported in association with Capgras (Christodoulou *et al.* 1995) and Frégoli syndromes (Wolff & McKenzie 1994), both of which are forms of delusional misidentification; Cotard's syndrome with nihilistic and hypochondriacal delusions (Wolff & McKenzie 1994); and other delusional syndromes such as *koro* (Westermeyer 1989) and de Clérambault's syndrome (Signer & Isbister 1987). Clearly, where one type of delusion is present, the emergence of another delusion becomes more likely and also the delusion that is shared may be a delusion for which there is a specific designation—such as delusional misidentification.

Distinction from other conditions

Usually it is not difficult for the clinician to separate *folie à deux* from the abnormal ideas seen in mass hysteria or in certain religious cults; however, the difference cannot be readily defined. Dewhurst and Todd (1956) report as an example of *folie à deux* the case of Sir William Cortenay who believed he was the 'Son of God' and led a group of 'yokels' in a series of riots in 19th-century England. More recently, Myers (1988) interviewed a dozen members and ex-members of an American sect, the 'League of Geniuses', and reviewed documents, speeches and other communications. He viewed the beliefs of the sect members as delusional, and suggested that the conditions of sect life generated and maintained a 'subculture-bound syndrome.' According to Myers, many (though presumably not all) sect members' delusional beliefs resolved once they were 'unbound' from the sect. The mass suicide in 1978 of 912 members of the People's Temple Cult, including Jim Jones, their leader, and 260 children, has been likened to *folie à deux* (Salih 1981), but the lack of evidence from contemporaneous clinical assessments leaves room for uncertainty. Rosen (1981), basing his view on transcripts of contemporaneous tape recordings, considers it unlikely that the cult members were deluded. The essential element which is usually lacking in these cases is the undisputed evidence of delusion rather than an alternative such as overvalued idea.

Substance abuse involving cannabis (Dalby & Duncan 1987) and methylphenidate (Spensley 1972) has been reported to precede the onset of *folie à deux*. While reports of such cases share many of the characteristics of the syndrome, they are excluded from the DSM-IV classification except, it would appear, in circumstances where the delusion of one subject, whose psychosis is the result of substance abuse, is shared by another, whose psychosis is not the result of substance abuse. This occurred in one of the cases reported by Spensley (1972). In ICD-10, more than one diagnosis may be appropriate.

Reports of psychosis occurring in twins reared apart (Craike & Slater 1945) cannot be considered as *folie à deux* unless the subjects are in close association. Psychoses occurring in families reported as *folie à deux* without evidence that the subjects share, accept and support the delusions of the other (Kallmann & Mickey 1946) are spurious.

Clinical epidemiology

Accurate figures for the incidence and prevalence of *folie à deux* are not available. A frequency of 29 individuals in 1700 consecutive admissions (1.7%) to an American state hospital has been reported (Spradley, in Grover 1937), but no detail is available on the methodology underlying this figure. The condition is not confined to Western societies and has been reported in countries including Nigeria and India (Ilechukwu & Okyere 1987; Pande & Gulabani 1990). The incidence in the population aged over 65 years appears to be the same as in the population as a whole (McNiel *et al.* 1972). *Folie à deux* may be more common than previously reported, and may go unrecognized because such patients rarely seek treatment, or because of the neglect of assessment of the families of patients who are recognized as psychotic (Sacks 1988).

Certain conditions may be more frequently associated with *folie à deux* than would be expected. Munro (1986) found nine cases in 50 patients suffering from monosymptomatic hypochondriacal psychosis (MHP). In delusional parasitosis, a subtype of MHP, a quarter may be involved in *folie à deux* (Macaskill 1987). The increased frequency in the latter may partly reflect the common observation that the symptom of itching is easily transmissible by suggestion.

The disorder may involve two, three (Fernando & Frieze 1985), four (Sims *et al.* 1977), five (Kamal 1965), six (Dippel *et al.* 1991), and even up to 12 people (Waltzer 1963). As might be expected, the condition becomes less common as the number of those involved increases. Glassman *et al.* (1987) found only 20 cases in the literature where whole families were involved.

Folie à deux is an uncommon condition or situation. Like most rare conditions, it is found to be not quite so uncommon when looked for assiduously. It is somewhat more common in isolated communities or alienated families. At this time no precise frequency can be given.

Relationship between subjects

Gralnick (1942) reported on 103 cases with a total of 238 subjects involved. The following relationships were found: two (or more) sisters, 34%; husband and wife, 22%; mother and child, 20%; two (or more) brothers, 9%; brother(s) and sister(s), 5%; father and child, 2%; fellow patients or friends, 8%. A number of cases involving twins has been reported (Gralnick 1942; Kendler *et al.* 1986; Lazarus 1986).

Mentjox *et al.* (1993) reported on 76 cases with 107 associates. The commonest relationship between principal and associate was mother–child(ren) with a frequency of 21%, followed by wife–husband, 19%; woman–sibling, 17%; husband–wife, 13%. Alternatively, the frequency of the relationships in the latter review could be considered as 'marital partners', followed by 'mother and child.' Reasons for the disagreement in reported frequencies in marital partners and sisters may include changes in domestic living arrangements and in social roles.

Sex distribution

Women are over-represented (Lasègue & Falret 1877; Gralnick 1942), constituting 72% of principals and 54% of associates in those cases where sex was reported (Mentjox *et al.* 1993). Reasons suggested to account for this include the restricted social roles of women leading to dependence in their relationships (Gralnick 1942), and the frequent caring role of women within relationships (Mentjox *et al.* 1993). Neither suggestion adequately explains the over-representation of women among principals. Another suggestion is a that women are more likely to seek hospital treatment (Sacks 1988).

Behavioural correlates

Theft, murder and suicide pacts have been reported in association with *folie à deux* (Greenberg 1956; Salih 1981) but are uncommon. Not all suicide pacts are associated with *folie à deux*. Nevertheless, at least one person in each pact is usually suffering from mental illness, most commonly depression. This, together with the mutually dependent nature of the relationship between those involved in such a pact, in a setting of social isolation (Rosen 1981; Brown *et al.* 1995), suggests *folie à deux* may occur in some pacts, but reliable evidence is difficult to obtain.

Diagnosis in the partners

The difficulties in the interpretation of the findings of the two most recent reviews of reported cases include the lack of standardized diagnostic criteria in the original reports. Soni and Rockley (1974) traced 163 cases reported in the English literature. In 109 cases, they considered there was adequate information to make a diagnosis. The diagnosis in the primary partner was usually of a functional psychosis; schizophrenia in 60%, paraphrenia in 28%, affective psychosis in 8%. Organic disorders were much less common; 'senile arteriopathic psychosis' was diagnosed in 4%. More than half of the secondary partners had schizophrenia or paraphrenia; very few had an affective psychosis. A significant number of the secondary partners had personality disorder, dementia, mental retardation, physical disability such as deafness or stroke, or a problem with language, either in addition to or without suffering a psychotic illness.

Mentjox *et al.* (1993) report findings broadly in agreement with these. Of principals, 58% suffer from schizophrenia or paranoid psychosis. Induced psychotic disorder was the only diagnosis in 60% of associates. Twenty-one per cent of associates were probably suffering from a psychotic illness before the onset of shared delusions, thus implying that the form of *folie à deux* was *folie induite*. In 20% of recipients, a non-psychotic psychiatric condition was diagnosed in addition to *folie à deux*; these included personality disorder, anxiety disorder, physical or mental handicap.

Phenomenology/psychopathology

Munro (1986) considers that those who are the recipients of an imposed notion (*folie imposée*) are highly impressionable rather than deluded. Lasègue and Falret (1877) said the same of the recipients in the condition they described, which was *folie imposée*. In *folie communiquée*, the secondary subject develops a true delusional disease in which the delusional content of a latent psychotic condition is shaped by the illness of the primary case. In *folie simultanée* and *folie induite*, those involved are also truly deluded. Greenberg (1956) and Sacks (1988) regard the associate in imposed and communicated psychosis as representing extremes of a continuum, from being highly impressionable to having a true delusional disorder. However, the experience of delusion is an all-or-none phenomenon; it does not readily lend itself to being viewed on a continuum. Having said this, it is not always easy to judge whether a belief is delusional or is understandable in the light of the subject's experience and therefore an overvalued idea. This does not mean that delusion and overvalued idea are continuous rather than categorical, merely that the psychiatrist has difficulty making the distinction. It can be difficult for a jury to decide on the guilt or innocence of a defendant, though whether a crime has been committed or not is clearly categorical in nature.

Greenberg (1956) raises the question as to whether an associate whose behaviour is so abnormal as to amount to murder can be regarded as psychotic on the grounds that to act on abnormal beliefs implies that the beliefs are of delusional intensity. This assumption is inaccurate and echoes the popular view that people who commit serious crimes must be 'sick'. Abnormal behaviour as well as abnormal ideas may be shared in the syndrome, regardless of the presence of psychosis in the associate. In the case reported by Greenberg (1956), no psychotic explanation was offered by the associate for his action, suggesting he was not truly psychotic and should receive a diagnosis of *folie imposée* and even casting doubt on the presence of *folie à deux*. This illustrates the importance of a thorough history and examination of the mental state in such cases.

THE CONTENT OF THE DELUSIONS

Gralnick (1942) reported on what he termed 'the principal type of delusion', although other delusions were present in the cases he reported. In nearly three quarters of instances, the delusional content was persecutory, the remainder being religious, grandiose, depressive, and of infidelity. The elderly do not appear to differ in this respect (McNiel *et al.* 1972). Mentjox *et al.* (1993) reported 'paranoid' delusions occurred in almost three quarters of inductors. Unfortunately, it is unclear whether 'paranoid' here refers incorrectly to persecutory delusions, or whether it is used in the correct sense, self-referent (Sims 1995). In addition, transmission of delusions of infestation, of body image and of hypochondriasis have been described (Munro 1986).

HALLUCINATIONS

Gralnick (1942) reported the presence of hallucinations, where this could be decided, in all subjects involved in 38% of cases; absent in all subjects in 48%; present only in the inducer in 12%; present only in the recipient in 1%. In the elderly, all subjects were known to experience hallucinations in almost a quarter of all cases (McNiel *et al.* 1972). These were usually auditory, but visual and tactile hallucinations also occurred. In both reviews, the presence or absence of hallucinations was uncertain in a substantial number of cases.

It is uncertain from the literature whether these phenomena represent true hallucinations in all instances. It would be logical to assume that in cases of *folie imposée* they are more likely to be experienced by the associate as not being concrete or real, or are experienced within the mind. Therefore, it may be better to regard them as pseudohallucinations.

Aetiology

The following aetiological factors relate specifically to the development of *folie à deux*. In addition there will be aetiological factors related to the underlying psychiatric disorder of the principal in *folie imposée*, and of all subjects involved in the other subtypes of the syndrome.

PREDISPOSING FACTORS

Gralnick (1942) wrote that those involved in *folie à deux* have a constitutional predisposition. Because few people in close association with deluded people acquire their delusions, it might reasonably be supposed that there must be some abnormalities of the associate which predispose to the acquisition of the principal's delusions. This argument, then, seems to be after the event.

Mental and physical illness

The range of psychiatric disorders, mental handicap and physical diagnoses in associates in the studies by Soni and Rockley (1974) and Mentjox *et al.* (1993) may contribute to the development of the syndrome. In the review by Mentjox *et al.* (1993), a large number of recipients were suffering from a psychotic illness before the onset of shared delusions and were presumed to be suffering *folie induite*. No systematic information is available as to whether the subjects may be predisposed by the experience of previous episodes of psychotic illness. Mentjox *et al.* (1993) report that an unspecified number of recipients were suffering from an anxiety disorder in addition to *folie à deux*. It seems likely that at least some patients will have experienced a neurotic disorder in the past. Whether this occurs with greater frequency than in the general population is unknown.

Physical handicap, partial deafness and language barriers may lead both to increased dependency on, and to an ambivalent attitude toward, the partner, together with increased social isolation. There is some evidence that hearing impairment may increase vulnerability to paranoid psychosis in general (Kendell 1993).

Dementia

McNiel *et al.* (1972) reported that dementia appears to have little or no aetiological role in reported cases in the elderly. Despite the reports of dementia in the cases they reviewed, they considered symptoms of poor memory and disorientation to be absent or mild. Soni and Rockley (1974) found a very small number of principals suffered senile arteriopathic psychosis and a slightly larger number of associates suffered dementia, including a small number of cases of presenile dementia. However, the degree of severity of dementia and any possible role in aetiology was not reported. Subsequent case reports suggest that dementia in one (Brooks 1987) or both (Fishbain 1987; Draper & Cole 1990) partners may be important.

Genetic contribution

Over 90% of cases of *folie à deux* occur within families (Gralnick 1942). In almost two thirds of cases, those involved are first degree relatives (Mentjox *et al.* 1993), and a small number involve identical twins (Lazarus 1986). These figures do not help to distinguish between the effects of heredity and the family environment. Scharfetter (1970) studied 215 reports of 'symbiontic' (sic), or induced psychoses, in 75 inducers and 140 induced. Using diagnoses based on the definitions of Eugen and Manfred Bleuler, he found an increased risk of schizophrenia in the families of the induced subjects compared with the general population. This was the case even when the induced and inducer were not genetically related. This suggests an increased genetic vulnerability to psychosis in the associate.

Social isolation

Social isolation was regarded as a necessary cause by Lasègue and Falret (1877). However, later writers, while in agreement that it is frequent in those who develop *folie à deux* (Glassman *et al.* 1987), consider that it is not universal (Soni & Rockley 1974). The role of social isolation has been the subject of speculation. In sensory deprivation, a state of intense longing for external stimuli has been described, together with increased suggestibility. In some cases, psychotic symptoms are said to occur. It has been suggested that social isolation in *folie à deux* may give rise to psychotic symptoms in the same way (Waltzer 1963; Lozzi *et al.* 1992). This would seem a less convincing explanation of the effect of social isolation than that intimacy between partners coupled with a desire to live in seclusion favours the domination of the weaker partner by the stronger, because the weaker is cut off from influences which might counterbalance the effect of the stronger. This is supported by the observation that in many cases a 'leader–follower' relationship existed between the partners before one becomes psychotic (Dewhurst & Todd 1956).

Premorbid personality

Lasègue and Falret (1877) commented on the passive personality of the secondary partner. Suggestibility is often said to be important (Gralnick 1942) and personality disorder with marked dependent, hysterical or paranoid traits have been reported (Soni & Rockley 1974). Scharfetter (1970) described the premorbid personality of inducers as 'sthenic', dominant and of normal intelligence; the induced are asthenic, 'infantile' and less intelligent.

Nature of the relationship between subjects

A relationship where one partner is dominant and the other submissive is seen by most writers as conducive to the development of the syndrome (Dewhurst & Todd 1956; Layman & Cohen 1957; Rioux 1963; Lozzi *et al.* 1992). Seniority in age, superiority in intelligence, education and 'drive' or aggressiveness are factors which may favour one partner becoming dominant (Dewhurst & Todd 1956). Gralnick (1942) noted the view of most writers up until that time that the first person to develop delusional beliefs was usually the dominant figure in the relationship, but considered that evidence of dominance and submission was not present in many cases. This view is shared by later writers (Mentjox *et al.* 1993). The onset of symptoms in the associate usually takes place when the principal is in the initial stage of illness, before he has lost contact with reality and is still able to exert authority over the associate (Coleman & Last 1939). This may be seen as supporting the role of dominance and submission.

Those involved in *folie à deux* are always closely associated, usually for a long time, but sometimes the length of association is relatively short (Gralnick 1942). Occasionally, *folie à deux* may arise after brief contact between subjects who have been closely associated in the past (Layman & Cohen 1957). This intimate association means that those involved share the same feelings, interests, apprehensions and hopes (Lasègue & Falret 1877), and thus have very similar psychological needs. It has been suggested that delusional beliefs which are formed by one partner to meet morbid psychological needs may be accepted by the other partner because they meet his own pre-existing psychological needs (Layman & Cohen 1957).

However, Gralnick (1942) refers to Deutsch, who indicated that the association *per se* was less important, and is merely the product of abnormal attachment. Viewed in this way, it is this abnormal attachment which results in the acceptance of delusional beliefs by the associate.

The much greater frequency of sister–sister associations than brother–brother (Gralnick 1942) and the overall over-representation of women (Mentjox *et al.* 1993) makes an interesting comment on the differences between female and male relationships.

Low intelligence

Lasègue and Falret (1877) observed the secondary case to be of low intelligence, but this may represent too literal a translation of the French word *'intelligence'*, used by Lasègue and Falret in the sense of 'logical and ethical capacity' (Evans & Merskey 1972). Gralnick (1942) refers to Tuke, who considered the secondary partner was 'feeble minded', and described a case where one partner was mentally subnormal. However, Gralnick stressed that in most cases the recipient was of normal intellect. Soni and Rockley (1974) reviewed the literature and found 'mental subnormality' reported in the associate in only five out of 123 series (4%). Few reports of *folie à deux* with unequivocal evidence of mental retardation in either partner have appeared since (Meakin *et al.* 1987; Ghaziuddin 1991). The latter case draws attention to the difficulty in distinguishing the principal from the associate even when one suffers mental retardation.

It would appear that some authors have not made a clear distinction between lower intelligence (which is present only in a minority of cases) and weak-willed or submissive personality traits which occurs in many, perhaps most, associates.

Poverty

Coleman and Last (1939) regarded poverty as the most potent reason for causing dissatisfaction with reality, and considered that it facilitated the development of *folie à deux*. They regarded any belief which brings real or imagined relief from poverty as more readily accepted. In support of this view, they cite the greater readiness to accept such economic and religious doctrines as communism and Christianity by those in poverty. Despite the speciousness of this argument, the association with poverty continues to be reported (McNiel *et al.* 1972). The balance of evidence in relation to schizophrenia is that poverty is the result rather than the cause of illness (Gelder *et al.* 1989), and this is likely to be the case in *folie à deux*.

The content of the delusions

Delusions are more likely to be accepted if they are plausible, and play on the hopes and fears of the secondary subject (Lasègue & Falret 1877). This touches both on the idea referred to above that the partners have similar psychological needs, and also that impressionable subjects are more likely to accept morbid beliefs if the beliefs are within the bounds of possibility.

Family dynamics

Glassman *et al.* (1987) think there are six typical features of families who develop *folie à famille*: (i) social isolation; (ii) family relationships tend to be mutually dependent and ambivalent; (iii) the families are repeatedly in crisis; (iv) there is often an underlying threat or presence of violence; (v) the family membership is stable over a long period of time; and (vi) there is a dominant family member, the inducer, around whom the delusional beliefs evolve. The induced are often less intelligent, female, passive, dependent, suggestible, or histrionic.

PRECIPITATING CAUSES

Few writers have commented on the role of stressors in precipitating the syndrome. Many cases reports refer to clear stressors preceding the syndrome, as might be expected. In view of the close relationship between those involved such stressors are likely to have an impact on both partners. In the elderly, when stressors can be identified they are those commonly found at this time of life: feelings of inferiority and failure, material losses and loss of physical health (McNiel *et al.* 1972).

Explanatory models

PSYCHODYNAMIC EXPLANATIONS

The psychological defence mechanism of identification, where characteristics of another are unconsciously adopted by oneself, has been invoked in several related explanatory psychodynamic models. The partners are dependent on each other, and the principal resents the dependence of the associate. The principal projects his hostility towards the associate onto outsiders, as persecutory delusions. The associate initially refuses to accept the delusions, and is subjected to hostility by the principal. The associate feels anxious, and guilty about the demands he has placed on the principal in the past. By a process of identification with this 'aggressor', the associate accepts the delusion, and the hostility of the partners toward each other is projected onto outsiders as persecutory beliefs (Pulver & Brunt 1961).

Using object-relation theory, a disturbance in the 'individuation-separation' process is seen as predisposing to *folie à deux* in the associate (Mentjox *et al.* 1993). During this phase, the child learns to distinguish himself from others, and develops his own feelings, wishes and thoughts. 'Magical thinking' at this stage is said to have similarities with psychotic thought disorder. In this phase the child may adopt the parent's experience of reality, even if this is psychotic. That is, *folie à deux* in children may result from incomplete or insufficiently consolidated individuation-separation.

In response to stress, adults who experienced difficulty at the individuation-separation stage may succumb to regression. The extent of regression is determined by the personality and severity of the stressor. If the degree of regression is sufficient, the associate can 'identify' with the psychotic ideas of the principal. Thus, the associate 'identifies' with non-threatening aspects of the principal, and attributes the threatening aspects to others (Sacks 1988; Mentjox *et al.* 1993). This, once again, is the defence mechanism 'identification with the aggressor'.

In practice, although magical thinking and delusions can occur coincidentally in the same subject contemporaneously, they are phenomenologically distinct.

IMPOSITION VS. ADOPTION

Many writers see the development of the syndrome as the 'imposition' of a delusional idea by a stronger person into the mind of a weaker one (Dewhurst & Todd 1956; Soni & Rockley 1974). The observation that delusions could be shared after a brief period of close reassociation, by those who had been closely associated in the past, has led some to propose that the delusions are instead 'adopted'. When people live closely, they may do so because they have similar psychological needs, or their needs become similar. Delusions develop in one subject because they meet his morbid psychological needs (which is undoubted). They are accepted by the other, who is already psychotic, because they meet his own morbid psychological needs; they are 'tailor made' and therefore retained on separation (Layman & Cohen 1957). This is more tenuous.

Others see imposition as of little importance because of the absence of clear dominant and submissive roles in many cases, and the apparent reversal of previously held dominance and submission during the course of the syndrome in some cases. The mechanism is seen as adaptive. That is, it helps to preserve the close relationship of mutually dependent subjects. If one subject developed a delusion which the other did not accept, this would threaten the relationship. If the subjects assume dominant and submissive roles, this may further strengthen their relationship because it reduces the chance of disagreement (McNiel *et al.* 1972).

OTHER MECHANISMS

Dewhurst and Todd (1956) see suggestion operating in a mechanism similar to that which occurs in hypnosis, but, in addition, the primary partner's beliefs are reinforced by feedback from the secondary. The establishment of a degree of dominance over the subject (associate), the use of a constant single stimulus, a voice (a delusional idea), together with relative deprivation of other sensory stimuli (social isolation), allows the hypnotist (principal) to induce the subject (associate) to accept suggestion without critical appraisal. This is close to the idea later put forward that the mechanism is similar to that occurring in brainwashing (Waltzer 1963). It is suggested that each consists of three phases. In the first, sensory deprivation (social isolation) leads to a breakdown of psychological defences. In the second, identification with the aggressor takes place, and the victim (associate) is shown kindness. In the third, the victim (associate) is exposed to constant stimulation on a single theme (a delusion) until it is incorporated by the individual. Such explanations seem to be an oversimplification of more complex issues.

Management

ASSESSMENT

The clinician must first consider the possibility of *folie à deux*. A psychiatrist who regards a patient as deluded may doubt his own judgement if the beliefs are apparently confirmed by a relative or close friend, which can clearly have an adverse effect on management (Munro 1986). It is important to decide which of the patients have a true psychosis, as the management of such patients will almost always involve medication. Where there is doubt, Sacks (1988) recommends hospitalizing both patients together or hospitalizing one and permitting frequent contact. Observing the two together will often clarify the distinction between an imposed and a communicated psychosis, and between the primary and secondary partners. An imposed psychosis with an underlying personality disorder in the secondary partner is suggested by an automatic quality in the recitation of the shared beliefs, or an absence of firm conviction in the secondary partner. A mutually supportive and interactive elaboration and maintenance of the delusion will suggest a communicated psychosis and that the secondary partner has a primary autonomous disease such as schizophrenia, or bipolar affective disorder. If there is doubt, temporary separation may help clarify the issue.

Rioux (1963), on the other hand considers that there is an automatic quality to the expression of the abnormal beliefs by both partners. That this feature cannot be given much diagnostic weight seems likely; an automatic quality may be a function of the duration of the beliefs and the number of occasions on which they are enquired about. However, the absence of firm conviction in one partner indicates the absence of a true psychosis and a diagnosis of *folie imposée* in that partner.

SPECIFIC TREATMENT OF THE PRINCIPAL

The treatment is that of the underlying psychiatric disorder, and may include a neuroleptic agent, antidepressant drug, lithium therapy and/or electroconvulsive therapy. Admission to hospital is often indicated, if necessary using a compulsory order. Maintenance and preventative medication should be considered on discharge. In *folie simultanée* and *folie induite*, where there is no principal, treatment should be along these lines for all subjects involved.

Rarely, the disorder may appear to respond to supportive psychotherapy alone (Macaskill 1987), but it is more likely that, in true psychotic states, such instances represent spontaneous remission in cases with a good prognosis regardless of the treatment.

SPECIFIC TREATMENT OF THE ASSOCIATE

In *folie imposée*, recovery will often accompany recovery of the principal. Specific treatment may be needed where learning difficulty, dementia, or physical disability, including sensory deficits, are contributing to the dependence of the recipient on the inducer. In *folie communiquée*, the associate will require treatment of the underlying or associated psychiatric disorder.

While treatment may be theoretically straightforward, in practice it may be very difficult if the patients refuse to cooperate with treatment, with each colluding in the other's beliefs. Even in *folie imposée*, both patients may be irrational and require compulsory admission and treatment, though only one may be truly psychotic (Munro 1986).

SEPARATION

Lasègue and Falret (1877) proposed separating the primary partner from the secondary partner, but were aware that this was not invariably effective. Later writers (Layman & Cohen 1957; Lazarus 1986) report the result is often ineffective. Mentjox *et al.* (1993) reviewed the result of separation in 58 case reports; separation of associate children from the inductor led to resolution of symptoms in 85% of cases, but was only successful in 55% of cases of adult associates. This suggests the degree of dependence may be important in determining the effect of separation.

Separating elderly associates seems to be less successful (McNiel *et al.* 1972; Fishbain 1987), and may appear contraindicated—for example, where an elderly couple depend on each other in order to continue to live at home, and separation may lead to irreversible institutional care (Draper & Cole 1990).

Dewhurst and Todd (1956) see the stability of the delusions in the secondary subject as being influenced by the duration of the condition, the nature of the delusions (those which are of value to the secondary in psychological terms being given up less readily), and the suggestibility of the secondary subject. Highly suggestible people acquire false notions more easily in *folie à deux*, but also shed them more easily. These factors may have a bearing on the degree of success of separation.

Opinion is divided on whether separation is effective when the recipient was already suffering from a psychosis. Mentjox *et al.* (1993) found seven such cases, and in four, separation resulted in some reduction in intensity of delusional beliefs. Brooks (1987) reports that separation in these cases 'produces an unfavourable reaction'. Gralnick (1942) refers to a case where separation after a long period of association was followed by a deterioration in the condition of the recipient.

Whatever the implications for treatment, separation may be undesirable in some instances, for example in a mother–child dyad. In other instances, foster care may be considered until the response of the parent to treatment is known (Sacks 1988).

It should be borne in mind that little or no evidence has been offered to support these suggestions, which may be tried on empirical grounds.

TREATMENT OF THE RELATIONSHIP

Once the inductor and recipient have been treated, whether by pharmaco-therapy, other specific treatments, and/or separation, attention should be directed towards the relationship between the two. Interventions aimed at separation in psychological terms may be more important than those aimed at physical separation (Rioux 1963; Mentjox *et al.* 1993). The general aim is to increase the autonomy of both the inductor and recipient, by providing alternative supports, activities and interests. This, it is hoped, will reduce the pathological enmeshment of the partners (Sacks 1988). This may require the involvement of a social worker.

In some instances, psychotherapy aimed at insight into issues of aggression, dependence, and separation may be useful (Sacks 1988). Others suggest joint psychotherapy with a male and female therapist, directed at exploring issues of hostility and dependence (Bankier 1988), or facilitating direct expression of feelings, exploring poor parental relationships, and encouraging modelling on the relationship of the therapists (Potash & Brunell 1974). Unfortunately, such therapy may be very lengthy, and its effectiveness is uncertain.

In a communicated psychosis, Porter *et al.* (1993) consider deliberately shifting dependency may be beneficial—for instance, from a deluded dominant figure to a sane one—but that for most patients the aim should be independence. They cite various reports of separation where they suggest shifts of dependency may have been responsible for resolution of psychosis in the dependent partner. That their own case report was of a patient whose treatment included separation, a neuroleptic, individual and group psychotherapy indicates the difficulties of attributing recovery to a single agent in such cases.

Prognosis

It might be supposed that the prognosis for the principal, and for the associate suffering from an underlying mental illness, is probably somewhat worse than for others with that core illness. However, little is known of long-term treatment results. Mentjox *et al.* (1993) hypothesize that in recipients, the degree of differentiation of the personality and the amount of stress to which he or she is exposed are determining factors for prognosis. Unfortunately, there is little evidence to support this sensible view. Relapse is said to be a danger in the recipient if the inducer relapses (Fernando & Frieze 1985). McNiel *et al.* (1972) state that there are no reports of recovery in the elderly, although this may be be due to some extent to the lack of follow-up reports.

Areas for future research

Little is certain about the management of *folie à deux*. In a comparatively uncommon disorder, single-case methodology may be the most useful approach to remedy this. This methodology includes establishing a baseline value for dependent variables, changing one independent variable at a time, and repeated measures of dependent variables. Detailed accounts may be found elsewhere (Barlow & Hersen 1984). Case reports in future should also make use of standardized diagnostic instruments, and rating scales, in place of vague and unrepeatable outcome measures.

References

American Psychiatric Association (1987) *Diagnostic and Statistical Manual of Mental Disorders*, 3rd edn, revised (DSM-III-R). American Psychiatric Association, Washington, D.C.

American Psychiatric Association (1994) *Diagnostic and Statistical Manual of Mental Disorders*, 4th edn (DSM-IV). American Psychiatric Association, Washington, D.C.

Bankier, R.G. (1988) Role reversal in folie à deux. *Canadian Journal of Psychiatry* 33, 231–232.

Barlow, D.H. & Hersen, M. (1984) *Single Case Experimental Designs: Strategies for Studying Behaviour Change*, 2nd edn. Pergammon Press, New York.

Brooks, S.A. (1987) Folie à deux in the aged: Variations in psychopathology. *Canadian Journal of Psychiatry* 32, 61–63.

Brown, M., King, E. & Barraclough, B. (1995) Nine suicide pacts: A clinical study of a consecutive series, 1974–93. *British Journal of Psychiatry* 167, 448–451.

Christodoulou, G.N., Margariti, M.M., Malliaras, D.E. & Alevizou, S. (1995) Shared delusions of doubles. *Journal of Neurology, Neurosurgery and Psychiatry* 58, 499–501.

Coleman, S.M. & Last, S.L. (1939) A study of folie à deux. *Journal of Mental Science* 85, 1212–1223.

Craike, W.H. & Slater, E. (1945) Folie à deux in uniovular twins reared apart. *Brain* 68, 213–221.

Dalby, J.T. & Duncan, B.J. (1987) Shared paranoid disorder preceded by cannabis abuse: Case report. *Canadian Journal of Psychiatry* 32, 64–65.

Dewhurst, K. & Todd, J. (1956) The psychosis of association: Folie à deux. *Journal of Nervous and Mental Disease* 124, 451–459.

Dippel, B., Kemper, J. & Berger, M. (1991) Folie à six: A case report on induced psychotic disorder. *Acta Psychiatrica Scandinavica* 83, 137–141.

Draper, B. & Cole, A. (1990) Folie à deux and dementia. *Australian and New Zealand Journal of Psychiatry* 24, 280–282.

Enoch, M.D. & Trethowan, W.H. (1991) *Uncommon Psychiatric Syndromes*, 3rd edn. Butterworth Heinemann, Oxford.

Evans P. & Merskey H. (1972) Shared beliefs of dermal parasitosis: Folie partagée. *British Journal of Medical Psychology* 45, 19–26.

Fernando, F.P. & Frieze, M. (1985) A relapsing folie à trois. *British Journal of Psychiatry* 146, 315–324.

Fishbain, D.A. (1987) Folie à deux in the aged. *Canadian Journal of Psychiatry* 32, 498–499.

Gelder, M., Gath, D. & Mayou, R. (1989) *Oxford Textbook of Psychiatry*, 2nd edn. Oxford University Press, Oxford.

Ghaziuddin, M. (1991) Folie à deux and mental retardation: Review and case report. *Canadian Journal of Psychiatry* 36, 48–49.

Glassman, J.N., Magulac M. & Darko, D.F. (1987) Folie à famille: Shared paranoid disorder in a Vietnam veteran and his family. *American Journal of Psychiatry* 144, 658–660.

Gralnick, A. (1942) Folie à deux: The psychosis of association—A review of 103 cases and the entire English literature: With case presentations. Part 1. *Psychiatric Quarterly* 16, 230–263.

Greenberg, H.P. (1956) Crime and folie à deux: Review and case history. *Journal of Mental Science* 102, 772–779.

Grover, M.M. (1937) A study of cases of folie à deux. *American Journal of Psychiatry* 93, 1045–1062.

Hunter, R. & MacAlpine, I. (1963) *Three Hundred Years of Psychiatry*, 1535–1860. Oxford University Press, London.

Ilechukwu, S.T. & Okyere, E. (1987) Folie à deux in two sisters: Case report from Nigeria. *Canadian Journal of Psychiatry* 32, 216–218.

Kallman, F.J. & Mickey, J.S. (1946) The concept of induced insanity in family units. *Journal of Nervous and Mental Disease* 104, 303–315.

Kamal, A. (1965) Folie à cinq: A clinical study. *British Journal of Psychiatry* 111, 583–586.

Kendell, R.E. (1993) Paranoid and other psychoses. In: *Companion to Psychiatric Studies* (eds R.E. Kendell & A.K. Zealley), 5th edn, pp. 459–471. Churchill Livingstone, Edinburgh.

Kendler, K.S, Robinson, G., McGuire, M. & Spellman, M.P. (1986) Late-onset folie simultanée in a pair of monozygotic twins. *British Journal of Psychiatry* 148, 463–465.

Lasègue, C. & Falret, J. (1877/1964) La folie à deux: ou folie communiquée (trans. R. Michaud). *American Journal of Psychiatry* 121(4) (Suppl.), 1–23.

Layman, W.A. & Cohen, L. (1957) A modern concept of folie à deux. *Journal of Nervous and Mental Disease* 125, 412–419.

Lazarus, A. (1986) Folie à deux in identical twins: Interaction of nature and nurture. *British Journal of Psychiatry* 148, 324–326.

Lozzi, B., Michetti, F., Alliani, D., Preziosa, P., Loriedo, C. & Vella, G. (1992) Relationship patterns in folie à deux. *Annali dell Instituto Superiore di Sanità* 28, 295–298.

Macaskill, N.D. (1987) Delusional parasitosis: Successful non-pharmacological treatment of a folie à deux. *British Journal of Psychiatry* 150, 261–263.

McNiel, J.N., Verwoerdt, A. & Peak, D. (1972) Folie à deux in the aged: Review and case report of role reversal. *Journal of the American Geriatrics Society* 20, 316–323.

Meakin, C.J., Renvoize, E.B. & Kent, J. (1987) Folie à deux in Down's syndrome: A case report. *British Journal of Psychiatry* 151, 258–260.

Mentjox, R., Van Houten, C.A. & Kooiman, C.G. (1993) Induced psychotic disorder: Clinical aspects, theoretical considerations, and some guidelines for treatment. *Comprehensive Psychiatry* 34, 120–126.

Munro, A. (1986) Folie à deux revisited. *Canadian Journal of Psychiatry* 31, 233–234.

Munro, A. (1987) Paranoid (delusional) disorders: DSM-III-R and beyond. *Comprehensive Psychiatry* 28, 35–39.

Myers, P.L. (1988) Paranoid pseudocommunity beliefs in a sect milieu. *Social Psychiatry and Psychiatric Epidemiology* 23, 252–255.

Pande, N.R. & Gulabani, D.M. (1990) Folie à deux: A socio-psychiatric study. *British Journal of Psychiatry* 156, 440–442.

Porter, T.L., Levine, J. & Dinneen, M. (1993) Shifts of dependency in the resolution of folie à deux. *British Journal of Psychiatry* 162, 704–706.

Potash, H. & Brunell, L. (1974) Multiple conjoint psychotherapy with folie à deux. *Psychotherapy: Theory, Research and Practice* 11, 270–276.

Pulver, S.E. & Brunt, M.Y. (1961) Deflection of hostility in folie à deux. *Archives of General Psychiatry* 5, 257–265.

Rioux, B. (1963) A review of folie à deux, the psychosis of association. *Psychiatric Quarterly* 37, 405–428.

Rosen B.K. (1981) Suicide pacts: A review. *Psychological Medicine* 11, 525–533.

Sacks, M.H. (1988) Folie à deux. *Comprehensive Psychiatry* 29, 270–277.

Salih, M.A. (1981) Suicide pact in a setting of folie à deux. *British Journal of Psychiatry* 139, 62–67.

Scharfetter, C. (1970) On the hereditary aspects of symbiontic psychoses: A contribution towards the understanding of the schizophrenia-like psychoses. *Psychiatria Clinica* 3, 145–152.

Signer, S.F. & Isbister, S.R. (1987) Capgras syndrome, de Clérambault's syndrome, and folie à deux. *British Journal of Psychiatry* 151, 402–404.

Sims, A. (1995) *Symptoms in the Mind: An Introduction to Descriptive Psychopathology*, 2nd edn. Saunders, London.

Sims, A., Salmons, P. & Humphreys, P. (1977) Folie à quatre. *British Journal of Psychiatry* 130, 134–138.

Soni, S.D. & Rockley, G.J. (1974) Socio-clinical substrates of folie à deux. *British Journal of Psychiatry* **125**, 230–235.

Spensley, J. (1972) Folie à deux with methylphenidate psychosis. *Journal of Nervous and Mental Disease* **155**, 288–290.

Waltzer, H. (1963) A psychotic family: Folie à douze. *Journal of Nervous and Mental Disease* **137**, 67–75.

Westermeyer, J. (1989) A case of koro in a refugee family: Association with depression and folie à deux. *Journal of Clinical Psychiatry* **50**, 181–183.

Wolff, G. & McKenzie, K. (1994) Capgras, Frégoli and Cotard's syndromes and Koro in folie à deux. *British Journal of Psychiatry* **165**, 842.

World Health Organization (1992) *The ICD-10 Classification of Mental and Behavioural Disorders. Clinical Descriptions and Diagnostic Guidelines.* World Health Organization, Geneva.

CHAPTER 9

Pseudodementia

BRICE PITT

Introduction

Dementia prevails in 5% of those aged 65 and upwards, and in 20% of those in their 80s (Jorm *et al.* 1987). The first sign is usually impairment of memory. But memory is always, at all ages, finite, and forgetting is a normal, everyday experience at all ages. However, as dementia is hardly ever seen in those under 50 (unless due to head injury), that diagnosis is most unlikely to be invoked for younger people. On the other hand, it is a ready catch-all for many vagaries of thinking and behaviour in later life.

Dementia is not only a devastating disorder but a devastating diagnosis. It is often a 'write-off', meaning that there's nothing more to do by way of investigation or treatment, only management of a person diminished by dwindling faculties.

Case No. 9.1

A professional man in his 50s learns, at about the same time, that his eyesight is threatened by glaucoma and his wife is being unfaithful. He is so distressed that he cannot cope with work and is admitted to a psychiatric unit. He is impervious to supportive counselling, makes no response to antidepressants and although there is a partial improvement in his mood after electroconvulsive therapy (ECT), he is on several occasions incontinent of urine. A computerized tomography (CT) brain scan shows cortical atrophy. He is given the diagnosis of a presenile dementia and transferred to a mental hospital for continuing care. His wife obtains an advantageous divorce settlement. After 3 years, a new clinical assistant notes that his mental state has not deteriorated. Postulating depressive pseudodementia, she resumes antidepressant treatment and encourages him and the ward and, occupational therapy (OT)

195

staff in a rehabilitation programme. Six months later he is back at work, and after another 6 months he is suing the original psychiatrists for the damage resulting from their misdiagnosis.
Moral: Put not your trust in a CT scan alone.

Case No. 9.2

An edgy old man is exasperating his wife by his agitated, irrational, controlling behaviour. He will not let her cook or even turn on the lights. He gives a very poor account of himself, appearing bleak and preoccupied. A clinical psychologist carries out the Wechsler's Adult Intelligence Scale (WAIS; Wechsler 1981) and reports that this shows a moderate dementia. However, as the deterioration is over a matter of months, and some of the old man's behaviour could be construed as agitated depression with delusions of poverty, he is given ECT. After 6 treatments he has recovered. Repeat WAIS testing 6 weeks later shows that he is performing normally.
Moral: Clinical psychological testing does not give the pathology of the dementia.

Case No. 9.3

A not very bright driver in his later 40s turns to selling ice-cream from a van after a business venture fails. He is impatient, hasty, makes misjudgements, gives the wrong change, abuses his customers and has a number of minor accidents; his wife refuses to travel with him any more. A neurologist finds a borderline score on the Mini-Mental State Examination (MMSE), and gets a history that the patient's mother died in mental hospital in her 60s, apparently with dementia. A clinical psychologist reports a pattern indicating dementia. A CT brain scan shows cortical atrophy. His wife is told that he has presenile dementia. They both give up work and are supported by a community psychiatric nurse. Three years later the wife sees that a university department is seeking subjects for a new antidementia drug. She refers her husband, who is seen by a psychiatrist who notes that there has been no deterioration over the years. His National Adult Reading Test (Nelson 1982) IQ is 80, his MMSE score (Folstein et al. 1975) is 23/30, his Cambridge Mental Disorders of the Elderly Cognitive Examination (CAMCOG; Roth et al. 1986) score is 85/107, while on the Brief Assessment Schedule Depression Scale Cards (BASDEC; Adshead et al. 1992) he scores 13/21. The psychiatrist alters the diagnosis to atypical depression with pseudodementia (it emerges that the patient's mother had a similar illness). Six months later, on

fluoxetine and after attending a psychiatric day hospital, he scores 25 on the MMSE, 90 on the CAMCOG and is seeking a driving job again.
Morals: As before; also, be wary of a low previous IQ and make sure you get the correct family history.

Definitions

This chapter is chiefly concerned with *depressive pseudodementia*, or the *dementia of depression* (Rabins 1983). However, it is appropriate first to consider how else 'dementia' may be wrongly applied.

Ageism (Butler 1975) may lead to the assumption that, because dementia becomes more and more common as people age, any forgetfulness or quirks of behaviour in an older person can be laid at its door. This error may be compounded by overlooking deafness, dysarthria (from cerebral vascular disease, Parkinson's disease or ill-fitting or absent dentures) and dysphasia as causes of impaired communication.

Dementia is overrepresented among old people in general hospital wards, prevailing in about a third of in-patients over 65 (Feldman *et al.* 1987; Johnston *et al.* 1987), but there are other causes for apparent confusion in such a setting, notably delirium. About 16% of older people are delirious on their admission to hospital (Seymour *et al.* 1980), and another 9% become so during their stay (Rockwood 1989). Without a history from an informant of a recent onset to the confusional state, without a very obvious underlying physical illness and without the characteristic but by no means always present clouding of consciousness, a misdiagnosis of dementia is readily made, with a consequent quest for 'disposal' rather than for causation and treatment. Old people in hospital may also give a poor account of themselves because they are apprehensive, bewildered, awed and uninformed rather than because of intrinsic cognitive impairment.

Dementia and depression are not the only mental illnesses of late life. Chronic schizophrenia, now more often managed in the community than the mental hospital, may present a dementia-like picture of self-neglect, peculiar talk and erratic behaviour which may mislead those who lack a history (Wright & Silove 1988). Paraphrenia and some stages of dementia share paranoid delusions about thefts and intruders, though in paraphrenia the delusions are more elaborate and sustained and better argued (Naguib & Levy 1987). Mania and hypomania, causing garrulity, circumstantiality, lability of mood, self-neglect or eccentricity and disinhibition can be mistaken for dementia or delirium (Wright & Silove 1988). Intoxication, from a variety of drugs, notably long-acting benzodiazepines prescribed as hypnotics and, occasionally, alcohol (Gurnack & Hoffman 1992), by impairing coherence and self-care, may masquerade as dementia. Learning disability (Patel *et al.* 1993)—say, when the parents have died very old and the surviving child does not quite know how to survive alone — may superficially resemble dementia, and eccentric personalities, notably those with the Diogenes or senile squalor syndrome (Cooney & Hamid 1995), may be misdiagnosed because of their unusual or frankly squalid lifestyle.

The term 'pseudodementia' was coined by Kiloh (1961). Wells (1979) made a detailed study and devised a checklist to distinguish pseudo- from true organic dementia (see below). Lishman (1987) describes pseudodementia as 'a number of conditions [in which] a clinical picture resembling organic dementia presents for attention yet physical disease proves to be little if at all responsible'. This is more elegant than Caine's (1981) somewhat laboured and tautologous 'intellectual impairment in patients with a primary psychiatric disorder, in which the features of intellectual abnormality resemble, at least in part, those of a neuropathologically induced cognitive deficit. This neuropsychological impairment is reversible, and there is no apparent primary neuropathological process that leads to the genesis of this disturbance.' Bulbena and Berrios (1986) remark that there is no consensus on the use and application of the diagnosis 'pseudodementia'. They used the criteria of 'cognitive impairment, of the type seen in dementia but with no relevant organic disorder and reversibility' in a retrospective study of psychiatric in-patients, and identified a group with depressed mood correlating with delusions, unipolar illness, past history of affective illness and positive outcome, and negatively with non-affective illnesses and confusion, whom they deemed to represent the syndrome of depressive pseudodementia. The term, however, or its equivalent, does not appear either in ICD-10 (World Health Organization (WHO) 1992) or DSM-IV (American Psychiatric Association (APA) 1994) so the concept may still be unaccepted; if it does not appear in the diagnostic 'bibles' it may well be missed by the inexperienced.

According to Marsden's (1978) definition, which (rightly) invokes neither progression nor irreversibility (a point endorsed by Mahendra 1985), depression could be one cause of dementia without the qualification 'pseudo': 'Global cognitive impairment in an alert patient of more than three months' duration'.

Probably, as has already been indicated, the likeliest misdiagnosis of depression as dementia is by the patient. Depressed people expect the worst, and weight themselves in the balance and find themselves wanting. They are unforgiving about memory lapses and take them as evidence of their senility (Kahn *et al.* 1975).

Case No. 9.4

A dentist aged 67 has felt that his memory is not as sharp as it was for some years. His mother-in-law has Alzheimer's disease — 'she's like a vegetable' — and he believes that he is heading the same way. He makes errors when setting his video to record future programmes, and his ritual for washing and dressing in the mornings is sometimes out of sequence. Though retired, he is not as well off as he should be, and relations with his wife are strained. He has had to return to part-time clinical work, but feels his performance is below par. Although neurological examination, including magnetic resonance imaging (MRI) brain scan, is normal and his general health is good, a clinical psychologist's report largely confirms his gloomy self-appraisal. He does not understand why the neurologist prescribes amitriptyline, and stops it after only 6 weeks. Yet, although still convinced that he has Alzheimer's disease, he still seeks treatment. He attends a memory clinic: his MMSE score is 30; his CAMCOG, 97; his BASDEC, 11. He is told that with so long a history, no family history and his current cognitive performance, he cannot have Alzheimer's or any other dementia. On the other hand, he is highly likely to be suffering from depression. He accepts a prescription for fluoxetine.

Moral: Listen to what the patient has to say, but be less ready to accept a self-diagnosis. Older people who complain of a bad memory are much likelier to be suffering from depression than dementia.

Mechanisms of depressive dysmnesia

Where there is objective evidence of depressive dysmnesia the possible mechanisms are:
- poor motivation;
- negativism — irritability, low expectation;
- response bias;
- overcaution;
- 'learned helplessness';
- anergy and retardation;
- preoccupation;
- agitated inattention;

- iatrogenic;
- altered brain function;
- language impairment.

These will now be considered in a little more detail.

POOR MOTIVATION

Depression saps enterprise and initiative and the will to engage in social activity. Conversation is an effort, and the demands of cognitive testing may seem excessive, especially for any effortful tasks. Apathy and readiness to give up prevail. There is a disinclination to try at all, and 'don't know' answers (often signifying 'can't be bothered') are much more likely than inaccuracies (Miller 1975).

NEGATIVISM

Surliness and contrariness are occasional features of depressive illness in later life, limiting cooperation and causing some questions to be answered, if at all, in a perverse and blatantly inaccurate way. There may be a 'will to fail', fulfilling low self-expectations: 'Can't think, won't think!'

RESPONSE BIAS

Depressed older people remember the bad things in their lives better than the good or indifferent. Lloyd and Lishman (1975) found that the higher patients scored for depression, the faster they produced unhappy personal memories in association with neutral words. Teasdale and Fogarty (1979) induced an unhappy mood in normal subjects who were then slower to evoke positive memories. Clark and Teasdale (1982) found that clinically depressed patients varied in their ability to repond to a cue word with a pleasant personal event according to the diurnal variation in their mood. Zuroff *et al.* (1983) found that more depressed subjects tended to apply more negative adjectives to themselves, and subsequently recalled negative rather than positive words, and on a recognition task recognized negative adjectives which they had not, in fact, been previously shown.

OVERCAUTION

A tendency in older subjects to hesitate before answering in case they should be wrong, or to play safe in, say, a recognition task by a bias to not recognizing words, names, pictures or faces shown previously when presented with previously unseen material, is often exacerbated by depression. O'Connor *et al.* (1990) found that depressed older people in the community complained of indecision, mental slowing and impaired concentration.

'LEARNED HELPLESSNESS'

Seligman's (1975) hypothesis that people, as well as dogs, trapped in situations in which whatever response they make to a stimulus has no bearing on the outcome, is appropriate for many older depressed people, especially those rendered dependent by infirmity or being in institutional care.

ANERGY AND RETARDATION

Stuporose patients are unable to communicate, and lesser degrees of retardation are associated with slow and scant answers. Any tests which have to be performed in limited time will therefore be compromised.

PREOCCUPATION

Brooding about doom, gloom and guilt is not conducive to registration or encoding new information, or to its recognition or recall ('cognitive interference', according to Miller (1975)).

AGITATED INATTENTION

This is, perhaps, an extreme form of preoccupation. The severely agitated depressive is too distraught to attend to tasks or questions and is likely instead to reiterate exclamations of anguish or beg for help.

IATROGENIC

The older, best-known and cheaper tricyclic antidepressants are powerfully anticholinergic and may cause confusion, especially in older patients with mild early dementia or minimal cognitive impairment.

ALTERED BRAIN FUNCTION

Late-onset depressive illness severe enough to come to psychiatric attention is associated with physical and physiological changes intermediate between those of normal old age and dementia. Jacoby *et al.* (1981) showed cortical atrophy and increased ventricular brain ratio intermediate between normality and dementia in late-onset depressed patients, and Abas *et al.* (1990) that the ventricular brain ratio correlated with measures of slowing. Pearlson *et al.* (1989) confirmed such findings in subjects with dementia syndrome of depression, but observed no significant cognitive deterioration after 2 years.

LANGUAGE IMPAIRMENT

While depressed older subjects perform language tasks much better than those with early dementia, they have problems with more complex tests compared with normal old people (Emery & Breslau 1989) which could affect their reporting of more involved happenings.

Distinguishing pseudo- from organic dementia

The following criteria (after Wells 1979) all favour depression.
- A short history (weeks or months).
- A previous or family history of affective illness.
- A definite time of onset ('It began last Easter').
- Misery, or lack of joy.
- Disparity between subjective and objective assessment (relatives say that the patient is exaggerating).
- Drawing attention to disability.
- Moderate cognitive impairment.
- 'Don't know' rather than wrong answers.
- No confabulation (Post 1975).
- No cortical features (e.g. no dysphasia or dyspraxia).
- No progression of disability.
- Response to a trial of antidepressants.

Conclusion

Depressed older people who 'show their age', complain particularly of their memories, show some cognitive impairment, present atypical pictures, fail to respond to initial treatment and whose brain scans show age-consistent cortical atrophy are at risk of being misdiagnosed as demented and denied further, more active treatment but are instead 'managed' as lastingly disabled.

Further hazards are assessment by a care manager who may recommend social or institutional care rather than medication, or by doctors who do not think of depression, or if they do consider it justified and withhold treatment or give too little for too long. This matters because depression is treatable, blights life and leads to debility and sometimes to suicide. A diagnosis of Alzheimer's disease is by exclusion, can only be confirmed by neuropathological examination of the brain, and should be kept under review until there is clear evidence of progression of the disease.

Finally, depression is a common accompaniment of dementia, and its treatment can significantly improve the quality of life, if not cognition.

References

Abas, M.A., Sahakian, B.J. & Levy, R. (1990) Neuropsychological deficits and CT scan changes in elderly depressives. *Psychological Medicine* 20, 507–520.

Adshead, F., Day Cody, D. & Pitt, B. (1992) BASDEC: A novel screening instrument for depression in elderly medical in-patients. *British Medical Journal* 305, 397.

American Psychiatric Association (1994) *Diagnostic and Statistical Manual of Mental Disorders*, 4th edn (DSM-IV). American Psychiatric Association, Washington, D.C.

Bulbena, A. & Berrios, G.E. (1986) Pseudodementia: Facts and figures. *British Journal of Psychiatry* 148, 87–94.

Butler, R.N. (1975) *Why Survive? Being Old in America*. Harper & Row, New York.

Caine, E.D. (1981) Pseudodementia: Current concepts and future directions. *Archives of General Psychiatry* 38, 1359–1364.

Clark, D.M. & Teasdale, J.D. (1982) Diurnal variations in clinical depression and accessibility of memories of positive and negative experiences. *Journal of Abnormal Psychology* 91, 87–95.

Cooney, C. & Hamid, W. (1995) Review: Diogenes syndrome. *Age and Ageing* 24, 451–453.

Emery, O.B. & Breslau, L.D. (1989) Language deficits in depression: Comparisons with SDAT and normal aging. *Journal of Gerontology* 44, M85–92.

Feldman, E., Mayou, R., Hawton, K. *et al.* (1987) Psychiatric disorder in medical in-patients. *Quarterly Journal of Medicine* 240, 301–308.

Folstein, M.E., Folstein, S.E. & McHugh, P.R. (1975) 'Mini-mental state': A practical method for grading the cognitive state of patients for the clinician. *Journal of Psychiatric Research* 12, 189–198.

Gurnack, A.M. & Hoffman, N.G. (1992) Elderly alcohol misuse. *International Journal of Addiction* 27, 869–878.

Jacoby, R.J., Levy, R. & Bird, J.M. (1981) Computed tomography and the outcome of affective disorder: A follow-up study of elderly depressives. *British Journal of Psychiatry* 139, 288–292.

Johnston, M., Wakeling, A., Graham, N. & Stokes, F. (1987) Cognitive impairment, emotional disorder and length of stay of elderly patients in a district general hospital. *British Journal of Medical Psychology* 60, 133–139.

Jorm, A.F., Korten, A.E. & Henderson, A.S. (1987) The prevalence of dementia: A quantitative integration of the literature. *Acta Psychiatrica Scandinavica* 76, 465–479.

Kahn, R.L., Zarit, S.H., Hilbert, N.M. & Niederehe, G. (1975) Memory complaint and impairment in the aged: The effect of depression and altered brain function. *Archives of General Psychiatry*, 32, 1569–1573.

Kiloh, I. (1961) Pseudo-dementia. *Acta Psychiatrica Scandinavica* 37, 336–351.

Lishman, W.A. (1987) *Organic Psychiatry* (2nd edn) Blackwell Scientific Publications, Oxford.

Lloyd, G.G. & Lishman, W.A. (1975) Effects of depression on speed of recall of pleasant and unpleasant experiences. *Psychological Medicine* 5, 173–180.

Mahendra, B. (1985) Depression and dementia: The multi-faceted relationship. *Psychological Medicine* 15, 227–236.

Marsden, C.D. (1978) The diagnosis of dementia. In: *Studies in Geriatric Psychiatry* (eds A. Isaacs & F. Past). Wiley, Chichester.

Miller, W.R. (1975) Psychological deficit in depression. *Psychological Bulletin* 82, 238–260.

Naguib, N. & Levy, R. (1987) Late paraphrenia: Neuropsychological impairment and structural brain abnormalities on computed tomography. *International Journal of Geriatric Psychiatry* 2, 83–90.

Nelson, H.E. (1982) *The National Adult Reading Test*. NFER-Nelson, Windsor.

O'Connor, D.W., Pollitt, P.A., Roth, M. *et al.* (1990) Memory complaints and impairment in normal, depressed and demented elderly persons identified in a community survey. *Archives of General Psychiatry* 47, 224–227.

Patel, P., Goldberg, D. & Moss, S. (1993) Psychiatric morbidity in older people with moderate and severe learning disability. 2. The prevalence study. *British Journal of Psychiatry* 163, 481–491.

Pearlson, G.D., Rabins, P.V., Kim, W.S. *et al.* (1989) Structural brain CT changes and cognitive defects with and without reversible dementia ('pseudodementia'). *Psychological Medicine* 19, 573–584.

Post, F. (1975) Dementia, depression and pseudodementia. In: *Psychiatric Aspects of Organic Disease* (eds D.F. Bensan & D. Blumer). Grune and Stratton, New York.

Rabins, P.V. (1983) Reversible dementia and the misdiagnosis of dementia: A review. *Hospital and Community Psychiatry* 32, 490–492.

Rockwood, K. (1989) Acute confusion in elderly medical patients. *Journal of the American Geriatrics Society*, 37, 150–154.

Roth, M., Tyms, E., MountJoy, C.Q. *et al.* (1986) CAMDEX: A standardised instrument for the diagnosis of mental disorder in the elderly, with particular reference to the early detection of dementia. *British Journal of Psychiatry* 149, 698–709.

Seligman, M.E.P. (1975) Depression and learned helplessness. In: *The Psychology of Depression: Contemporary Theory and Research* (eds R.J. Friedman & M.M. Katz). Winston-Wiley, New York.

Seymour, D.G., Henschke, P.J. & Cape, R.D.T. (1980) Acute confusional states in the elderly: The role of dehydration/volume depletion, physical illness and age. *Age and Ageing* 9, 137–146.

Teasdale, J.D. & Fogarty, S.J. (1979) Differential effects of induced mood on retrieval of positive and negative and neutral words. *Journal of Abnormal Psychology* 88, 248–257.

Wechsler, D. (1981) *The Manual for the Wechsler Adult Intelligence Scale* (revised). Psychological Corporation, New York.

Wells, C.E. (1979) Pseudodementia. *American Journal of Psychiatry* 136, 896–900.

World Health Organization (1992) *The ICD-10 Classification of Mental and Behavioural Disorders. Clinical Descriptions and Diagnostic Guidelines.* World Health Organization, Geneva.

Wright, J.M. & Silove, D. (1988) Pseudodementia in schizophrenia and mania. *Australia and New Zealand Journal of Psychiatry* 22, 109–114.

Zuroff, D.C., Colussy, S.A. & Wielgus, M.S. (1983) Selective memory and depression: A cautionary note concerning response bias. *Cognitive Therapy and Research* 7, 223–232.

CHAPTER 10

Deliberate Self-Harm
MICHAEL J. CROWE

Introduction

In this chapter I will be dealing primarily with the repetitive forms of self-harm which are seen in patients with personality disorders, although in introducing the topic it will be helpful to sketch in a more general perspective to include some of the other conditions in which self-harm also plays a part, including psychoses, genetic disorders and depression.

There are a number of ways in which psychiatric patients harm themselves, most of which do not present an immediate danger to life. These include fairly common acts such as cutting or burning the skin, scratching or biting oneself, hitting one's head against objects or walls, and self-poisoning without true suicidal intent. They also include more unusual acts such as cutting oneself internally, swallowing sharp objects, amputating fingers or genitals, gluing eyelids together or deliberately losing blood so as to become anaemic. The various acts of self-harm are quite widespread within psychiatry, and are by no means restricted to one diagnostic group. Certainly many of those who harm themselves are psychotic, but there is also a large group of self-harmers who display the characteristics of borderline personality disorder. Self-harm is also seen in those with learning difficulties, and there is a large, and probably increasing, incidence of self-harm among both male and female prisoners.

Deliberate self-harm is also, however, a common activity in many otherwise normal individuals. Many teenagers with acne will squeeze their spots to an excessive degree, and cause unnecessary scarring. Nail biting is also a common and relatively harmless form of self-harm, and dermatitis artefacta and many cases of lichen planus are probably caused by rubbing and pinching the skin.

Deliberate self-harm also occurs in many religious and social rituals, both in the present time and throughout history. Favazza (1996) has given examples of the widespread use of various forms of self-harm practised in ancient and modern civilizations. He includes such activities as mass flagellation in mediaeval Europe, religious self-abasement leading to injuries in Latin America and many other cases of self-mutilation for religious purposes. In addition, he cites many examples of bodily injury imposed by societies on their members, which, although interesting in themselves, do not involve self-harm as such. These include foot binding among the Chinese, genital mutilation and tribal skin scarring in Africa and head moulding in ancient Egypt. There are also various examples in the world of more serious self-mutilation such as self-castration in Russia and in India, which is carried out in the interests of gaining special religious status.

There are many examples in literature and in history of the more familiar types of self-mutilation which might be termed pathological. One of the earlier ones is the account in the New Testament (Mark 5:5) in which a man with an unclean spirit, whose name was 'Legion', was always 'in the mountains and in the tombs, crying, and cutting himself with stones'. When Christ finally cast out his devils, they entered a herd of swine, who threw themselves off a precipice and were drowned.

In other accounts there is a connection between self-mutilation and guilt, as in the Oedipus legend, in which he puts out his eyes when he realizes that he has killed his father and married his mother.

In the present day, there is a fashion in California and other places for decorative self-mutilation, as reported by Favazza (1996), and this is done sometimes by the individual himself or herself and sometimes by friends or by tattooists. The insertion of rings or other ornaments in parts of the body ranging from ears and nose to umbilicus and genitals is also widespread at the present time. There is thus a spectrum or gradation between those forms of self-harm which are acceptable either by the whole of society or by a subgroup (either religious or subcultural), and those which are seen as the result of psychiatric illness or personality disorder.

Deliberate self-harm is included in a number of diagnostic descriptions in both ICD-10 (World Health Organization (WHO) 1992) and DSM-IV (American Psychiatric Association (APA) 1994). In ICD-10, self-mutilation is included in the criteria for diagnosing emotionally unstable personality disorder (borderline type) and there are also specific entries under the categories of external causes of morbidity for 'intentional self-harm' using many different methods. In DSM-IV, self-mutilating behaviour is a criterion for the diagnosis of borderline personality disorder. In both publications, suicidal thoughts and behaviour are included in the descriptions of depression or dysthymia, but the type of self-harm and the degree of dangerousness are left unspecified.

It is rather unsatisfactory that the only diagnostic group to include self-harm as a criterion is that of a personality disorder, since in some cases it seems that the self-harm is really the patient's only major problem, and that there are few of the other signs of personality disorder. In addition, in some cases, the behaviour has occurred for only a short period in adult life, perhaps in the context of a depressive illness or after childbirth. In these cases the label of a personality disorder seems to be inappropriate, and it would be better to use a label which simply describes the self-harm alone, as suggested by Kahan and Pattison (1984).

The fact that the behaviour occurs in many different diagnostic groups suggests that, rather like a pyrexia, it is an indication that something is wrong rather than a diagnostic syndrome *per se*. However, there are a number of different patterns of self-harm which may be found in individuals with specific diagnoses, such as those with learning difficulties, those with borderline or dissociative personality disorder, those with psychosis, patients in prison and forensic units, and those who are using the behaviour as a means of obtaining medical attention (Munchausen's syndrome). These syndromes differ from each other in various ways, although there are also overlapping features. In this chapter the main focus for discussion will be the syndrome of self-harm occurring in those with unstable or borderline personality disorder.

Epidemiology

The syndrome of self-harm in the context of a personality disorder has been reviewed by Tantam and Whittaker (1992) in a wide-ranging article dealing with epidemiology, aetiology (as far as that can be determined), and treatment. They estimate from a variety of British studies that self-injury sufficient to take the patient to hospital occurs in 1 in 600 of the population, although this may be an underestimate, because, as they go on to say, some such acts may be concealed by the patient or by relatives. In the survey by Johnson *et al.* (1975) in Canada, which included many settings such as general practices, nursing homes and prisons as well as hospitals, the incidence was considerably higher, at approximately 1 in 200 of the population. The true incidence may be different between different countries, but the inclusion of populations with a propensity to self-injury, such as prisoners and those with learning difficulties, will reveal the true extent of the problem in the total population in a way which cannot be done by simply counting hospital admissions.

There is some controversy over the gender incidence of this form of behaviour. Psychiatric units probably see more women than men who harm themselves, and in some the proportion is as high as $3:1$. However, overall epidemiology (Robinson & Duffy 1989) shows a much more equal gender distribution, and this may reflect the wider catchment population covered by their survey.

Neither self-poisoning nor self-injury are necessarily carried out with suicidal intent, and many different rationales are given for the behaviour. Favazza (1989) interviewed a large number of self-harmers, and quotes widely varying explanations given, on the one hand by those patients (mainly psychotic or depressed) who carried out major but infrequent self-mutilation and on the other hand by those (personality disordered and neurotic) who regularly harmed themselves more moderately. The former were likely to use religious or sexual explanations, while the latter tended to blame anger against self or others, the need for relief of tension, the influence of multiple personalities or the wish to impress on others the degree of their own pain. In clinical practice, it is quite common for the repeated self-harmers to describe an almost addictive quality to the urge, which has prompted the speculation that endorphins may be involved in the mechanism which leads to repetition. This, however, according to Favazza, remains speculative.

Aetiology

The aetiology of repeated self-harm is clearly multifactorial, if only because it occurs in such a wide variety of conditions, from personality disorder and psychosis to mental handicap. The causative factors should properly be divided into predisposing and precipitating, and these too will differ from case to case. Among predisposing factors, the presence of guilt and self-blame is fairly common, and patients who harm themselves will often express self-hatred, whether from the process of their psychosis or through the almost universal finding, both in psychotic and non-psychotic patients, of low self-esteem. The self-harm may be associated with hallucinations which command the patient to carry out the behaviour, and other psychotic phenomena such as specific delusions may be part of the syndrome. In the non-psychotic cases, however, the predisposing factors are more varied. They may include depressive mood, and this is a common finding, whether the depression is primary or in response to a life crisis such as bereavement. In many of the patients, there is a history of abuse in childhood, either physical or sexual, and in a number of series this has been found to approach 80% (Briere & Zaidi 1989; Tantam & Whittaker 1992). This, however, does not mean that the abuse is the cause of the self-harm, because there may be other aspects of childhood deprivation which contribute to the syndrome, and there is by no means a one-to-one relationship between abuse and self-harm (Mullen *et al.* 1993). Other possible predisposing factors include inconsistent or broken parental relationships and time spent in foster care or children's homes. Psychodynamic explanations (Feldman 1988) include aggression turned inwards, the need to feel 'in control', the wish for self-punishment, a symbolic form of castration, a form of suicide avoidance, or a fusion of pre-Oedipal aggressive and sexual impulses. Many such patients may have a sense of unreality, and the self-harm may be a way of assuring themselves that they exist. In certain conditions, such as Lesch–Nyhan's syndrome, repeated self-harm, especially by biting and head banging, seems to be an integral aspect of the disorder, and this may be true of other developmental disorders such as some forms of childhood autism.

The precipitating and maintaining factors for self-harm are more numerous and better understood. I have already mentioned the addictive quality of much repeated self-harm. In addition, many of the patients say that they self-harm in order to relieve tension, and that the relief may last for up to 12 hours. Many patients feel no pain at the time of the injury, and only begin to feel pain when the wound stops bleeding or they are being sutured. Some patients are in an altered state of mind, sometimes amounting to a dissociation, at the time of the self-harm, only coming back into their normal state afterwards, and with no memory of the event. The act may be rewarding, as in one patient who described the 'exquisite pain' produced by her self-harm. In addition, some patients (though probably a minority) achieve some secondary gain from family or carers from the act, and may value the attention. In some settings, such as prisons and residential homes, the self-harm may be 'rewarded' by a move to more comfortable accommodation such as the prison hospital. In these settings, there may also be either epidemics of self-harm or even self-harming in groups. Once the urge to self-harm has been felt it is usually very hard to resist. A patient may be dissuaded from harming himself or herself for a time, but it is unusual for this to be successful in the long term without some more radical therapeutic input.

Among those patients with personality disorder who self-harm, there is often an admixture of other self-damaging behaviour. The association with bulimia nervosa is well documented (Lacey & Evans 1986), and these authors have suggested that self-harm could be seen as part of a 'multi-impulsive' disorder, including alcohol and drug abuse. These patients are also very likely, if they manage to form intimate relationships, to choose partners who treat them in an abusive manner, and the relationships are therefore often stormy and of short duration.

Course

The overall course of the self-harming behaviour has been studied by Tantam and Whittaker (1992). In their review of the literature, they concluded that the great majority of repeated self-harmers begin the behaviour in teenage years, though some cases have started in earlier childhood. There is a tendency for the behaviour, once begun, to be repeated many times, and a chronic pattern with multiple visits to accident departments is quite common. The repetition of the self-harming behaviour is associated with a forensic history, living alone, being unemployed, regular use of alcohol or drugs, and being out of contact with parents (Kreitman & Casey 1988). The link with actual suicide, however, is not very strong. Some patients, notably those with marked depression, express suicidal wishes, and most self-harmers would say that they are not greatly motivated to live, but in two studies cited by Tantam and Whittaker the suicide rate over 5 years was 13% and 16%, respectively. On the other hand, in the same two studies the 'improved' rate after 5 years was 50%, and this correlates with clinical experience, in that it is quite common to find that in their 30s and 40s many patients who had previously harmed themselves are now no longer doing so. This is not to say that their general adjustment is necessarily good, but at least the serious consequences of repeated self-harm are not in evidence.

Management

The management of repeated self-harm is not easy (Feldman 1988). It is not a subject which is well covered in traditional textbooks, and there is a tendency for reports on this topic to be combined with those on suicide and attempted suicide. The treatment of these patients is hampered by the fact that they are often articulate and assertive, and seem superficially to be able to make decisions for themselves, while at the same time carrying out acts of self-mutilation which horrify their carers and seem to require preventive measures. This contrast, and the extreme emotional strain imposed on those around them, make them often rather unpopular, particularly to the staff on the busy general psychiatric and accident units on which they are usually treated.

Feldman has emphasized the effect on staff and carers, whose feelings after a mutilating act are described as 'fluctuating among rage, sympathy, guilt, solicitude and the urge to retaliate'. There is also a tendency for the self-harming patient to become the centre of staff conflict, with disagreement as to the amount of supervision needed by the patient. These conflicts will often emerge most acutely in relation to night staff and emergency doctors who have to deal with a recent episode, and an 'in-group' and an 'out-group' among the staff may develop, with the patient's care suffering as a result.

The patient will often elicit the responses characterized by Main (1957) in his classic paper on the management of 'special' patients on general psychiatric wards. He specifically cites the ability of such patients to evoke an 'insincere goodness' in their carers, associated with splits between those staff members who have been taken into the patient's confidence and treated as special allies, and the rest of the staff who are trying to treat the whole patient group fairly and equally. He advocates the open discussion between staff members on the subject of disagreements about these 'special' patients and the avoidance of any secrets kept between the patient and one selected staff member.

Feldman suggests that excessive restrictions on self-harmers are seldom effective. These forms of control imply that the staff have the responsibility for preventing the patient's self-harm, and this leads to conflict with the patient and also to a general abdication of the patient's own sense of responsibility, and a probable delay in discharge and improvement. On the other hand, the self-harm may escalate sufficiently to lead to significant danger to life if it is allowed to continue, and in these circumstances the team may have to make the decision to detain the patient; this should normally be for the minimum necessary period. The difficulty is that, having once been detained, the patient may be willing to raise the 'stakes' again on a subsequent occasion, and a vicious cycle may ensue which is hard to break. There is a calculated risk to be taken in each case, which may occasionally lead to disaster, but which is probably better for the majority than automatic resort to detention.

For the individual patient, there are many forms of psychological therapy which have been advocated. Perhaps the most widely used is psychodynamic psychotherapy. Much of the improvement in patients who have had this type of therapy is attributed to their ability to understand the origins of the behaviour and their increased ability to verbalize their feelings. On the other hand, many authors (Feldman 1988) emphasize the need to be cautious about premature interpretation, and the need to concentrate on making the patient feel secure and safe in the therapy. Tantam and Whittaker (1992), however, suggest that these strictures apply more to traditional psychoanalysis, and less to the more modern types of psychodynamic therapy which emphasize the here-and-now rather than the historical origins of the conflict which has led to the self-harm. Kernberg (1987) suggests that intensive psychoanalytic therapy may be harmful, and advocates therapy no more often than twice per week.

There is also a recommendation in many of the papers for the therapist to be clear about boundaries and rules, because the borderline patient is particularly susceptible to develop a strong dependence on the therapist, and may wish to telephone out of hours, to know about the therapist's personal life and to have an exclusive relationship which may result in an alliance against others. In most cases this is inappropriate, but in some it may be helpful for a therapeutic team member to be available on rotation for emergencies, thus providing cover without breaking the normal boundaries of therapy. As in other types of therapy it should be remembered that the patient may become more disturbed as a result of a session, and that this may lead to more, rather than less, self-harm in the short term.

Modifications of the psychodynamic approach have been used with this group of patients, and in particular cognitive-analytic therapy (CAT) has been advocated (Ryle *et al.* 1989). This involves a 16-session structured course of therapy in which the patient explores the origins and maintenance of the problem, using a series of diagrams, writing letters and making specific contracts with the therapist. The clear boundaries around this type of therapy (including the strict 16-session limit) may be useful with this particular group of patients, but it has the disadvantage that the long-term support which they often need and crave is not possible, and termination at the 16th session may be traumatic.

A different form of psychodynamic therapy has been advocated by Kraupl Taylor (1969), under the title of *prokaletic therapy*. The therapist is encouraged to form a supportive and non-time-limited relationship with the patient, and within that relationship to use various forms of interpretation to 'countermanipulate' the manipulative side of the patient. Such interventions include the prediction of self-harm before the next session (leading to abstinence in order to prove the therapist wrong), a refusal to show optimism ('you are very ill and it will be a long hard struggle for you') in order to reassure the patient that he or she is being taken seriously, and the challenging interpretation, in which the self-wounding is said to be a masturbatory equivalent. This method was developed specifically for self-harming patients, and still has some important lessons for treatment today.

Cognitive approaches to therapy have been described by Salkovskis *et al.* (1990) in a group of patients who repeatedly attempt suicide. They used a 'problem solving' method, in which the negative thinking which led to the self-harm was replaced by more positive coping strategies, with an improvement in depression and a reduced rate of repetition in comparison with controls. Linehan (1993) has a composite form of treatment which involves extinction of the parasuicide threat, while at the same time working on encouraging alternative ways of signalling distress, and using 'dialectical behaviour therapy' to help the patient to adjust to life, to be more assertive, and to think positively. One of her more important injunctions is that as far as possible the self-harming behaviour should not be reinforced by excessive attention.

More traditional behavioural approaches are often used predominantly where the self-harm occurs in those with learning difficulties. In institutions where there is a behavioural approach to the general management of patients, the management of self-harm is on the same lines, with differential reinforcement of 'other' (non-self-harming) behaviour, withdrawal of social reinforcement of the self-harm, and in some cases punishment of the behaviour itself. Not many trials are reported of these approaches, but in one (Corter *et al.* 1971) it appeared that punishment was the most effective form of treatment, but the improvement was not able to be generalized outside of the experimental situation. Behavioural principles are often also applied in a general way to self-harm in the non-learning disabled population of patients, but strict behavioural management would be difficult here because of the need for a reasonable level of cooperation on the part of the patient, or at least no deliberate sabotage of the therapy, and this would probably not be possible in the majority of cases.

The treatment of self-harming patients in groups is another therapeutic possibility which has been proposed. In mixed groups on general psychiatric wards the self-harmer may become scapegoated, and will create difficulties for the leaders as well as themselves and the other group members. Group therapy exclusively for self-harmers has been presented as a method of treatment by Walsh and Rosen (1988). The type of therapy used is more rigid and prescriptive than conventional group therapy, and aims to inculcate interpersonal skills, to discuss the implications of self-harm as a means of obtaining intimacy and nurturance, and to develop better methods of obtaining the care the patient desires and needs.

The majority of patients with self-harm in a non-psychotic setting give a history of prior sexual abuse. There are, of course, many other apparent sequelae of such abuse, as evidenced by the statistical correlations in population surveys between a history of abuse and current symptoms (Mullen *et al.* 1993). These include eating disorders, anxiety, depression and substance abuse, as well as suicidal and (by implication) self-harming behaviour. It is therefore appropriate to consider what specific therapy may be given to a self-harmer who gives a sexual abuse history, although it is interesting that this possibility is relatively new to the management of this problem, and has not been raised in the earlier reviews of self-harming cited above. Sexual abuse can be seen as an example of post-traumatic stress, and the specific sequelae can be very similar to those, for instance, following a car crash or shipping disaster. These will include flashbacks and nightmares, and avoidance of situations similar to those in which the trauma occurred. In addition, in the survivors of abuse, as opposed to other forms of post-traumatic stress disorder, there may be major problems with relationships (especially those which involve some degree of trust), sexual phobias, and generally low self-esteem. The difference arises from the fact that the survivors of childhood abuse may have experienced many years of a very complex and ambivalent relationship with (usually) a trusted adult, and the effect on their development leads to a general disturbance of relationships and of self-image, as opposed to the rather briefer (albeit dangerous and overwhelming) experience of a sudden traumatic event such as an accident, which may lead to specific forms of avoidance and phobia.

In treating these problems, the first hurdle to overcome is the crisis of disclosure. This needs to be handled with understanding and sympathy, and without either premature calls for action against the abuser or any response which implies disbelief or blame. It is also important to balance the risks to the patient of confrontation (including the stress of possible court appearance and cross-questioning) and the opposite risks of keeping silent and perhaps exposing others to the risk of abuse by the same person. The best policy is to proceed at the patient's own pace, and to remain non-judgemental at all stages of the process.

There are many approaches to the therapy of post-traumatic stress, but in the management of sexual abuse survivors the method of Dolan (1991) is very useful. This is a combination of cognitive and solution-focused therapy (De Shazer *et al.* 1986). The general therapeutic stance is one of replacing negative, self-destructive expectations with a positive, yet realistic, vision of the future. A wide variety of techniques is employed, including the utilization of supportive family relationships, the management of feelings towards non-supportive family members and perpetrators, and ensuring safety in the current situation. Specific tasks are given, to help the patient to 'reclaim the body', to reduce dissociation and to write letters (not usually sent) to abusers and other significant figures. A similar package is recommended by Linehan (1993), who specifically avoids making too many connections with the past until the patient has developed the 'strength' to cope with the increased stress involved. In the latter stages of therapy, there is an encouragement to try to reduce self-hate and shame, and for patients to construct their own consistent version of what has happened to present to others in the future.

The use of medication in the management of self-harming patients is perhaps more controversial than the use of therapy. Feldman (1988) simply lists the types of drug used and reports both negative and positive results from their use. The drugs include many of the usual antidepressants and antipsychotics, but also lithium (as a mood stabilizer) and naloxone (presumably as a means of reducing any satisfaction from the self-harm). Tantam and Whittaker recommend antidepressants in those who have clear evidence of depression, and make the point that the newer preparations are to be preferred because of their lower toxicity in overdose. Of the specific serotonin reuptake inhibitors, in particular, fluoxetine was associated with a significant reduction in self-harming in a controlled study by Markovitz *et al.* (1991). Anecdotal support is given to the use of both lithium and carbamazepine in reducing self-harm, and the use of neuroleptics is also supported, in at least one controlled trial, particularly in those cases where there are definite psychotic symptoms.

Other measures can be taken, including the use of electroconvulsive therapy (ECT) (only for cases where there is clear evidence of depression unresponsive to antidepressant treatment), and various neurosurgical techniques, largely on an experimental basis, such as leucotomy and amygdalectomy. These should be approached with extreme caution, and the question should be asked whether in recommending such radical measures there might be some punitive aspect.

An in-patient unit for self-harmers

An in-patient unit for self-harmers was planned during 1991, and opened in 1992 (Crowe 1994). It began as one half of a general ward, sharing with a unit devoted to the care of psychiatrically ill health professionals. This produced some complicated relationships in which the health professional patients tried to 'mother' the self-harmers, and in some cases developed similar symptoms themselves. The combined unit remained together for 2 years, but in 1995 the self-harmers' unit moved to a smaller ward for its exclusive use. The unit is now known as the 'Crisis Recovery Unit', a title which was chosen by the in-patients themselves, who also prefer to be known as 'residents' rather than patients (though here for the sake of clarity I will use the term 'patient'). It is a 12-bedded unit, with a consultant psychiatrist, senior registrar and registrar, a clinical nurse leader and full nursing staff, psychologist, occupational therapist and social worker.

The management protocols of the unit have changed somewhat since it first opened, mainly through staff discussion and experimentation. From the beginning there was a policy of treating the self-harm itself in a matter of fact way, asking the patients in milder cases of self-harm to apply Steri-strips and to clean their own wounds, but bringing the junior doctors in to suture the deeper wounds, and sending the patient to an accident unit to deal with any life-threatening injury. There was, however, at first a policy of preventing self-harm by isolating those patients who were doing it most frequently, if necessary under Section 3 of the Mental Health Act (1983), and using close supervision to stop the behaviour. It was found that it was possible in this way to stop much of the behaviour, but at the price of the staff taking responsibility for the patient, and the patient doing everything he or she could to outwit the staff and obtain the materials for self-harm.

It was in response to this stand-off situation that the multidisciplinary group decided that it would be preferable to allow these very disturbed patients more freedom and responsibility, and this led to a slight increase in the frequency and severity of self-harm, but also to a greatly increased level of staff–patient cooperation and a greater degree of satisfaction among both groups. The 'retention of responsibility' approach which this led to has continued for 3 years, with a good deal of self-harm, but a general atmosphere of goodwill, which has worked to the benefit of the patients. The problems mainly arise in relation to patients who are very unmotivated to improve, and have such severe self-destructive wishes that they are actively suicidal much of the time. In these cases, we are sometimes forced to resort to detention under the Mental Health Act and to prevent self-harm by close supervision. This can, of course, only be sustained for a relatively short time, after which the patient may either be sufficiently recovered to be released from the Section, or has to be transferred to a more conventional unit where he or she can be nursed under close supervision.

The management of overdosage is also rather unconventional, especially with the very commonly used paracetamol. If a patient reports a paracetamol overdose, the staff will ask how many tablets have been taken. The duty doctor is then asked to see the patient, and if there is any clinical concern, he or she will be sent to the Accident and Emergency department. If, however, there is no worry about the patient's physical state, he or she may be given a course of methionine by mouth, blood will be taken (4 hours after the overdose) for laboratory analysis of paracetamol levels, and the patient observed. In most cases, this procedure is satisfactory, and in only a very few is it necessary to resort to a late referral to the Accident and Emergency department following blood tests.

The unit is open to patients aged between 17 and 40 years old, male or female (but in practice there is a predominance of females), and in general they are with us because of a history of self-harm which has become difficult for the referring psychiatric unit to manage. A high proportion of referrals are accepted, but there are some factors which lead to exclusion at the assessment interview. These are a history of recent fire setting or interpersonal violence, severe substance abuse, severe psychosis, a moderate or severe degree of learning difficulties, or poor motivation to attempt to work on the problem. Patients who are detained under the Mental Health Act may be accepted, but must become Informal (released from detention) before transfer to the unit.

At admission, there is a full history and mental state examination, and medication is usually continued, although with a general aim to reduce this as far as possible. There is a 3-week period of assessment, with more observation than active therapeutic input, and then a team decision is made whether to continue for the full 5-month admission period. Each patient has a primary team of three nurses. Throughout the admission, there are regular meetings with members of the team, who usually each have a particular role for the patient (for example, to deal with general fears of social situations, to help with memories of prior sexual abuse, or to discuss family problems). The psychologist or social worker may take on specific tasks in this area for some patients, and the junior doctor deals with medical issues. There are regular staff meetings, and all information about the patients is shared, while 'secrets' between a patient and a staff member are discouraged (see Main 1957). There is also a general rule that staff should not tell the patient that he or she is doing well, since in many patients this induces a sense of panic that people are expecting too much, and it may lead to another act of self-harm. Instead, it is customary to say that he or she has been 'working very hard' but that there is a long way to go. In a similar vein, it is better not to talk about 'cure' with this very damaged group of patients, but rather to state that the end of the admission on the unit will be 'another stepping stone' towards better adjustment.

There is a daily morning community group meeting, followed by a staff discussion. It is interesting that often there is a parallel 'post-group discussion' among the patients, at which no doubt equally valid comments and suggestions are made. There is an evening evaluation group, usually quite well attended, and on most evenings there is also an informal activity for patients and sometimes also the staff—for example, a visit to the cinema or a ball game in the hospital grounds.

In addition to the community groups, there is a weekly 'small group' run by the registrar and a senior nurse, which deals in more intimate detail with some of the difficult issues brought by patients. The group is attended also by recently discharged patients, who often bring a sense of reality to the discussions in helping the current patients to understand how it is out in the community as opposed to the ward.

There are a number of occupational therapy activities, including projective art sessions, assertiveness groups, living skills groups and the 'peer evaluation group', in which each attender evaluates progress over the last week and plans his or her activities for the next week.

When crises occur on the ward, and these are not rare events, there is usually an emergency group, attended by all available residents and staff, at which the situation is discussed. The group does not, however, decide the action to be taken, but often suggests specific ideas which may be taken up by the staff.

Much of the daily interactive work with the patients is done by their primary nurse, who is assigned to them as part of a three-nurse team (to cover shift work and annual leave) on a continuing basis. The primary nurse (or associate nurse) is the person to whom the patient will go in a crisis, and there are also planned meetings, weekly or more often. At these meetings any topic of importance is discussed, but in those who give a history of abuse, and are strong enough psychologically to manage the stress involved, abuse counselling is carried out. This is cognitive in nature, along the lines of post-traumatic counselling, but also uses some of the techniques advocated by Dolan (1991) (see above). These include the writing of letters to the abuser and other significant persons inside or outside the family, which are generally not sent but discussed with the primary nurse. Another useful approach is the appropriate attribution of blame and the reduction of guilt for what has happened. We try to utilize the patient's strengths to help them 'plan safety' with the primary nurse, and to try to dissociate themselves from negative emotions and attitudes which belong to the past rather than the present. There is a great deal of other discussion taking place in these planned sessions, depending on what is most important for the patient at that particular time, and when discharge approaches, the emphasis often changes to the topics of ending the therapeutic relationship and retaining the skills which have been learned while on the unit.

In some cases, the patient has continuing contact with the family of origin or with partner and children. In these cases it is often helpful to hold family or couple therapy sessions, usually led by the consultant or the social worker. In contrast to more traditional family sessions, however, these are more restricted in what can be discussed, and the patient will often ask the therapist not to raise certain issues (such as prior abuse) because of the painful emotions aroused. Typical themes which may be dealt with include the necessity of listening more carefully to the patient and giving them their own 'space' at home. It is also useful in these sessions to try to dispel high expectations of 'cure', and to help the parents to accept that small improvements are worth while.

In response to the general regime described here, many patients say that it is refreshing not to be treated by the staff as a freak, but rather as a normal human being. This is in contrast to what may be done on other units, where in general psychiatric wards they may be seen as attention-seeking or otherwise undeserving, and in Accident and Emergency departments they may be treated with little sympathy because they have caused their own injuries. The regime seems to be beneficial for some of the patients, who can build self-esteem while on the unit which they can maintain after discharge.

PATIENTS ADMITTED, 1992–1996

Details of the patients admitted to the unit from its commencement in July 1992 until the present are summarized in Table 10.1. It will be seen that they are a predominantly young group, and that females outnumber males. In the original referrals, the gender difference was not so marked, but our assess-

Table 10.1 Details of patients admitted 1992–1996.

No. of patients admitted: 74 (12 male, 62 female)
Mean age: 26 years (range, 17–48 years)
No. of patients giving a history of sexual abuse: 44 (59%)
No. of patients who had ever married or cohabited: 33
No. of patients who had carried out cutting or similar self-harm: 58
Self-harmers who gave a history of sexual abuse: 38 (63%)
No. of overdose takers (many of whom were also cutters): 49
Diagnoses
   Borderline personality disorder: 58
   Sociopathic personality: 3
   Schizoid personality: 1
   Schizophrenia: 3
   Temporal lobe epilepsy: 2
   Autism: 1

---

ment process seems to favour females, perhaps because of the greater tendency to interpersonal violence in males.

Self-mutilators make up more than half of the total, but proportionally they make a greater impact on the atmosphere of the ward than the other patients. There is often a sense of drama about them which is not seen with depressive or more conventionally suicidal patients. The degree of handicap with such patients is great, and many of them have been hospitalized for long periods in conventional units before coming to the present one. As will be seen from Table 10.2, 14 of the patients were unable to be discharged from in-patient status when they left the unit, and most of these 14 remained under Section 3 of the Mental Health Act when they left us. On the other hand, more patients were able to return to the community after discharge than had been admitted from the community, thus suggesting a degree of progress.

One source of disappointment is that, because of hospital policy and geographical distance, it is not possible to follow-up many of these patients following discharge. From the work of both the cognitive (Linehan 1993) and psychodynamic therapists (Feldman 1988), it appears that the best form of long-term management of such problems is by a reliable and non-threatening relationship with one person or one team of people. There is the possibility in our setting of continued out-patient care by the team, but this is only available in a minority of cases, again because of distance and policy in the present National Health Service. Those who do attain out-patient care after

Table 10.2 Progress of patients through the unit (mean length of stay, 4.6 months; range, 1 week to 18 months).

	No. of patients		
	In-patient unit	Out-patient unit	Prison
Admitted from	22	50	2
Discharged to	14	60	

Of the 58 self-mutilators, 32 had significantly reduced the frequency of this at the time of discharge, and 23 had made no change in frequency.

admission are, by definition, less severely ill than those who have to be transferred back to in-patient care, but in spite of this it seems that both groups take up less health service time and money in the year after discharge from our unit than in the year before admission.

EFFECTS ON THE STAFF OF WORKING WITH
THIS PATIENT GROUP

The staff members who show the greatest amount of stress on this unit are the nurses. Medical staff, psychologists, social workers and occupational therapists can all leave the ward more readily than nurses, and tend not to be excessively affected by the unit. Nurses, however, are not able because of their working practices to leave during their shift, and the stress resulting from this is shown in various ways. A survey done on the ward during a fairly stressful period (Ritter *et al.* 1995) compared our nurses with those on two more typical wards. The nurses on this unit had twice as much sick leave as the control nurses (15 days per year compared to 8), and noticed more symptoms of burnout, but were still able to show a high degree of empathy with the patients. There was also a generally high level of satisfaction with their work, as shown by discussion with the researchers.

There are three staff support groups per week, which mitigate some of the stress factors. The first is a 45-minute multidisciplinary staff discussion group, the second a 90-minute group led by an outside facilitator and attended mostly by nurses, and the third is a supervision group for those of all professions who are dealing with survivors of childhood sexual abuse. These groups provide a focus for the airing of problems and dissatisfactions among the staff, and they also facilitate the discussion of particular patients who are causing unusual degrees of stress. In the groups, and the less frequent general staff discussion days, it becomes possible to discuss new initiatives in the management of patients, and to suggest changes of policy.

Conclusions

The syndrome of deliberate self-harm is not a very common one, but it attracts more attention both from Accident and Emergency departments and from psychiatric units than many other conditions. There has been an increased degree of interest in these patients in recent years, partly because of the work of Favazza, who has devoted his working life to the condition, and perhaps because of a genuine increase in the incidence of the problem. Although the repeated self-harm seen in patients with personality disorder comes most readily to the notice of psychiatrists, self-harm is probably more common in absolute terms in learning difficulty and forensic settings than in personality disordered patients. The history of prior sexual abuse is seen in a high proportion of these patients, but it is not entirely clear whether the abuse by itself contributes to the problem or whether the emotional and other forms of deprivation in these families is a more powerful influence.

The behaviour seems to be maintained by its tension-relieving properties, by the continued low self-esteem of the patients, and perhaps by some sort of biological addiction to the consequences. It is a very difficult form of behaviour to eradicate, and may persist for years: on the other hand, there is a tendency for it to remit spontaneously after the age of about 40, and elderly self-harmers are very rare.

The management of the problem is not easy, and many different regimes have been suggested. General ward management should include a matter-of-fact approach to the self-harm, without too much attention, but encouragement for the patients to live as normal a life as possible. If possible, the patients should be allowed to self-harm to a limited extent without preventive measures or detention, but this depends on a strong and tolerant ward regime. Support for the nursing staff should be available, and a united multidisciplinary team will help in management. Many forms of medication may be used, for the various specific symptoms, but it may be that SSRI (specific serotonin reuptake inhibitors) antidepressants have a particular place in management. Psychotherapy of various sorts may be helpful, preferably with a medium to long-term course; psychodynamic, cognitive and other therapies have been advocated, and in cases of prior sexual abuse a post-traumatic counselling approach can be used.

With good general and specific management and the minimum of stigmatization it is possible to help even the most entrenched and self-destructive patients towards rehabilitation, and it is to be hoped that in future a more humane and less punitive attitude will emerge towards this unfortunate group of patients.

References

American Psychiatric Association (1994) *Diagnostic and Statistical Manual of Mental Disorders*, 4th edn (DSM-IV). American Psychiatric Association, Washington, D.C.

Briere, J. & Zaidi, L.Y. (1989) Sexual abuse histories and sequelae in female psychiatric emergency room patients. *American Journal of Psychiatry* 146, 1602–1606.

Corter, H., Wolfson, A. & Locke, B. (1971) A comparison of procedures for eliminating self-injurious behaviour of retarded adolescents. *Journal of Applied Behaviour Analysis* 4, 201–203.

Crowe, M. (1994) The multidisciplinary team in the management of patients with deliberate self-harm. Paper presented at the XI International Symposium for the Psychotherapy of Schizophrenia, June 12–16, 1994, Washington, D.C.

De Shazer, S., Berg, I., Lipchik, E. *et al.* (1986) Brief therapy: Focused solution developments. *Family Process* 25, 207–222.

Dolan, Y. (1991) *Resolving Sexual Abuse*. W.W. Norton & Co., New York.

Favazza, A. (1989) Why patients mutilate themselves. *Hospital and Community Psychiatry* 40, 137–145.

Favazza, A. (1996) *Bodies under Siege: Self-mutilation and Body Modification in Culture and Psychiatry*, 2nd edn. Johns Hopkins University Press, Baltimore, Md.

Feldman, M.D. (1988) The challenge of self-mutilation: A review. *Comprehensive Psychiatry* 29, 252–269.

Johnson, F., Frankel, B., Ferrence, R., Jarvis, G. & Whitehead, P. (1975) Self-injury in London, Canada. *Canadian Journal of Public Health* 66, 307–316.

Kahan, J. & Pattison, E. (1984) Proposal for a distinctive diagnosis: The deliberate self-harm syndrome. *Suicide and Life-threatening Behavior* 14, 17–35.

Kernberg, O. (1987) A psychodynamic approach. *Journal of Personality Disorders* 1, 344–346.

Kraupl Taylor, F. (1969) Prokaletic measures derived from psychoanalytic techniques. *British Journal of Psychiatry* 115, 407–419.

Kreitman, N. & Casey, P. (1988) Repetition of parasuicide: An epidemiological and clinical study. *British Journal of Psychiatry* 153, 792–800.

Lacey, J.H. & Evans, C.D.H. (1986) The impulsivist: A multi-impulsive personality disorder. *British Journal of Addiction* 81, 641–649.

Linehan, M. (1993) *Cognitive-Behavioural Treatment of Personality Disorder*. Guilford Press, New York.

Main, T.F. (1957) The ailment. *British Journal of Medical Psychology* 30, 129–145.

Markovitz, P., Calabrese, J., Schulz, S.C. & Meltzer, H.Y. (1991) Fluoxetine in the treatment of borderline and schizotypal personality disorders. *Americal Journal of Psychiatry* 148, 1064–1067.

Mullen, P.E., Martin, J.L., Anderson, J.C., Romans, S.E. & Herbison, G.P. (1993) Childhood sexual abuse and mental health in adult life. *British Journal of Psychiatry* 163, 721–732.

Ritter, S., Tolchard, B. & Stewart, R. (1995) Coping with stress in mental health nursing. In: *Stress and Coping in Mental Health Nursing* (eds J. Carson, L. Fergin & S. Ritter), pp. 161–179. Chapman & Hall, London.

Robinson, A. & Duffy, J. (1989) A comparison of self-injury and self-poisoning from the Regional Poisoning Treatment Centre, Edinburgh. *Acta Psychiatrica Scandinavica* 80, 272–279.

Ryle, A., Poynton, A. & Brockman, B. (1989) *Cognitive Analytic Therapy*. John Wiley, Chichester.

Salkovskis, P., Atha, C. & Storer, D. (1990) Cognitive-behavioural problem solving in the treatment of patients who repeatedly attempt suicide: A controlled trial. *British Journal of Psychiatry* 157, 871–876.

Tantam, D. & Whittaker, J. (1992) Personality disorder and self-wounding. *British Journal of Psychiatry* 161, 451–464.

Walsh, B.W. & Rosen, P.M. (1988) *Self-Mutilation: Theory, Research and Treatment*. Guilford Press, New York.

World Health Organization (1992) *The ICD-10 Classification of Mental and Behavioural Disorders. Clinical Descriptions and Diagnostic Guidelines*. World Health Organization, Geneva.

CHAPTER 11

Recurrent Brief Depression: 'Nasty, Brutish and Short'

DAVID S. BALDWIN AND
JULIA M.A. SINCLAIR

Introduction

Psychiatrists and general practitioners are well aware of the importance of distinguishing between depressive symptoms, syndromes and disorders. This awareness arises from clinical practice, but is also partly due to the development of operationalized criteria for making the diagnosis of depression, from early approaches such as the Feighner criteria (Feighner *et al.* 1972), and the Research Diagnostic Criteria (RDC) (Spitzer *et al.* 1978), to current schemes including the clinical descriptions included within the ICD-10 system of the World Health Organization (WHO 1992), and the DSM-IV classification produced by the American Psychiatric Association (APA 1994). The various diagnostic systems have employed somewhat differing definitions of depressive illness: for example, the criteria for 'major' depression vary with respect to the range and severity of symptoms, the duration of illness, and the social and occupational consequences of the disorder (Table 11.1).

However, psychiatrists see a rather unrepresentative sample of depressed patients, being particularly likely to see the most severely ill, and those with comorbid disorders (Shepherd *et al.* 1981). Because of this, definitions of depression which are exclusively derived from samples of psychiatric in-patients may have only little relevance in primary care settings, where many depressed patients do not fulfil the accepted criteria for major depression, either because their illness is too mild or too short, too long or without social consequences. As such, the more recent classifications have included a number of 'by-product' depressive disorders, in an attempt to describe and include these important groups of patients, who otherwise could not be allocated a diagnosis. For example, both the DSM-IV classification and the ICD-10 system include dysthymia (a chronic mild depressive state), and the

Table 11.1 Diagnostic criteria for 'major' depressive disorders. (From Angst *et al.* (1990); adapted to include ICD-10 and DSM-IV.)

	Feighner *et al.* (1972)	RDC (Spitzer *et al.* 1978) Major	RDC (Spitzer *et al.* 1978) Minor	DSM-III (APA 1980)	DSM-III-R (APA 1987)	ICD-10 (WHO 1992)	DSM-IV (APA 1994)
Low or dysphoric mood	+	+	+	+	+	−*	−†
Duration (weeks)	4	2	1	2	2	2‡	2
Symptoms§	5/8	5/8	2/16	4/8	5/9	4/10	5/9
Impairment	No	Yes	No	No	No	Yes	Yes
Recurrence¶	No	No	No	No	No	No	No

* ICD-10 depressive episode (F32) requires presence of at least two of three 'typical' symptoms (depressed mood, loss of interest and enjoyment, and reduced energy).
† DSM-IV major depressive episode requires presence of at least one of two symptoms (depressed mood, loss of interest or pleasure).
‡ ICD-10 depressive episode can be diagnosed earlier than 2 weeks, if symptoms are unusually severe and of rapid onset.
§ Refers to minimum number of symptoms required for diagnosis.
¶ Recurrence required to make diagnosis.

ICD-10 also incorporates recurrent brief depression depressive disorder (RBD) within the group of mood disorders.

Historical background: development of the concept of recurrent brief depression

Recurrent brief depression is not a 'new' disorder. Short and mild depressive and hypomanic states were subsumed within the nosological category of manic depressive illness by Kraepelin in 1889 (Kraepelin 1921). Transient episodes of severe affective disturbance were described over 80 years ago (Strohmeyer 1914; Gregory 1915). A disorder similar to modern conceptions of RBD was delineated by 1929 (Paskind 1929), and was regarded as being of particular importance in primary-care settings. Patients were described as suffering from depressive episodes that were short-lived (lasting from a few hours to a few days), but which tended to recur over the course of many years. Further early accounts of this condition emphasized both the personality characteristics of the patients and the increased risk of suicide (Read 1929; Buzzard *et al.* 1930).

Despite its early recognition, and obvious clinical importance, the syndrome of RBD was not subject to extensive investigation over the next 40 years. The Research Diagnostic Criteria (Spitzer *et al.* 1978) included a category that recognized the existence of depressions that were intermittent but classified them as a form of 'minor' depression in contrast to 'major' depression, implying that it was a mild disorder, of lesser clinical importance.

Although many studies of the prevalence of patients with mild or transient affective disturbances in the general population have been performed, investigations of the longitudinal incidence and course of these disorders have been rather uncommon. In recent years, however, this situation has changed. The Zurich Study (Angst *et al.* 1984), a prospective epidemiological investigation of depressive, neurotic and psychosomatic syndromes, was the first to lead to a renewed and increased awareness of the clinical importance of short-lived but recurring and often severe episodes of depression.

THE ZURICH STUDY

In this investigation, a sample of young people from the Canton of Zurich in Switzerland has been interviewed repeatedly over a period of over 15 years. The design of the study and characteristics of the sample have been described fully elsewhere (Angst *et al.* 1984). People within the cohort have been examined on many separate occasions, using a specially designed interview schedule known as the SPIKE (Illes 1991). This instrument covers a range of psychological and somatic syndromes, each of which is assessed according to the presence and number of its component symptoms, their duration, frequency and consequences, the treatment received, and the presence of any family history.

Using the SPIKE data, Professor Angst and his colleagues showed that approximately half of those subjects who received treatment for depression do not fulfil DSM-III (APA 1980) criteria for major depression. These patients tended to experience depressive episodes that were rather short-lived, but otherwise indistinguishable from episodes of major depression. Furthermore, around half of this group of subjects suffered from brief depressions that recurred at least monthly and were associated with significant social and occupational impairment.

The Zurich Study indicates that some 5.0–9.5% of the general population experience intermittent brief depressions within any one year (Angst & Hochstrasser 1994). The period-prevalence over the 10-year period when the sample were aged between 20 and 30 years was approximately 11% (Angst 1992). The recognition of this important group of depressed patients has subsequently led to the development of diagnostic criteria for RBD.

Diagnostic criteria for recurrent brief depression

The 'Zurich criteria', as proposed by Professor Angst (Angst & Dobler-Mikola 1985; Angst *et al.* 1990), stipulate that RBD is akin to DSM-III major depression in respect of symptoms: and similar to the Research Diagnostic Criteria (Spitzer *et al.* 1978) with respect to occupational impairment (Table 11.2). However, RBD differs from these two disorders, in that the depressive episodes last less than 2 weeks, but recur at least monthly over 1 year.

Broadly similar criteria for RBD are included within the ICD-10 (Table 11.3). Depressive episodes must last less than 2 weeks, and should occur approximately monthly over a period of 1 year. The DSM-IV places RBD within Appendix B, which represents a group of proposed mental disorders, worthy of further investigation (Table 11.4).

Table 11.2 Recurrent brief depression: Zurich criteria. (From Angst & Dobler-Mikola 1985.)

---

1 Dysphoric mood or loss of interest or pleasure
2 Four out of eight symptoms as listed for DSM-III major depression
   • poor appetite or significant weight loss (when not dieting) or increased appetite or significant weight gain
   • insommia or hypersomnia
   • psychomotor agitation or retardation
   • loss of interest or pleasure in usual activities, or decrease in sexual drive
   • loss of energy, fatigue
   • feelings of worthlessness, self-reproach, or excessive or inappropriate guilt
   • diminished ability to think or concentrate, slowed thinking or indecisiveness
   • recurrent thoughts of death, suicidal ideation, wishes to be dead, or suicide attempts
3 Present less than 2 weeks but recurring at least monthly over 1 year
4 Reduced subjective capacity at work

Table 11.3 Recurrent brief depressive disorder (ICD-10 F38.10) (WHO 1992).

Recurrent brief depressive episodes, occurring once a month over the past year. The individual depressive episodes all last less than 2 weeks (typically 2–3 days, with complete recovery) but fulfil the symptomatic criteria for mild, moderate, or severe depressive episode (F32.0, F32.1, F32.2)

Differential diagnosis
In contrast to those with dysthymia (F34.1), patients are not depressed for the majority of the time. If the depressive episodes occur only in relation to the menstrual cycle, F38.8 should be used with a second code for the underlying cause (N94.8, other specified conditions associated with female genital organs and menstrual cycle)

Table 11.4 Research criteria for recurrent brief depressive disorder (APA 1994).

A   Criteria, except for duration, are met for a major depressive episode
B   The depressive periods in Criterion A last at least 2 days but less than 2 weeks
C   The depressive periods occur at least once a month for 12 consecutive months and are not associated with the menstrual cycle
D   The periods of depressed mood cause clinically significant distress or impairment in social, occupational, or other important areas of functioning
E   The symptoms are not due to the direct physiological effects of a substance (e.g. a drug of abuse, a medication) or a general medical condition (e.g. hypothyroidism)
F   There has never been a major depressive episode and criteria are not met for dysthymic disorder
G   There has never been a manic episode, a mixed episode or a hypomanic episode and criteria are not met for cyclothymic disorder. *Note*: This exclusion does not apply if all of the manic-, mixed-, or hypomanic-like episodes are substance or treatment induced
H   The mood disturbance does not occur exclusively during schizophrenia, schizophreniform disorder, schizoaffective disorder, delusional disorder, or psychotic disorder not otherwise specified

RESULTS OF FURTHER EPIDEMIOLOGICAL STUDIES

The results of the recent World Health Organization study (Weiller *et al.* 1994) of the psychological disorders seen in primary-care settings provide further evidence for the existence of RBD. From a group of 9697 consecutive general practice attenders, a sample of 1911 underwent a structured psychiatric interview. The point prevalence of RBD was found to be 3.7%, with women being more frequently afflicted. Comorbidity with other psychiatric disorders was widespread, being especially common with major depression and generalized anxiety disorder. The lifetime rate of suicidal behaviour in this primary-care sample was 14%.

Further epidemiological investigations have been able to confirm the validity of the diagnosis of RBD. For example, a sample of 300 patients in primary care was assessed with respect to the number of symptoms they experienced, and the length of any depressive episodes. Brief depression was defined according to the Zurich criteria, and minor depression was regarded as being a 'sub-threshold' condition, characterized by the presence of only three or four depressive symptoms. The point prevalence of brief depression in this sample was found to be 30%, strictly defined RBD having a point prevalence of 5.4%. The validity of brief depression, as assessed by demographic and clinical variables, appeared greater than that of minor depression (Maier *et al.* 1994).

A fourth investigation (Altamura *et al.* 1995), performed in both urban and rural areas of Sardinia, Italy, has also found that RBD is not uncommon in the general population. Using a structured interview, the lifetime prevalence of RBD was found to be 6.9%, being similarly common in men and women, and showing little variation with age. Once again, RBD was associated with an increased risk of suicidal behaviour (9.1%), and comorbidity with other forms of mental disorder was common, particularly with major depression. Subjects with 'combined' depression (i.e. major depression and RBD) appeared to be at particular risk of suicidal behaviour.

Recurrent brief depression and major depression: differences, similarities, overlap

The results of the Zurich Study suggest that RBD is as stable a diagnosis as major depression. Some 20% of people with RBD report episodes of major depression when followed up, with a similar proportion showing a change in the opposite direction, i.e. from major depression to RBD (Angst *et al.* 1990; Angst & Hochstrasser 1994). The term 'combined depression' has been suggested as being suitable to describe the group of patients whose depressions vary in length, with prolonged episodes becoming superimposed on an underlying pattern of intermittent brief depressive episodes. The Zurich Study therefore allows a comparison of subjects who fulfil criteria for 'pure' RBD, with those who are recognized as suffering from either major depression, or from combined depression (Angst *et al.* 1990).

The 1-year prevalence of RBD is approximately 7%, which is greater than that of major depression. The three forms of depression (RBD, major, combined) all have a female predominance, this being especially marked in the group of patients with combined depression. There are no significant differences between RBD and major depression in terms of social class, although the social class of father and level of education of the proband were higher among cases of combined depression. Adults with RBD report a significantly greater mean number of childhood emotional and behavioural problems than that described by adults with major depression. The increased rates of childhood anxiety among adults with RBD is particularly notable. More than half of subjects with RBD and 70% of people with combined depression describe themselves as being more anxious and fearful than their peers throughout childhood. All three groups of patients report a similarly increased number of somatic disorders, when compared to the general population, with increased rates of gastrointestinal, cardiac and circulation syndromes, and sexual and eating problems (Angst *et al.* 1990).

The clinical characteristics of RBD, major depression and combined depression are rather similar. Although 'difficulty in thinking' is more frequent in patients with major depression, the clinical features of the two conditions are otherwise hard to distinguish. For example, the mean age of onset of illness, rates of family history of depression, and the proportion of subjects presenting for treatment do not differ (Angst *et al.* 1990). RBD shows a greater degree of comorbidity with panic disorder than does major depression, but a lesser association with dysthymia (Angst & Hochstrasser 1994).

The Zurich Study indicates that subjects with RBD have an increased risk of suicidal behaviour (11.4%) when compared to the general population. The lifetime risk of attempted suicide in RBD is similar to that for major depression. The risk is even greater in combined depression, where approximately 30% of patients had attempted suicide by the age of 28 years (Angst *et al.* 1990).

Investigations in clinical samples

Epidemiological investigations of RBD are now being supplemented by the results of clinical studies. For example, in two early double-blind placebo-controlled investigations of the effects of psychotropic drugs in the secondary prevention of suicidal behaviour (Montgomery *et al.* 1979, 1983), the reappearance of short-lived but severe episodes of depression was found to be significantly associated with subsequent deliberate self-harm. A number of more recent prospective studies have attempted to examine the length, severity and periodicity of brief depressive episodes with rather more accuracy than was possible in these earlier investigations.

Regular and frequent assessments of a large number of psychiatric out-patients, performed over a number of years, have revealed that the duration of brief depressive episodes shows an approximately 'normal' distribution, around a median length of 3–4 days (Montgomery *et al.* 1990). Approximately 90% of episodes resolve within 2 weeks, and therefore do not fulfil the duration criterion for major depression. The severity of the depressive episodes has been measured in a variety of ways but mainly through use of the Montgomery–Asberg Depression Rating Scale (MADRS; Montgomery & Asberg 1979). The mean severity of depression as measured by the MADRS is around 30, but with substantial variation from one episode to the next. The episodes are of similar severity to those in patients with major depression (Montgomery *et al.* 1990). The recurrence rate (the time from the onset of one episode to the onset of the subsequent one) is variable, with a median interval of approximately 18 days. The periodicity of the episodes is irregular, with some 95% occurring more frequently than every 8 weeks, but with only two thirds showing a monthly recurrence. Depressive symptoms are present for only 15–20% of the total period of follow-up (Montgomery *et al.* 1989, 1990).

Distinction from bipolar illness, cyclothymia and dysthymia

Depressive episodes in patients with RBD are usually sudden in onset, last a few days only, and then resolve rapidly. This rapidly shifting picture suggests a possible link with bipolar illness or rapid cycling affective disorder. However, data from epidemiological investigations and clinical observations indicate that such a link, if present at all, is not strong. The Zurich Study found that subjects with RBD had lower rates of mania or hypomania (2.2%) than subjects with either major depressive episodes (5.9%) or no depressive disorder (5.0%) (Angst *et al.* 1990; Angst & Hochstrasser 1994). In the clinical sample, only a small proportion of patients with RBD developed manic or hypomanic episodes during follow-up. Mania or hypomania was seen in 3.0% of the 'pure' RBD group, the rate being somewhat higher in patients with combined depression (D.B. Montgomery *et al.* 1992).

Other differential diagnoses to consider when assessing patients with probable RBD include cyclothymia and dysthymia. In the ICD-10 system, cyclothymia is described as a persistent instability of mood involving numerous periods of mild depression and mild elation. The instability develops in early adult life and tends to persist for many years, despite lengthy periods of normal mood. In clinical samples, there is minimal overlap with cyclothymia, for two reasons. First, when followed up over many months and years, very few patients with brief depression experience episodes of elation. Secondly, episodes of depression in subjects with RBD are simply too severe to be understood as manifestations of cyclothymia, which often goes unnoticed because the underlying mood changes are not as obvious as changes in activity and self-confidence. By contrast, RBD is a serious and disruptive illness (S.A. Montgomery *et al.* 1992).

Patients suffering from RBD may sometimes be misdiagnosed as suffering from dysthymia. Recollection of affect is often poor, particularly after a few months, and it is possible that patients and doctors tend to merge discrete short episodes of depression into chronic dysthymia. However, there is little overlap between RBD and dysthymic disorder, both in epidemiological samples (Angst *et al.* 1990) and in clinical samples. As depressive symptoms are present for only 15–20% of the total period of follow-up in prospective investigations, patients with RBD do not fulfil the diagnostic criteria for dysthymia (Montgomery *et al.* 1989, 1990).

Furthermore, RBD does not appear to be linked to either premenstrual or menstrual difficulties. As a condition, RBD is not uncommon in men (4.2% 1-year prevalence, compared to 10.3% in women), and in women is no more linked to the menstrual cycle than is major depression (Angst *et al.* 1990). Furthermore, prospective investigations in clinical samples have not been able to find any obvious relationship with the menstrual cycle (Montgomery *et al.* 1989, 1990).

Pharmacological treatment

Recurrent brief depression has been formally recognized only recently, and as yet no treatment is established. Most patients seem to recognize the intermittent nature of their disorder, but some present to doctors whilst acutely depressed, demanding treatment. It is probably misguided to attempt to manage acute episodes of RBD with psychotropic drugs, as the episode will usually have resolved before any agent has become effective. However, it seems sensible to advise patients to limit their consumption of alcohol and to avoid benzodiazepines, in view of the reported tendency for these drugs to cause disinhibition.

Few formal investigations of the long-term treatment of patients with RBD have been published. However, the results of a number of double-blind placebo-controlled studies of the secondary prevention of suicidal behaviour in other diagnostic groups, such as patients with 'emotionally unstable character disorder', offer some limited guidance (Baldwin *et al.* 1991). Amitriptyline, for example, appears no different to placebo in reducing either suicidal thoughts or aggressive behaviour in patients with borderline or schizotypal personality disorder (Soloff *et al.* 1986). By contrast, the monoamine oxidase inhibitor tranylcypromine has been found helpful in reducing the affective instability and impulsivity that is seen in most patients with DSM-III borderline personality disorder (Cowdry & Gardner 1988), and monoamine oxidase inhibitors (MAOIs) may prove beneficial in the management of certain patients with RBD. Flupenthixol seems efficacious in reducing suicidal behaviour in subjects with suicidal behaviour and brief depressive episodes (Montgomery *et al.* 1983), and significant reductions in 'suicidality' have been seen in patients with borderline personality disorder, treated with trifluoperazine (Cowdry & Gardner 1988). Lithium is effective in reducing impulsivity and self-harm in a variety of patient groups (Wickham & Reed 1987), and may possibly prove helpful in the long-term treatment of RBD.

Fluoxetine has not been found helpful in the prevention of brief depressive episodes in patients prone to suicidal behaviour but not suffering from major depression (Montgomery *et al.* 1994) (Table 11.5). Fluoxetine, at a dosage of 60 mg twice weekly, was found to be no different to placebo in preventing brief depressive episodes and associated suicidal behaviour. Fluoxetine neither raised nor lowered the suicide rate, providing no evidence to support the role of fluoxetine in suicide prevention — or indeed the provocation of attempted suicide — in this group of patients (Montgomery *et al.* 1994). Treatment studies with paroxetine have also proved disappointing, preliminary findings revealing no clear benefit with active treatment (Kasper 1995).

Table 11.5 Secondary prevention of suicidal behaviour with fluoxetine: recurrence rate of brief depressive episodes. (From Montgomery *et al.* 1994.)

	Fluoxetine ($n = 54$)	Placebo ($n = 53$)
Number of episodes	159	157
Interval (days)	18.7	17.6
Suicide attempts	18	18
Suicide attempt rate	33.3%	34.0%

Psychological therapies

In the absence of established effective pharmacological treatments, it seems likely that the most helpful treatment approach for patients with RBD is to strengthen coping mechanisms. Non-directive psychodynamic or confrontational behavioural approaches may be viewed as vague and unhelpful or alternatively intrusive and counter-therapeutic (Montgomery 1994). Patients report some success with supportive approaches and non-intrusive advice, aimed at avoiding confrontation during episodes of depression. As many patients are irritable and sensitive to criticism whilst depressed, it seems sensible for them to avoid important meetings and emotionally charged situations, delaying them whenever possible until after the episode has resolved (Montgomery 1994). Other than this, it is not currently possible to recommend any form of psychological treatment, as no studies of psychotherapeutic approaches in RBD have been performed. Training in problem solving skills may be of value in preventing repetition of suicidal behaviour, and in theory at least could be helpful in the overall management of RBD.

Future research

The inclusion of RBD within the group of mood disorders in ICD-10 and the limited inclusion within DSM-IV is certain to lead to an increase in research activity. As the diagnosis is now accepted, there is a particular need for well-conducted prospective pharmacological treatment studies, particularly with lithium or anticonvulsants, which will necessarily involve a double-blind placebo-controlled design. Unfortunately, although the Zurich criteria are suitable for making the diagnosis in community samples, they are probably inadequate for treatment studies. For example, the requirement of a monthly recurrence rate leads to the exclusion of a number of severely ill patients, who may experience more than 12 episodes per year, but in an irregular fashion. Furthermore, as the retrospective recollection of affective symptoms is often poor, the stipulation that there should have been 1 year's worth of brief depressive episodes is rather unrealistic. For these reasons, a set of diagnostic criteria for efficacy studies in patients with RBD have been proposed (Montgomery *et al.* 1989) (Table 11.6).

In addition to well-designed treatment studies, future research activities should also attempt to elucidate the underlying pathophysiology of RBD. Epidemiological observations and clinical investigations suggest that RBD and major depression are similar in many respects. Those 'biological' investigations which have been undertaken tend to suggest that the two disorders

Table 11.6 Diagnostic criteria for efficacy studies in recurrent brief depression. (From Montgomery *et al.* 1989.)

---

1 Three or more short-lived (1 week or less) depressive episodes in the previous 3 months
2 Recurrent pattern (unspecified) of intermittent short episodes of depression over the previous year
3 At least two of the episodes in the previous 3 months should satisfy criteria for major depression according to DSM-III-R diagnostic system without the 2-week duration criterion
4 At least two of the episodes in the previous 3 months should be of moderate severity
5 No episode of major depression in the previous 6 months

---

have a similar pathophysiology. For example, patients with RBD or major depression do not differ with respect to non-suppression on the dexamethasone challenge test, blunting of the thyroid-stimulating hormone response to challenge with thyrotrophin-releasing hormone, or on shortening of rapid eye movement sleep latency (Staner *et al.* 1992). Longitudinal investigations and studies of the value of phototherapy should also be performed, as there may be a seasonal concentration of brief depressive episodes in some patients (Kasper *et al.* 1992).

Research should also be undertaken to investigate the inter-relationships and degree of overlap between RBD and personality disorder. The overlap between RBD and DSM-IV borderline personality disorder includes affective instability, impulsivity and self-damaging behaviour. Clearly, these phenomena can be understood either as manifestations of underlying maladaptive personality traits, or as features arising from a primary disorder of mood. Many patients with RBD may receive the diagnosis of 'personality disorder' as a result of the failure of doctors to recognize an important and serious disorder of mood. Further studies should attempt to investigate the inter-relationships of personality and mood, both during and between depressive episodes.

Conclusions

Detailed epidemiological investigations and painstaking clinical observations, performed over a 15-year period, have resulted in the recognition and acceptance of RBD as a distinct medical condition. Recurrent brief depression is a common and serious disorder, associated with significant morbidity and mortality. Unfortunately, there is at present no established treatment for patients with this damaging and disruptive illness. Without such a treatment, brief depressive episodes remain 'nasty, brutish and short', and patients suffering from RBD will continue to experience a sometimes protracted but often dangerous condition.

Acknowledgements

Many thanks to Professor Chris Thompson, Daniel Inman-Meron and Mrs Marie Carter of the University Department of Psychiatry in Southampton, and Dr Dinesh Bhugra of the Institute of Psychiatry in London.

References

Altamura, A.C., Carta, M.G., Carpinello, B. *et al.* (1995) Lifetime prevalence of brief recurrent depression (results from a community survey). *European Neuropsychopharmacology* 5 (Suppl.), 99–102.

American Psychiatric Association (1980) *Diagnostic and Statistical Manual of Mental Disorders*, 3rd edn (DSM-III). American Psychiatric Association, Washington, D.C.

American Psychiatric Association (1987) *Diagnostic and Statistical Manual of Mental Disorders*, 3rd edn, revised (DSM-III-R). American Psychiatric Association, Washington, D.C.

American Psychiatric Association (1994) *Diagnostic and Statistical Manual of Mental Disorders*, 4th edn (DSM-IV). American Psychiatric Association, Washington, D.C.

Angst, J. (1992) Epidemiology of depression. *Psychopharmacology* 106, S71–S74.

Angst, J. & Dobler-Mikola, A. (1985) The Zurich Study: A prospective study of depressive, neurotic and psychosomatic syndromes. IV. Recurrent and non-recurrent brief depression. *European Archives of Psychiatry and Neurological Sciences* 234, 408–416.

Angst, J. & Hochstrasser, B. (1994) Recurrent brief depression: the Zurich study. *Journal of Clinical Psychiatry* 55(4) (Suppl.), 3–9.

Angst, J., Dobler-Mikola, A. & Binder, J. (1984) The Zurich Study: A prospective epidemiological study of depressive, neurotic and psychosomatic syndromes. I. Problem, methodology. *European Archives of Psychiatry and Neurological Sciences* 234, 13–20.

Angst, J., Merinkangas, K., Scheidegger, P. & Wicki, W. (1990) Recurrent brief depression: A new subtype of affective disorder. *Journal of Affective Disorder* 19, 87–98.

Baldwin, D.S., Bullock, T., Montgomery, D.B. & Montgomery, S.A. (1991) 5-HT reuptake inhibitors, tricyclic antidepressants and suicidal behaviour. *International Clinical Psychopharmacology* 6, 49–55.

Buzzard, E.F., Miller, H.E., Riddoch, G. *et al.* (1930) Discussion on the diagnosis and treatment of the milder forms of the manic-depressive psychosis. *Proceedings of the Royal Society of Medicine* 23, 881–895.

Cowdry, R. & Gardner, D. (1988) Pharmacotherapy of borderline personality disorder: Alprazolam, carbamazepine, trifuoperazine, tranylcypromine. *Archives of General Psychiatry* 45, 111–119.

Feighner, J.P., Robins, E., Guze, S.B. *et al.* (1972) Diagnostic criteria for use in psychiatric research. *Archives of General Psychiatry* **26**, 57–63.

Gregory, M.S. (1915) Transient attacks of manic-depressive insanity. *Medical Record* (New York) **88**, 1040–1044.

Illes, P. (1991) Validierung des Fragebogens SPIKE an Diagnosen der Krankengeschichten des Sozialpsychiatrischen Dienstes Oerlikon. *Med Diss.* Zurich.

Kasper, S., Ruhrmann, S., Naase, T. & Moller, H.J. (1992) Recurrent brief depression and its relationship to seasonal affective disorder. *European Archives of Psychiatry and Clinical Neurological Sciences* **242**, 20–26.

Kasper, S., Stamenkovic, M. & Fischer, G. (1995) Recurrent brief depression. Diagnosis, epidemiology and potential pharmacological options. *CNS Drugs* **4**(3), 222–229.

Kraepelin, E. (1921) Manic depressive insanity and paranoia. In: *Eighth German Edition of the Textbook of Psychiatry*, Vols 3 and 4 (trans. M. Barclay). E. & S. Livingstone, Edinburgh.

Maier, W., Herr, R., Garsicke, M., Lichtermann, D., Kousharg, K. & Benkert, O. (1994) Recurrent brief depression in general practice: Clinical features, co-morbidity with other disorders, and needs for treatment. *European Archives of Psychiatry and Clinical Neurological Sciences* **244**, 196–204.

Montgomery, D.B., Green, M., Bullock, T., Baldwin, D.S. & Montgomery, S.A. (1992) Has recurrent brief depression a different pharmacology? *Clinical Neuropharmacology* **15** (Suppl. 1), 13a–14a.

Montgomery, D.B., Roberts, A., Green, M., Bullock, T., Baldwin, D.S. & Montgomery, S.A. (1994) Lack of efficacy of fluoxetine in recurrent brief depression and suicidal attempts. *European Archives of Psychiatry and Clinical Neurological Sciences* **244**, 211–215.

Montgomery, S.A. (1994) Recurrent brief depression. In: *Psychopharmacology of Depression* (eds S.A. Montgomery & T.H. Corn), pp. 129–140. Oxford Medical Publications, Oxford.

Montgomery, S.A. & Asberg, M. (1979) A new depression scale designed to be more sensitive to change. *British Journal of Psychiatry* **134**, 382–389.

Montgomery, S.A., Montgomery, D.B. & Bullock, T. (1992) Brief unipolar depressions: Is there a bipolar component? *L'Encephale* **18**, 41–43.

Montgomery, S.A., Roy, D. & Montgomery, D.B. (1983) The prevention of recurrent suicidal acts. *British Journal of Clinical Pharmacology* **13**, 183s–188s.

Montgomery, S.A., Montgomery, D.B., Baldwin, D.S. & Green, M. (1989) Intermittent 3-day depressions and suicidal behaviour. *Neuropsychobiology* **22**, 128–134.

Montgomery, S.A., Montgomery, D.B., Baldwin, D.S. & Green M. (1990) The duration, nature and recurrence rate of brief depressions. *Progress in Neuropsychopharmacological and Biological Psychiatry* **14**, 729–735.

Montgomery, S.A., Montgomery, D.B., McAuley, R., Rani, S.J., Roy, D.H. & Shaw, P.J. (1979) Maintenance therapy in repeat suicidal behaviour: A placebo controlled trial. In: *Proceedings of the 10th International Congress for Suicide Prevention and Crisis Intervention*, pp. 222–227.

Paskind, H.A. (1929) Brief attacks of manic-depressive depression. *Archives of Neurology and Psychiatry* (Chicago) **22**, 123–134.

Read, C.F. (1929) Discussion. *Archives of Neurology and Psychiatry* (Chicago) **22**, 133.

Shepherd, M., Cooper, B., Brown, A.C. & Kalton, G. (1981) *Psychiatric Illness in General Practice*, 2nd edn. Oxford University Press, London.

Soloff, P., George, A. & Nathan, S. (1986) Progress in pharmacotherapy of borderline disorders: A double blind study of amitriptyline, haloperidol and placebo. *Archives of General Psychiatry* **43**, 691–697.

Spitzer, R.L., Endicott, J. & Robins, E. (1978) Research Diagnostic Criteria: Rationale and reliability. *Archives of General Psychiatry* **53**, 731–785.

Staner, L., de la Fuente, J.M., Kerkhofs, M., Linkowski, P. & Mendlewicz, J. (1992) Biological and clinical features of recurrent brief depression: A comparison with major depressed and healthy subjects. *Journal of Affective Disorders* **26**, 241–245.

Strohmeyer, W. (1914) *Manisch-depressives Irresein*. Bergman, Wiesbaden.

Weiller, E., Lecrubier, Y., Maier, W. & Ustun, T.B. (1994) The relevance of recurrent brief depression in primary care. *European Archives of Psychiatry and Clinical Neurological Sciences* **244**, 182–189.

Wickham, B. & Reed, J. (1987) Lithium for the control of aggressive and self-mutilating behaviour. *International Clinical Psychopharmacology* **2**, 181–190.

World Health Organization (1992) *The ICD-10 Classification of Mental and Behavioural Disorders. Clinical Descriptions and Diagnostic Guidelines*. World Health Organization, Geneva.

CHAPTER 12

Paraphilias
PADMAL DE SILVA

Introduction

The term 'paraphilia' is a relatively new one, and it was introduced to replace the term 'sexual deviation' (Money 1984; American Psychiatric Association (APA) 1987). The latter term had itself been introduced by professionals and researchers to replace an even earlier term, 'sexual perversion', which was seen as derogatory and judgemental. Some authors have also used the term 'sexual variation' (e.g. Wilson 1987) as a synonym of these. There are thus political reasons and political considerations that have determined the terminology in this area; understandably so, as the liberal attitudes in Western society in recent decades have led to a questioning of the rights and wrongs of identifying as marginal groups, those that are different from the majority in their practices, desires, and preferences.

Essentially, a paraphilia is an attraction (*philia*) to something that is outside the normal range (*para*), in the sphere of sex. The person with a paraphilia is not necessarily seen as someone with a problem, and in need of treatment. As with most other psychiatric phenomena, the clinical diagnosis is made only if the person's behaviour or desires cause significant distress and/or impairment in important areas of functioning. In clinical practice, these problems are encountered only in a limited way (see Abel & Osborn 1992). It is clear that many people have paraphiliac desires and practices (e.g. fetishes) which do not lead to problems either for themselves or others. For this reason, clinicians see only a minority of paraphilias, and this is one of the reasons why the phenomenon is underdiagnosed. The ways in which paraphilias present in clinical settings will be discussed later in this chapter.

History and culture

It is important, at this point, to note that paraphilias have been recorded in
the literature over many centuries, across a diversity of cultures. Cultures
and subcultures have had different perspectives on what is a paraphilia. Bullough and Bullough (1995), among others, have discussed in some detail this
cultural—and historical—variability:

> There is a tremendous variety out there. The ancient Greeks, for
> example, not only tolerated but encouraged the love of adolescent
> boys by older men. In parts of New Guinea, males are initiated into
> manhood by sucking the penis of an older man. In India, male
> members of a cult that worships Radha, the favourite consort of the
> God Krishna, dress like women and affect the behaviour, movements
> and habits of women, including menstruation. Many of them in the
> past emasculated themselves and all are supposed to play the part of
> women during intercourse. (p. 41)

Some of the phenomena are discussed more fully in Bullough and Bullough (1976). They have also discussed the influence of religious views
and rules on what was considered acceptable and what was seen as deviant
in sex, a key concept in this realm being that of certain sexual practices
being against nature (Bullough & Bullough 1995). This also led to some
behaviours being described as criminal, as religion often determined what a
society should and should not accept as lawful. Discussions of aspects of this
matter are found in several early sources, including Russell and Greaves
(1877).

In the literature of Buddhism, there are numerous references to paraphiliac behaviours among the monastic community over two and a half millen-
nia ago. These come in the texts on discipline for the monks and nuns
(*Vinaya Pitaka*). The behaviours include bestiality, necrophilia, fetishism
and others.

Early clinical accounts

In the clinical literature, and in clinical traditions, the subject of paraphilias
had already begun to be extensively discussed by the second half of the 19th
century. The classic example, and in many ways the major pioneering work,
is of course Richard von Krafft-Ebing's *Psychopathia Sexualis*. This book,
with the subtitle *With Especial Reference to the Antipathic Sexual Instinct*,
was first published in 1887, and was translated from the German into

English within a decade. It was then revised in many later editions. In this book, the author, a neuropsychiatrist, discusses numerous sexual problems in detail, using copious case material. He details, among others, fetishism, which he called 'fetichism', flagellation, sadism, lust-murder, necrophilia, sadistic acts with animals, masochism, coprolagnia, exhibitionism, bondage, paedophilia ('violation of individuals under the age of fourteen'), sodomy, pederasty, bestiality and incest. To cite a case example of fetishism:

> Z began to masturbate at the age of 12. From that time he could not see a woman's handkerchief without having orgasm and ejaculation. He was irresistibly compelled to possess himself of it. At that time he was a choir boy and used the handkerchiefs to masturbate within the bell-tower close to the choir. But he chose only such handkerchiefs as had black and white borders or violet stripes running through them. At fifteen he had coitus. Later on he married. As a rule, he was only potent when he wound such a handkerchief around his penis. Often he preferred coitus between the thighs of a woman where he had placed a handkerchief. Whenever he espied a handkerchief, he did not rest until he was in possession of it. He always had a number of them in his pockets and around his penis. (Krafft-Ebing 1965, p. 169)

An example of bestiality is given below:

> In a provincial town a man was caught in intercourse with a hen. He was twenty years old, and of high social position. The chickens had been dying one after another, and the man causing it had been 'wanted' for a long time. To the question of the judge, as to the reason for such an act, the accused said that his genitals were so small that coitus with women was impossible. (Krafft-Ebing 1965, p. 375)

A final example from Krafft-Ebing:

> Mr X, forty-seven years of age, of high social position, came to me for advice on account of a troublesome anomaly of his sexual life. He was about to be married and in his present condition considered it morally impossible to enter upon matrimony. X was evidently heavily tainted—his father, two of his sisters and one brother were highly neurotic. The mother was presumed to have been a healthy woman. The sexual instinct awoke early in X; he began to masturbate spontaneously at the age of eleven. He was decidedly hypersexual, practiced masturbation with passion, and at the age of fourteen he forgot himself so far as to sodomise bitches, mares and

other female animals. He ascribed these acts to excessive sexual desire and to want of opportunity to satisfy his cravings in the normal way—he spent his childhood and boyhood in a lonely part of the country and later on he visited a boarding school. X admitted that he was quite conscious of the abomination of his acts, and said that he fought with all his will power against these bestial impulses. But the greed, the lust, the pleasure which they gave, always overpowered him. When grown up to manhood he never had homosexual desires, nor did he feel an inclination for women . . . [W]hen at the age of twenty-five he sought to improve his condition by coitus with a woman, he derived not the slightest satisfaction from it, although he was quite potent and the girl pleasing and sympathetic . . . The mere sight of animals excited him wildly. The society of ladies caused him *ennui*. When he was with a girl, she had to resort to all sorts of manipulations to prepare him for the act. (Krafft-Ebing 1965, pp. 379–380).

As can be seen, paraphilias as a clinical problem have been noted and discussed for some time, essentially for over a century. These historical accounts are of much interest, both as evidence that the phenomena and their clinical significance were recognized by our professional predecessors, and as providing insights into the problem behaviours themselves. In fact, some of Krafft-Ebing's observations are of much value even today, and his work is still frequently cited.

Current classifications of paraphilias

The following are the classes of paraphilias recognized in the *Diagnostic and Statistical Manual* (DSM-IV) of the American Psychiatric Association, in its latest version (APA 1994).

EXHIBITIONISM

The person has recurrent, intense, sexually arousing fantasies, urges or behaviours involving exposure of one's genitals to an unsuspecting stranger. Typically, exhibitionists are post-pubescent males who obtain high levels of excitement from exposing their genitals to one or a few females, most commonly strangers at or just past puberty. Exhibitionism is among the most common of the paraphilias (McConaghy 1993). It is found mostly in men. Sometimes the man masturbates while exposing.

VOYEURISM

The person has recurrent, intense, sexually arousing fantasies, sexual urges or behaviours involving the act of observing an unsuspecting person who is naked, in the process of disrobing, or engaged in sexual activity. There may be masturbation during the act. Voyeurism appears to be exclusively carried out by men.

PAEDOPHILIA

The person has recurrent, intense, sexually arousing fantasies, sexual urges or behaviours involving sexual activity with a prepubescent child or children. To meet the diagnostic criteria, the person must be at least 16 years of age, and at least 5 years older than the child or children. The majority of paedophiles are men, but there are also female paedophiles (McConaghy 1993).

SEXUAL MASOCHISM

The person has recurrent, intense, sexually arousing fantasies, sexual urges or behaviours involving the act of being humiliated, beaten, bound or otherwise made to suffer. The acts considered within this category include being forced to crawl, kept in a cage, bondage, being blindfolded, being whipped or spanked, pinched, beaten, bruised, cut, raped, stabbed or tortured.

SEXUAL SADISM

The person has recurrent, intense, sexually arousing fantasies, sexual urges or behaviours involving acts in which the psychological or physical suffering, including humiliation, of the victim is exciting to the person. Sometimes the act is with a consenting partner, who has sexual masochism.

FETISHISM

This involves recurrent, intense, sexually arousing fantasies, sexual urges or behaviours, involving the use of inanimate objects, such as leather and rubber garments, women's underwear, stockings, bras, shoes and boots. If the desire is focused on a part of the body, such as feet, the DSM-IV regards this not as fetishism, but as 'partialism'. However, most clinicians would consider such desires as a type of fetishism (cf. de Silva 1993). When the fetishes are confined to female clothing that the person uses to cross-dress, this is called 'transvestic fetishism' (see below). A particular kind of fetishism, although it is hardly ever a clinical problem, is the erotic attraction to uniforms. This has been discussed recently by Bhugra and de Silva (1996) in some detail.

TRANSVESTIC FETISHISM

This refers to recurrent, intense, sexually arousing fantasies, sexual urges or behaviours involving cross-dressing. The DSM-IV confines its definition of this paraphilia to heterosexual males.

FROTTEURISM

This involves recurrent, intense, sexually arousing fantasies, sexual urges or behaviours, including touching and rubbing against a non-consenting person. The behaviour usually happens in crowded places.

PARAPHILIAS NOT OTHERWISE SPECIFIED

The DSM-IV lists several paraphilias as examples under this category. These include necrophilia (sexual desire for corpses), zoophilia (sexual desire for animals), telephone scatologia (lewdness), and interest in enemas (klismaphilia), faeces (coprophilia) and urine (urophilia). Those with such paraphilias are rarely seen in clinics nowadays.

HYPOXYPHILIA

The DSM-IV includes this under masochism, but this paraphilia needs to be recognized as separate. This involves attempts to enhance the pleasure of orgasm by a reduction of oxygen intake — for example, by placing a tight noose around one's neck. These behaviours can and often do lead to fatalities (e.g. Hazelwood *et al.* 1983). There are many more cases of hypoxyphilia than commonly believed (Money *et al.* 1991).

The other major classifactory system, the *International Classification of Diseases* (ICD-10; World Health Organization (WHO) 1992) uses the term 'disorders of sexual preference' to refer to paraphilias. It lists fetishism, fetishistic transvestism, exhibitionism, voyeurism, paedophilia, and sadomasochism (as one category). The ICD-10 also notes, correctly, that often more than one paraphilia may occur in an individual. It is stated that the commonest combination is fetishism, transvestism and sadomasochism. There is much evidence for the occurrence of multiple paraphilias (Flor-Henry 1987).

A clinical case example where fetishism and masochism co-occurred is given by de Silva (1993). Mr G, 36 years old, referred himself to a sexual dysfunction clinic. He was strongly attracted to the feet of women, and would achieve strong erections while fondling and kissing the partner's feet. He also had a desire to be 'humiliated' by women. The main form of humiliation was for him to be made to lie on the floor and the partner to stand on his body. He would often go to prostitutes and get them to treat him in this way. This was his main mode of sexual satisfaction.

Unusual or bizarre paraphilias

Clinically, one sometimes comes across a paraphilia which is not part of an established category, but which has all the features and significance of well-described paraphilias. Dewaraja and Money (1986) reported a case from Sri Lanka: a Buddhist man derived sexual pleasure from the tactile sensations produced by small creatures, such as snails and ants, creeping and crawling on his body. He masturbated while having these experiences. The authors named this paraphilia 'formicophilia'.

An equally unusual paraphilia was reported by de Silva and Pernet (1992). The young man concerned, who sought treatment for his problem, had a strong sexual preoccupation with a particular make and model of car. Gratification occurred though masturbation in the family car, which exemplified this make and model, and which was the main focus of his desires. He also masturbated to fantasies of it, and at times he masturbated squatting behind the car while the engine was running. He had a large collection of photographs of the car concerned, and he often masturbated while looking at these. His concern was that this desire had come to dominate his life, and he feared that he might not be able to develop normal sexual relations with females in the future. A somewhat similar case had been reported in 1947 by Bergman. This was an adolescent male who had a strong, fetishistic interest in the exhaust pipes of cars (Bergman 1947).

An even more unusual paraphilia has been reported more recently: a fetishistic interest in sneezing. The man concerned was sexually aroused both by his own sneezing and by the sneezing of others (King 1990).

Hypoxyphilia, also known as asphyxiophilia, was noted above. The forensic literature shows that various bizarre methods are used by some in their attempt to reduce oxygen intake for sexual pleasure. In one case reported in 1984, a 36-year-old man had died accidentally while using a novel method of producing asphyxia, i.e. submerging himself in water and achieving stimulation by partial drowning (Sivaloganathan 1984). The case of a young man who died through suffocation, using several articles of female clothing and a plastic bag, has been reported from Japan (Ikeda *et al.* 1988). The items of clothing were three skirts, a pinafore dress, and a pair of panty hose. These were used, in addition to a plastic bag, to cover the face and thus induce hypoxia. The fetishistic element that coexisted with the hypoxyphilia in this instance is obvious.

Necrophilia was mentioned in passing in earlier paragraphs. This bizarre paraphilia, which involves sexual contact with corpses, is clearly rare, but there are authentic reports of its occurrence (Smith & Dimock 1983). Prins (1990) gives an account of historical instances of necrophiliac behaviour. Sometimes it was socially sanctioned or was part of a ritual. In some, it was a genuine paraphiliac act. As noted in an earlier paragraph, this behaviour is noted in the early disciplinary texts of Buddhism, which reflect monastic life in ancient Northern India.

Development of paraphilias

Why do paraphilias develop? There is no agreed single answer to this question, and various theories have been put forward to explain their origins. In the psychodynamic tradition, the problem behaviour is usually seen as a manifestation of real or fantasy experiences, desires and/or conflicts, going back to the person's early psychosexual development (cf. Stoller 1975). The person has, it is assumed, got fixated at a particular stage, and the nature of the paraphilia is determined by this. Various psychological mechanisms, including ego defence mechanisms, are also said to play a part. In the behavioural tradition, an explanation has been offered in learning theory terms. The paraphilia (for example, a fetish) is seen as arising from the association of a previously neutral object with a sexually arousing object, and/or a sexually reinforcing experience. McGuire *et al.* (1965) put forward the view that the repeated reinforcement of the fantasies of the paraphiliac act or stimulus by orgasm achieved through masturbation was the key factor. Rachman (1966), in an experimental study, demonstrated how a sexual response could be conditioned to the picture of a pair of boots. This was achieved by presenting a slide of the boots repeatedly with slides of a sexually arousing nude woman. Rachman and Hodgson (1968) reported a more sophisticated experimental paradigm which was successful in establishing a conditioned sexual response to a photograph of a pair of knee-length boots, with five normal subjects. The learning model offers at least a partial explanation of the acquisition of paraphilias, but it is clear that cultural factors and cognitions, including symbolic meanings, may also have a part to play. Social learning is clearly a key factor, as witnessed by the practice of specific paraphilias in subcultural groups. Other psychological models, such as the addiction model and the behaviour completion model, have been considered at some length by several authors; for example, McConaghy (1993). Almost certainly, there are multiple factors involved in the establishment of a paraphilia. There is, in many cases, not only a deviant arousal (sexual arousal centred on a non-normal object or stimulus), but also a deficiency in normal (i.e. non-paraphiliac) arousal. There may also be anxiety in relation to more normal sexual behaviour and potential partners. There may, also, be skills deficits, either in terms of general social skills needed for dating, courtship, etc., or specific sexual skills. A multifaceted model of aetiology seems to be the most plausible. There is also the need to take note of possible biological factors, such as brain damage and genetic influences (e.g. Flor-Henry 1987; Marshall & Barbaree 1990).

The clinical presentation of paraphilias

Paraphilias seen in clinical settings are only a proportion of the cases where such behaviours and/or the urges exist. There are, broadly speaking, four classes of clinical referral.

1 Those sent for clinical intervention by the law enforcing authorities. These are sex offenders who are asked to have treatment to help them get over their problem behaviour. They often come with little or no motivation to change. Many are seen in correctional settings.

2 Those who seek help for their paraphilias because they are distressed by them. These include those who worry that they might commit law-breaking or embarrassing acts. Many are genuinely distressed by acts they see as an 'unnatural' behaviour, or are disturbed that they may imperil their life, career, etc. Many of these wish, at some level, to develop more normal desires and behaviours.

3 Those who come for help because their partners are distressed by the paraphilia. They are themselves distressed as a result of their partner's distress. These are people with stable or near-stable relationships. The para-

philia may be a part of the couple's sexual repertoire, or more likely, may have been so in the past and the partner has become increasingly unhappy about it. So help is sought.

4   Those who present with frank sexual dysfunction. These report erectile difficulties or other dysfunctions and this is usually secondary to the person's strong paraphiliac desires and his reliance on the paraphilia for his arousal. For example, a man may find that he is increasingly unable to sustain an erection for sexual intercourse with his partner unless he has contact with his paraphiliac stimulus, e.g. a leather garment. In these cases, the partner is also distressed and the couple decide to seek help.

The final category noted above can be deceptive at clinical presentation, and the clinician needs to be alert and skilled to extract relevant information about the real difficulty. The referral may be simply for 'erectile problems' and the person may not be able or willing to admit the related paraphiliac complication. This may be particularly so if the partner is not aware of this latter problem. For example, the individual may not be able to get an erection sufficient for penetration without recourse to strong fantasies of a paraphiliac nature, and/or he may find the obtaining of such fantasies increasingly hard, in the context of his sexual activity with the partner. In such cases, it is possible to completely miss the underlying paraphilia, or at least not to elicit it until well into several sessions of conventional sex therapy.

Clinical assessment

Once a paraphilia is presented for help clinically, or is detected as a key aspect of the presenting problem, the clinician needs to undertake a comprehensive assessment. The need is for a multifaceted assessment in order to get a clear understanding of the problem (see Barlow 1977; Gudjonsson 1986), so the following areas need to the elucidated:

1   deviant arousal;
2   whether there is a problem in arousal in relation to conventional stimuli (e.g. consenting adult partners);
3   anxiety about conventional sexual activity;
4   anxiety about social interactions with adults, especially those of the same age group and who are potential sexual partners;
5   skills deficits in social interactions;
6   skills deficits specifically in the sexual sphere, in the context of conventional adult sex; and

7   whether the person has a gender role identity problem.

This approach to the evaluation of paraphilias fully recognizes the complexity of the problem, and acknowledges the links and overlap that may exist between the paraphilia and sexual dysfunction. Thus, it provides the basis for an informed intervention.

A further key aspect of the assessment is the need to get a full, detailed analysis of the typical paraphiliac behaviour of the individual. In the case of an exhibitionist, for example, details of the setting conditions and triggers for the behaviour, internal state and cognitions at the time, the nature of the behaviour itself, and what follows the behaviour, need to be enquired about. Taking the person through the last real occasion when the problem behaviour took place is usually a good way of obtaining this information. One needs to be able to derive a functional analysis of the problem behaviour in this way.

It is equally important to elicit detailed information about the person's sexual fantasies. The person may need patient encouragement to talk in detail about his fantasies.

Needless to say, part of the assessment should be directed at an evaluation of the person's motivation. Unmotivated clients, especially those seen through coercion by the law-enforcing agencies, are rarely able to benefit properly from any form of treatment offered. Some time needs to be devoted to the issue of motivation, including considering ways to enhance the person's motivation to change.

Treatment

AIMS OF THERAPY

The aims of treatment need to be carefully considered, and the therapist and the client need to arrive at an agreed goal. Twenty years or so ago, most paraphiliacs were treated with one aim only: to eliminate their deviant sexual arousal. The main technique used was electrical aversion therapy (see Rachman & Teasdale 1968). These attempts were largely unsuccessful in terms of the maintenance of treatment gains. The problem behaviour was often suppressed through the electrical aversion treatment, but it re-emerged later. What the aversion therapy did was merely to suppress, not eliminate, the behaviour. If the goal is the elimination of the paraphilia, one needs to recognize that the success may be limited. Control may be achieved, but one needs to supplement this with gains in other, more acceptable, sexual behaviours. In practice, this means that any treatment programme which includes an attempt to get rid of the unconventional paraphilia must also include enhancement of other outlets. If the person has anxieties or skills deficits which hamper non-paraphiliac sex, then these need to be addressed. This entails an ambitious and time-consuming therapeutic endeavour.

TECHNIQUES OF CONTROL

Assuming the goals include control of the paraphilia, what techniques are available? Electrical aversion has already been mentioned, which involves the repeated pairing of the paraphiliac stimulus (e.g. on slides) with an unpleasant stimulus (electric shock). Quite apart from the limited success, this does raise ethical questions, as the infliction of pain is involved. A related aversion procedure is Cautela's covert sensitization (e.g. Cautela & Wisocki 1971). Here, the aversion is covert and imaginal, unlike electric shock. In this paradigm, the person is asked to fantasize a sequence of events involving his paraphiliac behaviour, and—at a crucial point of the sequence—he is asked to imagine a powerful aversive scene. For example, a paedophiliac might be asked to imagine the appearance of a police officer, at the point of his approaching a prepubertal child, in his sequence of images. The aversive scenes are selected and agreed on in advance, and typically more than one aversive consequence is used. A major advantage of covert sensitization is that it can be used, by a motivated client, as a self-control technique. In real life situations, he can resort to his aversive imagery and gain some control over the problematic urges.

Orgasmic reconditioning, also called masturbatory reconditioning, has been used since the 1970s (Marquis 1970). The main feature of this approach is the reinforcement of non-paraphiliac arousal and desires. Typically, the person is asked to masturbate with his paraphiliac fantasies. Then, when orgasm is imminent (the point of no return), the person switches to a fantasy of a more conventional sexual stimulus and/or behaviour. The ensuing orgasm then powerfully reinforces the non-paraphiliac desire. In each succeeding session (which the client carries out in privacy), the point at which the switching is made is brought forward so that, eventually, the entire sequence takes place to non-paraphiliac fantasies (Laws & Marshall 1991).

In practice, clients report that the switching of fantasies is not easy. In order to overcome this difficulty, external stimuli may be used. For example, pictures of attractive nude females may be placed on a side, and all the person has to do at the crucial moment is to turn his head 75 or 90 degrees, so that he can see the picture. This external prompting has been found to be much easier than reliance on fantasy switching.

A further technique used is satiation therapy (e.g. Marshall 1979; Quinsey & Earls 1990). In this, of which several variants have been used, the person is instructed to fantasize the paraphiliac act for a very long time, perhaps an hour. He would masturbate during this time, whether or not he reached an orgasm. It is said that the erotic value of the paraphilia would diminish as a result.

Cognitive therapies have also been used, mainly with paraphiliacs who are also sex offenders. These would include exploring and modifying faulty cognitions, techniques for enhancing empathy for the victims, and so on (e.g. Murphy 1990).

Some clinics operate group therapy programmes. These are most commonly used for sex offenders (e.g. Maletzky 1991). Group processes and group learning are exploited in these settings. In many programmes, this is undertaken in addition to individual work.

INCORPORATION AS A GOAL

Elimination of the paraphilia need not always be the treatment goal. In fact, given that the attempts at total elimination are often not very successful, a legitimate treatment goal would be to incorporate the paraphilia in a controlled way into the person's sexual repertoire. This is especially so in the case of those with partners who are distressed by the dominant role of the paraphilia in their sexual behaviour. It is also sensible for those who present with a sexual dysfunction which is linked to a paraphilia.

Obviously, this approach is untenable if the paraphilia is inherently an unacceptable one, such as paedophilia. It is also important that the paraphilia is something the partner can tolerate, in a limited, controlled way. Provided these two conditions are met, this approach provides perhaps the best option in the treatment of the paraphilias. In practice, the therapist will treat the couple with a multifaceted therapy programme. One aspect of such a programme is conventional sex therapy, aimed at enhancing the sexual relationship (see de Silva 1994). This will involve sensate focus, ban on intercourse in the initial stages, graded steps in touching, etc. Individual sessions with each partner may be needed in addition, to discuss views and attitudes about the paraphilia. In these sessions, cognitive techniques might be used for attitude change, as needed. In further joint work, the couple are helped to actively and systematically reduce the role of the paraphilia in their sexual relationship. For example, a man with a rubber/leather fetish may be asked to wear only a leather arm band during sex (de Silva 1995). Similarly, temporal control may be introduced, using a negotiated timetable approach (e.g. Crowe & Ridley 1990). In this latter approach, the couple agree, for example, to use the fetish object in their sexual relations on certain days of the week only. On other days, sex could take place without this being involved in any way. In clinical work with fetishists, the approach of incorporating the paraphilia in a controlled way has met with success (e.g. de Silva 1993).

CHEMICAL CONTROL

For paraphiliacs who are seriously problematic (for example, those with repeated offending), chemical treatment is sometimes considered. Reduction of the sex drive through drugs will, of course, reduce the problem behaviour, but its effectiveness is not selective: that is, the drive is dampened down *in toto*, not just the desire for the paraphiliac behaviour. However, in more sophisticated recent work (e.g. Bradford 1990; McConaghy 1990), medication has been used to help the patient by reducing the strength of the urges, including the paraphiliac urges, and then he is helped to control these latter urges in the presence of triggers and cues that provoke the desires. Over a period of time, this would enable the person to get control over the paraphiliac behaviour. When the drug regime is ended, it is claimed that at least some would retain their gains—i.e. not return to their paraphiliac behaviours. The use of Depo-Provera (medroxyprogesterone acetate) has been strongly recommended by some authorities in the treatment of potentially fatal hypoxyphilias (e.g. Money *et al.* 1991).

The treatment of paraphilias is neither a simple nor a simplistic matter. After careful assessment, treatment goals need to be established. In order to achieve the treatment goals, a multifaceted comprehensive therapeutic package is usually needed. Focusing on the paraphiliac arousal is only one aspect of the treatment, and therapy is rarely successful if this is taken as the sole focus.

Conclusions

Paraphilias present a fascinating set of disorders, and are often a challenge to the clinician. Not all paraphiliac urges and behaviours are problematic. Of those that are problematic, and are therefore in need of clinical intervention, only a proportion are referred for help. The person's lack of motivation to change is one reason for this. Another is the embarrassing nature of the difficulty. When paraphiliacs do come to clinics, the paraphilia many not always be the presenting problem. The problem complained about may well be a frank sexual dysfunction. There are also instances where a couple present for help with marital distress, but with an underlying, often unacknowledged, paraphiliac problem. Clinical skill and perceptiveness are needed to detect the underlying problem in cases like this. Once the problem is identified, a comprehensive assessment is needed, followed by the setting of realistic treatment goals. Therapy often requires a package consisting of many elements, flexibly and imaginatively combined. In every way, this is a field that offers the clinician an exacting challenge.

References

Abel, G.G. & Osborn, C. (1992) The paraphilias: The extent and nature of sexually deviant and criminal behavior. *Psychiatric Clinics of North America* 15, 675–686.

American Psychiatric Association (1987) *Diagnostic and Statistical Manual of Mental Disorders*, 3rd edn, revised (DSM-III-R). American Psychiatric Association, Washington, D.C.

American Psychiatric Association (1994) *Diagnostic and Statistical Manual of Mental Disorders*, 4th edn (DSM-IV). American Psychiatric Association, Washington, D.C.

Barlow, D.H. (1977) Assessment of sexual behaviour. In: *Handbook of Behavioral Assessment* (eds A.R. Ciminero, K.S. Calhoun & H.E. Adams), pp. 461–508. Wiley, New York.

Bergman, P. (1947) Analysis of an unusual case of fetishism. *Bulletin of the Meninger Clinic* 11, 69–75.

Bhugra, D. & de Silva, P. (1996) Uniforms: Fact, fashion, fantasy and fetish. *Sexual and Marital Therapy* 11, 393–406.

Bradford, J.M.W. (1990) The antiandrogen and hormone treatment of sex offenders. In: *Handbook of Sexual Assault* (eds W.L. Marshall, D.R. Laws & H.R. Barbaree) pp. 297–310. Plenum, New York.

Bullough, V.L. & Bullough, B. (1976) *Sexual Variance in Society and History*. University of Chicago Press, Chicago, Ill.

Bullough, V.L. & Bullough, B. (1995) *Sexual Attitudes: Myths and Realities*. Prometheus, Buffalo, N.Y.

Cautela, J.R. & Wisocki, P.A. (1971) Covert sensitization for the treatment of sexual deviations. *Psychological Record* 21, 37–48.

Crowe, M.J. & Ridley, J. (1990) *Therapy with Couples*. Blackwell Scientific Publications, Oxford.

de Silva, P. (1993) Fetishism and sexual dysfunction: Clinical presentation and management. *Sexual and Marital Therapy* 8, 147–155.

de Silva, P. (1994) Psychological treatment of sexual problems. *International Review of Psychiatry* 6, 163–179.

de Silva, P. (1995) Paraphilias and sexual dysfunction. *International Review of Psychiatry* 7, 225–229.

de Silva, P. & Pernet, A. (1992) Pollution in 'Metroland': An unusual paraphilia in a shy young man. *Sexual and Marital Therapy* 7, 301–305.

Dewaraja, R. & Money, J. (1986) Transcultural sexology: Formicophilia, a newly named paraphilia in a young Buddhist male. *Journal of Sexual and Marital Therapy* 12, 139–145.

Flor-Henry, P. (1987) Cerebral aspects of sexual deviation. In: *Variant Sexuality* (ed. G. Wilson). Croom Helm, London.

Gudjonsson, G.H. (1986) Sexual variations: Assessment and treatment in clinical practice. *Sexual and Marital Therapy* 1, 301–306.

Hazelwood, R.R., Dietz, P.G. & Burgess, D.W. (1983) *Autoerotic Fatalities*. D.C. Heath, Lexington, Mass.

Ikeda, N., Harada, A., Umetsu, K. & Suzuki, T. (1988) A case of fatal suffocation during an unusual auto-erotic practice. *Medicine, Science and the Law* 28, 131–134.

King, M.B. (1990) Sneezing as a fetish object. *Sexual and Marital Therapy* 5, 69–72.

Krafft-Ebing, R. von (1965) *Psychopathia Sexualis* (trans. F.S. Klaf). Stein and Day, New York.

Laws, D.R. & Marshall, W.L. (1991) Masturbatory reconditioning: An evaluative review. *Advances in Behavior Research and Therapy* 13, 13–25.

Maletzky, B.M. (1991) *Treating the Sexual Offender.* Sage, Newbury Park, Calif.

Marquis, J.N. (1970) Orgasmic reconditioning: Changing sexual object choice through controlling masturbation fantasies. *Journal of Behavior Therapy and Experimental Psychiatry* 1, 263–271.

Marshall, W.L. (1979) Satiation therapy: A procedure for reducing deviant sexual arousal. *Journal of Applied Behavior Analysis* 12, 10–22.

Marshall, W.L. & Barbaree, H.E. (1990) Outcome of comprehensive cognitive-behavioral treatment programs. In: *Handbook of Sexual Assault* (eds W.L. Marshall, D.R. Laws & H.E. Barbaree). Plenum, New York.

McConaghy, N. (1990) Assessment and management of sex offenders: The Prince of Wales program. *Australian and New Zealand Journal of Psychiatry* 24, 175–181.

McConaghy, N. (1993) *Sexual Behavior: Problems and Management.* Plenum, New York.

McGuire, R., Carlisle, J.M. & Young, B.G. (1965) Sexual deviations as conditioned behaviours. *Behaviour Research and Therapy* 2, 185–190.

Money, J. (1984) Paraphilias: Phenomenology and classifications. *American Journal of Psychotherapy* 38, 164–179.

Money, J., Wainwright, G. & Hingsburger, D. (1991) *The Breathless Orgasm.* Prometheus Books, Buffalo, N.Y.

Murphy, W.D. (1990) Assessment and modification of cognitive distortions in sex offenders. In: *Handbook of Sexual Assault* (eds W.L. Marshall, D.R. Laws & H.E. Barbaree). Plenum, New York.

Prins, H. (1990) *Bizarre Behaviours.* Tavistock/Routledge, London.

Quinsey, V.L. & Earls, C.M. (1990) The modification of sexual preferences. In: *Handbook of Sexual Assault* (eds W.L. Marshall, D.R. Laws & H.E. Barbaree). Plenum, New York.

Rachman, S. (1966) Sexual fetishisms: An experimental analogue. *Psychological Record* **16**, 293–296.

Rachman, S. & Hodgson, R. (1968) Experimentally induced 'sexual fetishism': Replication and development. *Psychological Record* **18**, 25–27.

Rachman, S. & Teasdale, J. (1968) *Aversion Therapy and the Behaviour Disorders.* Routledge and Kegan Paul, London.

Russell, W.O. & C. Greaves (1877) *A Treatise on Crimes and Misdemeanours*, 9th edn. T. & J.W. Johnson, Philadelphia.

Sivaloganathan, S. (1984) Aqua-eroticum: A case of auto-erotic drowning. *Medicine, Science and the Law* **24**, 300–302.

Smith, S.M. & Dimock, J. (1983) Necrophilia and anti-social acts. In: *Sexual Dynamics of Anti-Social Behaviour* (eds L.B. Schlesinger & E. Revitch). Charles Thomas, Springfield, Ill.

Stoller, R.J. (1975) *Perversion.* Pantheon, New York.

Vinaya Pitaka (1879–1883) (5 vols) (ed. H. Oldenberg). Pali Text Society, London.

Wilson, G. (1987) *Variant Sexuality.* Croom Helm, London.

World Health Organization (1992) *The ICD-10 Classification of Mental and Behavioural Disorders. Clinical Descriptions and Diagnostic Guidelines.* World Health Organization, Geneva.

CHAPTER 13

Pseudoseizures: A Semantic and Clinical Muddle

MICHAEL R. TRIMBLE

Introduction

It is common in clinical practice for patients to present to physicians with physical complaints for which seemingly no underlying somatic cause can be identified. In many settings, particularly in the community, these complaints reflect on mild degrees of psychopathology (e.g. anxiety and depression) and are short-lived. In certain specialist settings, however — for example, in gynaecology, gastroenterology and neurology—such patients are frequently encountered. This chapter is primarily concerned with the presentation of pseudoneurological symptoms, especially seizures.

Modern classification systems recognize this group of patients, although there is not good conformity between ICD-10 (World Health Organization (WHO) 1992) and DSM-IV (American Psychiatric Association (APA) 1994) in this regard. The term 'somatoform disorders' has been popularized through the DSM classifications, which recognize a number of subcategories, including somatization disorder and conversion disorder (Table 13.1; also see Chapter 6). In this classification, somatoform disorders are distinctly separate from dissociative disorders, and the diagnosis of conversion incorporates presentation with both additional motor and sensory symptoms which includes seizures.

In contrast, the ICD-10 places dissociative convulsions under the subheading 'dissociative (conversion) disorders', noting a difference between this and 'somatoform disorders' (see Table 13.1).

We have then the strange situation that ICD-10 views what will be referred to as 'non-epileptic (pseudo) seizures' as dissociative phenomena, while DSM-IV places them without this category.

Much of this reclassification reflects upon a disinclination to use the term 'hysteria', of which, while most people acknowledge it is one of

258

Table 13.1 Classification of dissociative and somatoform disorders.

ICD-10 (WHO 1992)	DSM-IV (APA 1994)
Dissociative (conversion) disorders	*Dissociative disorders*
Dissociative amnesia	Dissociative amnesia
Dissociative fugue	Dissociative fugue
Dissociative stupor	Dissociative identity disorder
Trance and possession disorders	Depersonalization disorder
Dissociative disorders of movement and	Dissociative disorder not otherwise
sensation	specified
• Dissociative motor disorders	
• Dissociative convulsions	
• Dissociative anaesthesia and sensory loss	
• Mixed dissociative (conversion)	
Other dissociative (conversion) disorders	
Somatoform disorders	*Somatoform disorders*
Somatization disorder	Somatization disorder
Hypochondriacal disorder	Undifferentiated somatoform disorder
Somatoform autonomic dysfunction	Conversion disorder (includes seizures)
Persistent somatoform pain disorder	Pain disorder
Other somatoform disorders	Hypochondriasis
Undifferentiated somatoform disorder	Body dysmorphic disorder
	Somatoform disorder not otherwise
Other neurotic disorders	specified
Neurasthenia	
Depersonalization–derealization syndrome	

the oldest conditions described in medicine (Veith 1965), definitions are hard to find.

Terminology

The term 'pseudoseizures' itself is problematic. The *Oxford English Dictionary* gives us the definition of 'pseudo' as 'false, counterfeit, pretend or spurious'. Thus, the term 'pseudoseizures' is misleading, in that the seizures that are being discussed are none of these: they are real, and experienced by patients, and observed by bystanders or physicians.

It is accepted that alternative terms, including 'hysterical pseudoseizures', 'pseudoepileptic seizures', 'hysteroepilepsy', and 'psychogenic seizures' are all inadequate, as they often lead to a pejorative inference about the nature of the episodes or are frankly misleading, as is the term 'psychogenic seizures'. This last term logically should be used to imply a form of reflex seizures induced by mental activities (Fenwick 1981). Unfortunately, it is commonly used by those who do not understand, or try not to understand, the meaning of the term 'psychogenic', in reference to the phenomena described in this chapter.

Table 13.2 Non-epileptic conditions leading to pseudoseizures.

NON-PSYCHIATRIC DISORDERS
Hypoglycaemia
Vasovagal
Cardiac (TIA)
Migraine
Vestibular disorders
Narcolepsy
Dystonias, tics, stimulus-sensitive myoclonus

SLEEP DISORDERS

Parasomnias
REM
  Nightmares
  Sleep behaviour disorder
Non-REM
  Somnambulism
  Night terrors

Hypersomnias
Cataplexy
Narcoleptic automatic behaviour
Sleep drunkenness

PSYCHIATRIC DISORDERS
Anxiety
  GAD
  Panic disorder (hyperventilation: depersonalization)
Depression (fugues)
Schizophrenia
Conversion disorder
Somatization disorder
Episodic dyscontrol
Malingering

GAD, generalized anxiety disorder; REM, rapid eye movement; TIA, transient ischaemia attack.

The author's preferred term for what is discussed here is 'non-epileptic seizures'. This term acknowledges that these phenomena are different from those of epilepsy, but also that the patient has had a sudden paroxysmal experience that may be interpreted as being epileptic-like.

More recently, the term 'non-epileptic attack disorder' has been popularized (Betts 1996). Betts has chosen to subdivide non-epileptic attack disorder into various groupings, potentially related to the clinical presentation and possible aetiological factors. Kalogjera-Sackellares (1996) classifies pseudoseizure syndromes into post-traumatic and developmental types, which has both aetiological and treatment implications.

There are a number of non-epileptic conditions that lead to such attacks, shown in Table 13.2, including psychiatric conditions.

Incidence

One important reason to include this topic in a book on troublesome disguises is the frequency with which this diagnosis is missed. There are a number of reasons for this, which are discussed further below.

Pseudoseizures obviously occur most commonly in neurological settings, and are frequent in patients with conversion symptoms. Ljungberg (1957) reported seizures as occurring in 25% of males and 41% of females in a large sample of patients with conversion disorder. Purtell *et al.* (1951) give a figure of 12% of women with Briquet's syndrome presenting pseudoseizures, and Trimble (1981) in reviewing the diagnosis of hysteria at the National Hospitals for Nervous Diseases throughout three decades (1950s, 1960s and 1970s), gave figures for seizures of 11.1%, 13.2% and 13.8% respectively.

The incidence of pseudoseizures in these selected populations is undoubtedly increasing. In a more recent report from the same hospital (Wilson-Barnett & Trimble 1985), seizures were reported in 34% of a consecutively referred sample of 79 patients with conversion symptoms. In this sample patients were not included if an alternative neurological diagnosis was apparent: in other words, these were not patients in whom a diagnosis of both epilepsy and hysteria would be acceptable. This emphasizes an important clinical point: although patients with epilepsy may have pseudoseizures, the latter frequently occur in the absence of epilepsy, and it is not necessary to entertain both diagnoses in the same patient. Lesser (1985) cautioned against making a double diagnosis, noting definite epilepsy in only 12% and possible epilepsy in 24% of over 300 reported cases of pseudoseizures.

More recent estimates of the frequency of patients having pseudoseizures amongst patients attending clinics with treatment-resistent seizures give estimates of prevalence at between 10 and 20% (Ramani 1986; Gates 1989).

If such figures are correct, many patients with pseudoseizures carry with them a diagnosis of epilepsy, and most of these patients take anticonvulsant drugs chronically, until such a time as the diagnostic error has been corrected, if it ever is. Clearly, at some stage in their history, a diagnostic pitfall was encountered and an inappropriate diagnosis was given.

A number of reasons are apparent as to why such diagnostic errors occur. There is a pressure on all of us to make an instant diagnosis in our patients, intensified by the insistence of managerial systems in some settings on providing diagnostic categories before reimbursement for medical treatment can be forthcoming. Further, in a diagnostic setting in which symptoms, rather than a patient's history, are often given primary importance, there seems to be a need to concentrate primarily on the phenomenology of the attacks themselves, and in the case of seizures often relying on a third-party description of the episodes in order to seek a diagnosis.

It is clearly preferable, in cases of difficult seizure disorders, to accept that the patient is a diagnostic conundrum, to note that there are alternative diagnoses to epilepsy that might apply to the patient, and to follow the patient over time with the expectation that the appropriate diagnosis will reveal

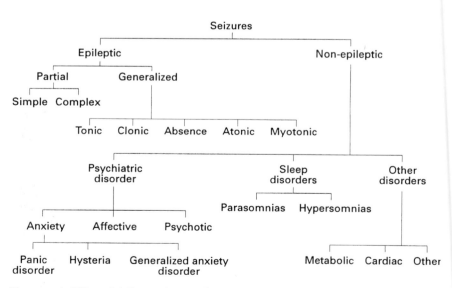

Fig. 13.1 A differential diagnostic tree of seizures.

itself as further information is gathered. A differential diagnostic tree is given in Fig. 13.1.

Seizure phenomenology

The presentation of patients with pseudoseizures is highly variable, but in general, if the condition is going to be mistaken for epilepsy, the patterns reported are going to be similar to those found in an epilepsy population. Thus, patients are either going to present with a partial seizure type, or a generalized seizure type, or a mixture of the two.

One of the problems in terms of diagnosis is that in many settings still, and certainly before the advent of videotelemetry monitoring, description of the patients' seizure was dependent upon what the patients themselves said, or upon third-party descriptions. These are known in many cases to be highly inaccurate. The latter may be particularly fallacious in coming to a decision about whether a diagnosis of epilepsy is appropriate or not, since one is dealing mainly with a lay interpretation of abnormal muscular movements, which the physician then fits into his own preconceived conception of what a description of epileptic seizures ought to sound like.

From the psychiatric point of view, careful attention to the patient's phenomenology, however, is very relevant. So often simple cases of panic disorder are missed because of failure to ask appropriate probing questions; likewise, depressive illness may not be enquired about.

It is often forgotten by investigating physicians that 'loss of consciousness' means different things to patients and doctors, and many patients with pseudoseizures actually present with an alteration of consciousness, rather than loss of consciousness. None the less, this is reported as loss of consciousness by patients when asked as a direct question.

Patients are often amnesic for their attacks, and this is thought to be a hallmark of the epileptic seizure. However, amnesia is also a hallmark of dissociation, and to equate amnesia for the episode as an attack of epilepsy is a fundamental clinical error. Many patients with partial epileptic seizures do not have alteration of consciousness (simple partial seizures). Further, on close questioning, patients who say they are unconscious during an episode may actually report a variety of sensory impressions which they experience, which are much more in keeping with dissociation than unconsciousness in the neurological sense.

Betts and Boden (1991) related seizure phenomenology to aetiology, dividing their seizure types into emotional attacks, swoons, tantrums and abreactive types. The frequency of sexual abuse was greatest in patients with swoons and abreactive seizure types. In the latter attack, patients present the well-described *arc en cercle*, with arching of the back and pelvic thrusting. It has been suggested that this relates to 'the acting out of an abuse flashback' (Betts 1996).

Differential diagnoses

HISTORY

The main conditions that may be mistaken for epilepsy are given in Table 13.2. In this chapter only the psychiatric variants are described, alternative references to the other disorders being readily available (e.g. Vossler 1995).

It should at the outset be reinforced that although textbooks for over a century have given advice as to how to distinguish between epileptic and non-epileptic seizures, all such listings are unreliable. Access to videotelemetry, where the patient's seizure can be viewed at the same time as the electroencephalographic (EEG) record, is an important method of suggesting the diagnosis of non-epileptic seizures in many patients but has only been widely available for some 10 years. However, reliance on videotelemetry alone is another clinical pitfall, and history taking, particularly in terms of exploring underlying potential psychopathology, is a vital component of the diagnostic process.

In patients with seizure disorders, a purely symptom-orientated approach, concentrating solely on the phenomenology of the seizures, may lead to wrong conclusions. An essential part of the investigation is the history with an understanding of the patient in whom the symptoms are presenting. In addition, information regarding such obvious factors as seizure precipitating events should be sought, paying particular attention to the setting and timing of the first attack.

It is a truism that seizures occurring many times a day in the presence of a normal interictal EEG are most likely to be non-epileptic, and that talking, screaming, or displays of emotional behaviour during or immediately after the attack are likely to lead to a similar conclusion.

A history of *status epilepticus*, where the patient is rushed to hospital, and has an attack which goes on 'for hours', should always be viewed with suspicion. *Status epilepticus* is a medical emergency, but it is estimated that perhaps 50% of patients admitted to emergency care with a diagnosis of *status epilepticus* do not actually have this condition (Betts 1996). The history of *status epilepticus*, with a normal interictal EEG, is highly unlikely to represent epilepsy, and simply because patients have been taken to an intensive care unit and given sedative medications, the diagnosis of epilepsy need not be reinforced. Indeed, iatrogenic damage is common in patients with pseudoseizures, some patients going as far as having respiratory arrest following inappropriate sedation and then having tracheostomies performed quite unnecessarily.

ELECTROENCEPHALOGRAMS

The EEG can be the most misleading of investigations. Non-specific interical EEG abnormalities are reported in up to 74% of patients with non-epileptic seizures (Wilkes *et al.* 1990; Lelliot & Fenwick 1991).

The presence of paroxysmal abnormalities on the EEG does not mean a diagnosis of epilepsy, and the only clear setting where epilepsy can be confirmed is when classical discharges associated with the seizure are viewed and captured on videotelemetry.

Paroxysmal discharges, even generalized spike wave complexes, can be found in up to 3% of healthy people (Fenton 1982). Certain rhythmic abnormalities on the EEG are associated with psychopathology. For example, rhythmic midtemporal discharges (paroxysmal theta activity maximally seen in midtemporal regions) and small sharp spikes (which are brief, small-amplitude spikes, again often exclusively temporal in location) have been associated with affective disorders, and a tendency towards suicide (Small 1970; Hughes & Hermann 1984). Often these variants can have a sharp appearance, leading the electroencephalographer to refer to them as 'epileptiform'. Unless the clinician is experienced in understanding EEG information, this is rapidly translated into 'epileptic', and the patient's seizure diagnosed as epilepsy.

It is now accepted that some 70% of patients respond to standard anti-convulsant drugs by becoming seizure free, and that patients who go on to have intractible seizure disorders usually will show signs of continued cerebral irritability through EEG abnormalities, focal, polyfocal or generalized. Thus, the patient who fails to respond to anticonvulsant drugs, but has a persistently normal EEG, should again arouse suspicion as to the diagnosis of epilepsy.

As emphasized, one way round this trap is to place only minimal reliance on the interictal EEG, and to examine where possible the ictal EEG using videotelemetry, or rather less satisfactory, ambulatory monitoring. In the latter, patients are connected to a portable EEG, and can therefore roam freely about in their daily lives. However, there is no direct viewing of the seizure. One only has the EEG record, and artefacts are readily provoked, particularly during the seizure episode itself. Again, it requires an experienced electroencephalographer to interpret such data. It is even possible to mistake artefacts on videotelemetry for epileptic seizures, unless care is taken.

SOME MORE FALLACIES

The diagnosis can also be mistaken if a number of clinical fallacies are not heeded. One of these relates to self-injury, another to incontinence.

Self-injury is just as likely to occur in epileptic as in non-epileptic seizures, although the site of the injury may be different. Patients with epilepsy often damage under the chin or alongside bones of prominence. Patients with non-epileptic seizures, whose injuries may be quite horrific, may present, for example, with carpet burns on the cheeks or on the surface of the brow. Carpet burns are virtually never seen in association with epilepsy, being pathognomonic of pseudoseizures.

Patients with non-epileptic seizures may fracture bones, dislocate joints, and have head injuries which in themselves may lead to a period of unconsciousness.

Incontinence occurs frequently in non-epileptic seizures, and is of no diagnostic value whatsoever.

Other fallacies include the relationship of the attacks to head injury, and also to a family history. The characteristics of head injury that lead to seizures have been well laid down (Jennett & Teasdale 1981) and the relatively minor head injuries of everyday life simply are not associated with an increased incidence of epilepsy. With regard to genetics, there are some well-known epilepsy syndromes that have a genetic base (for example, juvenile myoclonic epilepsy), but the genetic component to most epileptic disorders is not strong, and at present poorly characterized. Thus, a history of minor head injury or a family history of epilepsy should not allow the physician immediately to bias a diagnosis in favour of epilepsy.

SPECIFICALLY ASSOCIATED PSYCHIATRIC CONDITIONS

A variety of psychiatric disorders are found in patients with pseudoseizures (see Table 13.2). The commonest are anxiety disorders, which are linked to panic attacks, with or without agoraphobia, episodes of depersonalization and derealization, and to dissociative states.

A common underlying psychopathology is a depressive illness, and, more rarely, schizophrenia. In the latter condition, patients with sudden-onset catatonic behaviour are mistakenly diagnosed as epilepsy.

Non-epileptic seizures can be linked with malingering. This is a diagnostic entity of dubious validity, but none the less one which has to be considered in certain settings, particularly where financial compensation may be involved.

A number of authors have emphasized the importance of seeking underlying affective disorder, particularly major affective disorders. In some cases this is most obvious when the seizures are presenting as a new problem, and, at first, the affective disturbance may not be readily apparent. However, once initiated as a clinical pattern, the non-epileptic seizures may continue for a considerable period of time, well beyond receiving treatment for the depression. Once a patient is on the roundabout of receiving polytherapy with anti-convulsant drugs, the situation may be compounded, since a number of these drugs themselves may provoke or exacerbate depressive symptoms (Trimble 1996).

Briquet's syndrome, a form of stable hysteria, originally defined by Guze and Perley (1953), is also an important consideration (Woodruff *et al.* 1982). In DSM-IV this is referred to as somatization disorder.

Patients with this condition can often present with pseudoneurological problems, which include faints and convulsions, visual symptoms, weakness, headaches, pain, anaesthesias and paralyses. To the experienced eye, the past history of abnormal illness behaviour is usually readily apparent, but a purely symptom-orientated approach to seizures will miss the rich variety of complex somatization that these patients bring with them to the clinical investigation. Since by definition the condition is intractable, and difficult to treat, recognition of these patients is of paramount importance to avoid unnecessary surgical and medical intervention, which must include the prescription of anticonvulsant drugs.

Of the psychiatric symptoms most confused with epileptic seizures, panic attacks and rage attacks are the most frequent. The former usually occur in settings of stress, although stress can also of course precipitate some epileptic seizures. Distinguishing the aura of panic in a patient with temporal lobe epilepsy from panic disorder in the absence of epilepsy can be diagnostically difficult. The clue to the aura of epilepsy may be in the more stereotyped nature of the panic, and their more fleeting nature, with a greater paroxysmal quality. There is an absence of a build-up of anxiety sometimes hours before the attack, and a lack of the continuing presence of anxiety after the attack, which tend to accompany the panic attack of anxiety.

The unpleasant fear-like aura of temporal lobe epilepsy is often initially an epigastric feeling, with a very clear quality, rising up the midline of the chest into the throat, before the patient loses consciousness. In panic disorder, the feeling is often epigastric in origin but the pattern of radiation is more diffuse, spreading to involve the whole body. Further, hyperventilation, tachycardia, sweating, shortness of breath, and other autonomic manifestations of anxiety are often reported by the patient.

The episodic dyscontrol syndrome (Mark & Ervin 1970) is a condition of repeated paroxysmal episodes of violence, which often seem to come out of the blue, and are relatively short-lived, for which afterwards patients feel intense remorse. This may be confused with epilepsy, particularly if it is associated with a history of head injury, and an abnormal EEG with temporal lobe abnormalities is noted.

DISSOCIATION

Dissociative states are a heterogeneous group of psychosensory and psychomotor events in which 'a partial or complete loss of the normal integration between memories of the past, awareness of identity and immediate sensations, and control of bodily movements' occur (ICD-10, p. 151). The categorization suggests a relationship to psychological aetiology, related to 'trauma, insoluble or intolerable problems or disturbed relationships' (ICD-10, p. 152).

Dissociative mechanisms have a role in a variety of disorders, most notably with acute and chronic post-traumatic stress disorders, but also in affective disorder, and as a feature of certain personality disorders. Further, certain conditions, especially temporal lobe epilepsy, seem more linked to the reporting of dissociative phenomena (Schneck & Bear 1981). Twilight states, short of delirium, but with behaviour disorders and amnesia, are seen postictally, as well as in association with complex partial seizure status. Other neurological conditions that may be associated with dissociation include head injury, migraine, encephalitis, and a variety of drug intoxications from alcohol to psychodelic agents.

Dissociation is noted in many patients presenting with non-epileptic seizures, and this group are readily misdiagnosed as having epilepsy. Two main reasons for this are the reporting of amnesia, and the high incidence of

EEG abnormalities in patients with dissociative convulsive attacks (Jarwad *et al.* 1995).

Dissociative amnesia is one variant of psychogenic amnesia, and it is the reporting of the amnesia by the patient that often leads to the mistaken diagnosis of complex partial seizures. It is a clinical fallacy to assume that loss of awareness of and an amnesia for an episode leads to an automatic diagnosis of epilepsy.

Fugue states are prolonged episodes of amnesia associated with wandering. They are interlinked with a variety of psychopathologies. The amnesia lasts hours, weeks, or occasionally years, and, if related to psychiatric disability such as depression, is usually seen as in the setting of escape from some difficult or intolerable circumstances. These are quite unlike epileptic automatisms, which are briefer. The patients usually remain in contact with their environment, manipulating it successfully, often failing to draw much attention to themselves or others. This is also unlike episodes of transient global amnesia, which tend to be short-lived, and during which the patient often behaves inappropriately, asking repeatedly the same questions and appearing in some state of confusion.

Somnambulism implies sleep walking; this is one of the parasomnias, and usually arises out of non-REM sleep. There may be only brief wandering or lengthier episodes, with a completion of quite complex but semi-purposeful tasks for which there is amnesia. Its onset in adulthood is usually associated with emotional trauma, and is a further reflection of a patient's ability to dissociate.

Although not strictly among the DSM-IV diagnostic criteria for post-traumatic stress disorder, pseudoseizures may occur in this setting. The seizure may be the most dramatic aspect of the clinical presentation, leading to a line of enquiry which fails to detect the other underlying criteria which would allow diagnosis of this syndrome. Obviously, the precipitating trauma is a significant criterion for entry, but in many cases this may reflect upon previous trauma, perhaps reactivated by recent events. The similarity between post-traumatic stress disorder and non-epileptic seizure disorder has been commented on by Betts (1996), and even the hyperekplexia of post-traumatic stress disorder may be mistaken for myoclonic seizures.

Finally, a number of quite common psychiatric symptoms, which actually are not so common in epilepsy, may lead to a mistaken diagnosis. Derealization, and the related depersonalization, refer to a disturbance of feeling about the surrounding world, or about the self, respectively. The self is felt as unreal, dead: the world is seen as flat, two-dimensional or alien. Some patients feel that objects are new, or startling, and want to touch them to test their reality. These phenomena are usually distressing, and associated with high levels of anxiety, and are frequent accompaniments of states of dissociation. In autoscopy, patients report that they can stand outside of their body and look down upon it.

Déjà vu is an associated state, as is *jamais vu* and *déjà vécu*. These essentially represent mnestic dislocations. The commonest medical association of *déjà vu* is with an anxiety disorder, in which setting the experience fails to have the vivid, and often clearly repetitive, nature that an aura of temporal lobe epilepsy brings.

INVESTIGATIONS

The emphasis of this chapter has been on the clinical evaluation of patients with seizure disorders, demonstrating how difficult it can be to distinguish epileptic from non-epileptic seizures in some patients. It also emphasizes the great frequency with which diagnostic errors are made. Clinical evaluation can be enhanced by laboratory and biochemical assessments, and neuro-imaging. It is not the purpose of this chapter to review these, but a few comments will be made.

Aside from the EEG, measurement of serum prolactin comparing a baseline level to a postictal one is helpful, particularly in distinguishing seizures which have a generalized tonic–clonic expression, levels rising dramatically in patients with epilepsy. This can sometimes be helpful also with partial seizures, although it appears not to be useful in patients either in *status epilepticus*, or in patients with frontal seizures (Trimble 1978; Meierkord *et al.* 1992). A postictal rise to greater than 1000 i.u. per litre is highly suggestive of an epileptic seizure in the presence of a normal baseline.

High-resolution magnetic resonance imaging (MRI) scanning is also proving helpful in detecting relatively discrete lesions, particularly in medial temporal structures, which may be the site of epilepsy in many patients. Imaging with single-photon emission computerized tomography (SPECT) or positron emission tomography (PET) may reveal areas of hypometabolism, usually concordant with the site of abnormality of any EEG focus or MRI scan abnormality. Normal findings on structural or functional brain imaging does not, of course, rule out an epileptic cause for a seizure, but, taken in conjunction with other findings, may be helpful in the differential diagnoses of epileptic from non-epileptic attacks.

Conclusions

Amongst the conditions that come under the heading of troublesome diagnoses, seizure disorders must rate very high. It has been the purpose of this chapter to show that many patients diagnosed as having epilepsy do not have that condition, and that a wide variety of psychiatric and related conditions can lead to patients' presenting with a seizure disorder which is mistaken for epilepsy. Inevitably, these patients receive anticonvulsant medications, usually in the form of polytherapy, as their seizures simply do not respond to those treatments. Patients may be treated for epilepsy for many years, and suffer the social problems that patients with epilepsy face in society.

Patients with a seizure disorder that proves intractable to all treatments, and where there is suspicion that an alternative diagnosis other than epilepsy may be appropriate, should be referred for reassessment. Modern investigation of seizures involves sophisticated EEG monitoring, brain imaging, and a neuropsychiatric perspective which goes far beyond the simplistic view that all episodes of reported loss of consciousness are epileptic seizures, and that all seizures represent epilepsy.

References

American Psychiatric Association (1994) *Diagnostic and Statistical Manual of Mental Disorders*, 4th edn (DSM-IV) American Psychiatric Association, Washington, D.C.

Betts, T. (1996) Psychiatric aspects of nonepileptic seizures. In: *Epilepsy: A Comprehensive Textbook* (eds J. Engel & T.A. Pedley). Raven Press, New York.

Betts, T. & Boden, S. (1991) Pseudoseizures (nonepileptic attack disorder). In: *Women and Epilepsy* (ed. M.R. Trimble), pp. 243–258. J. Wiley & Sons, Chichester.

Fenton, G.W. (1982) Hysterical alterations of consciousness. In: *Hysteria* (ed. A. Roy), pp. 229–246. J. Wiley & Sons, Chichester.

Fenwick, P. (1981) Precipitation and inhibition of seizures. In: *Epilepsy and Psychiatry* (eds E.H. Reynolds & M.R. Trimble), pp. 306–321. Churchill Livingstone, Edinburgh.

Gates, J.R. (1989) Psychogenic seizures. In: *Nonepileptic Seizures* (eds J.A. Rowan & J.R. Gates). Butterworth-Heinemann, Boston, Mass.

Guze, S.D. & Perley, M.J. (1953) Observations on the natural history of hysteria. *American Journal of Psychiatry* 119, 960–965.

Hughes, J.R. & Hermann, B.P. (1984) Evidence for psychopathology in patients with rhythmic midtemporal discharges. *Biological Psychiatry* 19, 1623–1634.

Jarwad, S.S.M., Jamil, N., Clark, E.J. *et al.* (1995) Psychiatric morbidity and psychodynamics of patients with convulsive pseudo-seizures. *Seizure* 4, 201–206.

Jennett, B. & Teasdale, G. (1981) Assessment of head injuries. In: *Management of Head Injuries*, pp. 301–316. F.A. Davis, Philadelphia, Penn.

Kalogjera-Sackellares, D. (1996) Psychological disturbances in patients with pseudo-seizures. In: *Psychological Disturbances in Epilepsy* (eds J.C. Sackellares & S. Berent), pp. 191–217. Butterworth-Heinemann, New York.

Lelliott, P.T. & Fenwick, P. (1991) Cerebral pathology and pseudo-seizures. *Acta Neurologica Scandinavica* 83, 129–132.

Lesser, R.P. (1985) Psychogenic seizures. In: *Recent Advances in Epilepsy*, Vol 2 (eds T. Pedley & B.S. Meldrum), pp. 273–296. Churchill-Livingstone, Edinburgh.

Ljungberg, L. (1957) Hysteria. *Acta Psychiatrica Scandinavica* (Suppl. 112).

Mark, V.H. & Ervin, E.R. (1970) *Violence in the Brain*. Harper Row, London.

Meierkord, H., Shorvon, S., Stafford Lightman, S. & Trimble, M.R. (1992) Comparison of the effects of frontal and temporal lobe partial seizures on prolactin levels. *Archives of Neurology* 49, 225–230.

Purtell, J.J., Robins, E. & Cohen, M.E. (1951) Observation on clinical aspects of hysteria. *Journal of the American Medical Association* 146, 902–910.

Ramani, S.V. (1986) Intensitive monitoring of psychogenic seizures, aggression and dyscontrol syndromes. In: *Advances in Neurology* (ed. R.J. Gumnit), pp. 203–217. Raven Press, New York.

Schneck, L. & Bear, D. (1981) Multiple personality and related dissociative phenomena in patients with temporal lobe epilepsy. *American Journal of Psychiatry* 133, 1311–1316.

Small, J.G. (1970) Small spikes in a psychiatric population. *Archives of General Psychiatry* 22, 277–284.

Trimble, M.R. (1978) Serum prolactin in epilepsy and hysteria. *British Medical Journal* 2, 1682.

Trimble, M.R. (1981) *Neuropsychiatry*. J. Wiley & Sons, Chichester.

Trimble, M.R. (1996) *Biological Psychiatry*, 2nd edn. J. Wiley & Sons, Chichester.

Veith, I. (1965) *Hysteria: The History of a Disease*. University of Chicago Press, Chicago, Ill.

Vossler, D.G. (1995) Nonepileptic seizures of physiologic origin. *Journal of Epilepsy* 8, 1–10.

Wilkes, R.J., Thompson, P.M. & Vossler, D.G. (1990) Bizarre ictal automatisms: Frontal lobe epileptic or psychogenic seizures. *Journal of Epilepsy* 3, 297–313.

Wilson-Barnett, J. & Trimble, M.R. (1985) An investigation of hysteria using the Illness Behaviour Questionnaire. *British Journal of Psychiatry* 146, 601–608.

Woodruff, R.A., Goodwin, D.W. & Guze, S.D. (1982) Hysteria (Briquet's syndrome). In: *Hysteria* (ed. A. Roy), pp. 117–143. J. Wiley & Sons, Chichester.

World Health Organization (1992) *The ICD-10 Classification of Mental and Behavioural Disorders. Clinical Descriptions and Diagnostic Guidelines*. World Health Organization, Geneva.

CHAPTER 14

Atypical Illnesses

IAN W. COFFEY AND EVE C. JOHNSTONE

Introduction

The term 'atypical illnesses' has been taken to mean psychiatric disorders in which the clinical presentation is unusual and where therefore there may be a degree of diagnostic confusion. This issue is particularly important in psychiatric practice because in the great majority of cases the diagnosis depends upon the clinical picture and the course of the illness. There is as yet no diagnostic test for more than a very few psychiatric conditions, although there have been some promising preliminary findings to do with, for example, markers for those with a susceptibility to major depressive disorders (Ogilvie *et al.* 1996). Atypical illnesses are important because the diagnostic confusion with which they may be associated may give rise to inappropriate plans of management and inaccurate prognoses.

Here, atypical presentations have been classified as follows.
1 'Functional' disorders (principally affective and schizophrenic illnesses) which have a presentation suggestive of some other disorder, either another 'functional' condition or an organic disorder.
2 'Organic' disorders which present in a way that is suggestive of a 'functional' psychosis.

Atypical presentations of affective disorder

Essentially, atypical presentations are those which differ from classical presentations of depression, mania or mixed affective states. In these presentations, the disorder may be apparently affective but lack classical features or may resemble either physical disease, some psychiatric disorder other than affective illness, or a behavioural disturbance which is not recognized as representing illness at all. These presentations are most easily described in relation to depressive illness.

ATYPICAL DEPRESSION: DEPRESSIVE ILLNESS WITHOUT CLASSICAL FEATURES

The concept of 'atypical depression' was introduced into the literature in 1959 (West & Dally 1959). It describes depressive disorder which is characterized by complaints suggestive of depression but where the classical features are not those considered typical of depressive illness. The features of this condition are listed in a rating scale (Asnis *et al.* 1995) which has been devised for its assessment, and these include the presence of emotional reactivity during the depressive episode, hypersomnia, hyperphagia and rejection sensitivity.

MASKED DEPRESSION: DEPRESSIVE ILLNESS RESEMBLING PHYSICAL DISEASE

The concept of 'masked depression' refers to the situation where the patients present their symptoms in terms of complaints which are not apparently related to depression at all but which are physical in nature, for example 'atypical facial pain' (Lascelles 1966; Feinmann *et al.* 1984; Lesse 1993). The patient does not actually concede to feeling 'depressed' or having 'low mood' as such.

It has been claimed that a positive response to antidepressant therapy in such patients is evidence *per se* that the illness is depressive in nature (Paykel & Norton 1982). These claims highlight one of the underlying themes of the concept of atypical affective disorders, namely that conditions which do not initially appear to represent affective disorder are in fact manifestations of such and will benefit from treatments tried in affective illness. Such an idea cannot really be tested out at present as there is no currently available diagnostic test for any form of affective disorder. Clinical response of, for example, symptoms of pain to antidepressants or mood stabilizers (Magni 1991) could only be considered as evidence for the basically affective nature of such pain, if the view that the effects of those drugs were specific to affective illness could be sustained. Ideas of specificity cannot really be supported and the validation of these disorders as forms of affective illness must await the availability of some diagnostic test genetic or otherwise, but the practical issue of the value of antidepressant treatment in cases of 'masked depression' remains debatable.

What has been described as 'smiling depression' or 'depression *sine depressione*' is not the same as masked depression but refers to the situation where the depressed patient successfully conceals the intensity of his melancholia from the doctor (Sims 1995).

PSEUDODEMENTIA: DEPRESSSIVE ILLNESS RESEMBLING DEMENTIA

The term 'pseudodementia' is used here to refer to depressed patients who are cognitively impaired, but where cognition is restored when their depression improves. Depressed patients can perform very poorly on cognitive testing (Frith 1983) having difficulties resulting from poor attention, concentration, retardation, or severe agitation.

Although the validity of the term 'pseudodementia' has been questioned by some (Folstein & Rabins 1991), long-term follow-up supports the concept. One longitudinal study followed up 19 patients diagnosed as having pseudodementia over a 10-year period. In only one patient was the earlier diagnosis of pseudodementia revised to dementia (Sachdev *et al.* 1990; also see Chapter 9).

DEPRESSIVE ILLNESS PRESENTING AS BEHAVIOURAL DISTURBANCE

The presentation of depressive illness as difficult behaviour which is not recognized as illness has been described in elderly people and shown to respond to antidepressants (Monfort 1995). Such behavioural disturbance is more often said to be a manifestation of occult bipolar affective disorder (Tyrer & Brittlebank 1993) and it is the episodic nature of the behaviour which provides the clue to the relationship with affective disorder. Recent years have seen a growing interest in the identification of mild or subsyndromal forms of the major affective disorders, namely cyclothymia and dysthymia. These may pose a dilemma for the clinician, not least as to whether or not what is being presented actually represents psychiatric illness or a variant of 'normal' human behaviour.

Dysthymia—that is, persistent low mood of insufficient severity to merit the diagnosis of major depression—has been an important recent issue in the psychiatric literature (Freeman 1994). Kahlbaum (cited in Jelliffe 1931) coined the term 'dysthymia' and distinguished it from the fluctuating mood of cyclothymia. The primary distinction between dysthymia and major depressive disorder is that dysthymia is chronic, but symptomatically less severe. The extent to which the treatments used in major depressive disorder can be usefully extended to the treatment of this condition and the length of time for which they should be maintained are matters for debate (Tyrer *et al.* 1993; also see Chapter 11).

Cyclothymia is described (World Health Organization (WHO) 1992) as 'a persistent instability of mood, involving numerous periods of mild depression and mild elation'. How this shades into normal behaviour is unclear. ICD-10 specifies that one must know the patient for a long time or have particularly detailed information about their behaviour before definitively making the diagnosis.

While under this definition, numerous hypomanic episodes occur over at least 1 year. 'Marked impairment' is not present and, in addition, numerous periods of depressed mood or loss of interest or pleasure that did not meet all the criteria for a major depressive episode occur over the same period.

As with dysthymia, issues regarding treatment in cyclothymia are unclear. Some preliminary open studies have suggested that sodium valproate, the anticonvulsant, may be useful in patients with a primary diagnosis of cyclothymia (Freeman *et al.* 1992). Recent reconsideration of the placebo-controlled trials conducted in the 1970s has promoted the view that the long-term benefits of lithium in bipolar illness is unclear (Moncrieff 1994). Not all agree with this view (Goodwin 1994a), but the findings suggest that the benefits of lithium in manic-depressive patients may only be evident if the treatment is maintained for at least 2 years (Goodwin 1994b). These conclusions promote the view that it may be unwise to treat cyclothymic patients with this drug.

Atypical presentations of elevated mood

Atypical presentations of elevated mood are less well described. Subsyndromal elevation of mood does not normally present to the medical services. Patients generally feel well and have no reason to complain in either physical or psychological terms. Of course, subsyndromic elevation of mood need not be a disadvantage to the affected person.

ELEVATED MOOD RESEMBLING A PSYCHIATRIC DISORDER OTHER THAN MANIA

The principal relevant condition is schizophrenia. As there is no diagnostic test for either schizophrenia or affective psychosis, disputes as to whether or not any episode of functional psychosis is 'really' due to either condition cannot be definitively resolved. None the less, neither of these illnesses generally takes the form of a single episode. The generally adverse outcome of schizophrenia is often used as a validating criterion for the disease (Johnstone *et al.* 1992) and the phenomenology of subsequent episodes may also be used as a guide to overall diagnosis. Most experienced clinicians are familiar with a schizophrenic disorder which has been preceded by a manic or depressive episode. The more cynical among them may consider that such an occurrence is the result of reluctance to diagnose schizophrenia in a first episode but this phenomenon was described by Lewis and Pietrowski (1954), who found such a change in half of their 122 cases and pointed out that it was very rare for a schizophrenic patient to be 'reclassified ' as a 'manic-depressive psychotic'.

Sheldrick *et al.* (1977), studying extensive case-note material, were able to find 12 cases in which such a change of diagnosis occurred. Examining the follow-up of the International Pilot Study of Schizophrenia (WHO 1973), the same authors found a change from a diagnosis of schizophrenia to one of affective illness in a later sample in 3 % of the cohort. It may be that affective episodes occur in the course of some schizophrenic illnesses. None the less, in the material of Sheldrick *et al.* (1977), the sequence was unidirectional in that there was no single instance of a patient reverting to a schizophrenic syndrome after having relapsed with affective symptoms. These data are therefore perhaps less consistent with the possibility of one 'disease entity' being replaced by another than with an illness which subsequent events would clarify as affective, initially having features which supported a diagnosis of schizophrenia.

ELEVATED MOOD PRESENTING AS
BEHAVIOURAL DISTURBANCE

Disturbed and disinhibited behaviour is a common feature of hypomania and manic illnesses but it can generally be clearly seen as secondary to underlying mood change. Cases do, however, occur in which recurrent behavioural disturbance is present without obvious features of mood disorder.

Tyrer *et al.* (1993) describe two female patients who were diagnosed as having a personality disorder after several admissions to hospital but who subsequently developed bipolar affective disorder. Since treatment with lithium and adjunctive mood-stabilizing drugs, neither patient has required further admissions to hospital over the subsequent 5 years.

ELEVATED MOOD MANIFESTING AS CREATIVE BEHAVIOUR

The term 'behavioural disturbance' is generally used to describe behaviour of a negative detrimental kind. Unusual behaviour may have positive aspects and this is certainly true of that which occurs in association with elevated mood. Much has been written concerning the link between creativity and manic-depressive illnesss. It is particularly well described by Kay Jamison (1993) in her book *Touched with Fire: Manic Depressive Illness and the Artistic Temperament*. There are many examples of gifted individuals who are particularly creative in the setting of morbidly elevated mood. A frequently cited example is that of the composer Robert Schumann who, it is claimed, had severe manic episodes during which he described music pouring into him. He also described episodes of psychosis where he heard music which he subsequently was able to use in his compositions (Dowley 1982).

The issue of the relationship between creativity and illness and its treatment was formally studied by Schou (1979), who studied artists and writers who were manic-depressive and enquired about the effects of lithium upon their artistic productivity. Interestingly, in a recent review by Post (1996), it has been found that writers have an increased risk of affective disorders and alcohol abuse, but this pattern is not found among other artists, such as poets.

Mixed affective states

Mixed affective states are perhaps by their very nature somewhat atypical. In 1919, Kraepelin (1971) first observed that in manic patients who, as it were, 'turned depressed', features of both depression and mania could be displayed simultaneously. The same held true for the reverse situation—that is, where a patient who was depressed was becoming manic. Himmelhoch *et al.* (1976) took this further, naming six individual states (Table 14.1) where mood was either elated or depressed, thought tempo was either increased with racing thoughts or there was poverty of thought, and where there was agitation and motor overactivity or conversely motor retardation.

Up to 30% of first presentations of bipolar affective disorder may present as a mixed affective state (WHO 1992) but those mixed symptoms which occur in the first episode are usually transitory.

In established cases, knowledge of the previous history will clarify the diagnostic difficulty which may be presented by, for example, a case of manic

Table 14.1 The six mixed affective states described by Himmelhoch *et al.* (1976).

State	Mood	Thought tempo	Motor activity
1 Manic stupor	Elated	Racing	Retardation
2 Agitated depression	Depressed	Decreased	Agitation
3 Anxious mania	Elated	Racing	Agitation
4 Unproductive mania	Elated	Decreased	Agitation
5 Depression with flight of ideas	Depressed	Racing	Retardation
6 'Inhibited mania'	Elated	Decreased	Retardation

stupor. If, however, the history is not known and there is no collateral informant, the diagnosis may not be obvious and the possibility of these mixed states should be borne in mind in considering unusual mental states, particularly where marked retardation is a feature.

Functional psychosis and learning disability

Diagnosis may be difficult when a patient with a learning disability develops a comorbid psychotic state. Both affective and schizophrenic psychoses occur in the learning disabled population—indeed, the frequency of schizophrenia in the learning disabled—is three times that in the general population (Turner 1989). It has been shown (Sturmey *et al.* 1991) that diagnosis of schizophrenia can be reliably made in patients with IQs of 50 and over, although persons with a more severe diagnosis of learning disability are not able to describe the symptoms adequately to allow the diagnosis to be made reliably.

Difficulties may also occur in establishing a diagnosis of affective illness in the learning disabled. Classic features of pressure of speech, flight of ideas and so forth may not be present. None the less, one review (Sovner & Hurley 1983) concluded that patients with learning disability could be reliably identified as manic using DSM-III criteria (American Psychiatric Association (APA) 1980). Features which have been identified as being helpful in making the diagnosis of psychosis in the learning disabled patient include cyclical changes in behaviour, increased vocalization, activity and aggression. Although the patient may be unable to report auditory or visual hallucinations, it may be possible to infer their presence objectively from the patient's behaviour.

Atypical presentations of schizophrenia

In a similar way to that which we considered in relation to affective disorder, atypical presentations of schizophrenia may be classified as those apparently or probably schizophrenic but without classical features of the condition, those where the condition resembles some disorder other than schizophrenia, and those where the presentation is of behavioural disturbance which is not recognized as representing illness at all.

SCHIZOPHRENIA WITHOUT CLASSICAL FEATURES

It is nowadays customary to diagnose schizophrenia on the basis of clinical features which fulfil operational definitions such as those of DSM-IV (APA 1994). When this is done, patients without classical features are excluded. In the past, such operational definitions were not used. The varying concepts of the disorder which came to be adopted in the US and Europe were demonstrated in the US–UK diagnostic project (Cooper *et al.* 1972) which showed that schizophrenia was much more often diagnosed in the US where the concept of schizophrenia was much wider than in the UK and that this expansion of the concept of schizophrenia had occurred at the expense of affective disorders.

In the 1960s, especially in the US, patients were diagnosed as having forms of schizophrenia when they did not have classic symptoms. An example of this diagnostic practice is the concept of 'pseudoneurotic schizophrenia' (Hoch & Polatin 1949) where patients had a wide range of neurotic symptoms ranging from phobias, obsessions and depersonalization to hysterical conversion and hypochondriasis. It was stated that there might be severe anxiety and that the course of the illness might be punctuated by attacks of psychotic disturbance lasting days, hours or perhaps only minutes. Such patients would not often be diagnosed as having schizophrenia now and there was never any satisfactory evidence that they did suffer from that illness; on the other hand, in the absence of any diagnostic marker for schizophrenia, it cannot unequivocally be said that they do not.

The mode of onset of schizophrenia is very variable. It is sometimes very sudden but insidious onsets in which the illness gradually develops over months or even years also occur (Johnstone *et al.* 1986). During this prodromal period, a number of symptoms which are not clearly indicative of psychosis may develop and the situation only becomes clear when the psychosis becomes manifest. Symptoms of a non-schizophrenic nature may occur during the course of established or chronic illness. The occurrence of depressive symptoms is very well established (Siris *et al.* 1988). These respond to antidepressant treatment and in a similar way the obsessional symptoms which have been said to occur in up to 255 of patients with established schizophrenia may be relieved by clomipramine (Berman *et al.* 1995).

SCHIZOPHRENIA RESEMBLING ANOTHER PSYCHOSIS

The main source of diagnostic confusion is drug-induced psychosis. It has long been known that amphetamine and other dopamine-releasing drugs, if taken by non-psychotic individuals, could induce a schizophreniform psychosis that is a schizophrenia-like paranoid state (Connell 1958). More recent work has focused on marijuana (cannabis). The possibility that cannabis psychosis may be an entity separate from schizophrenia or manic-depressive psychosis has been considered (Imade & Ebie 1991) and certainly this is a diagnosis that has been widely made.

To a degree, the thinking underlying this, in some cases, seems to have been that a cannabis psychosis might be less serious and the outlook less pessimistic than in the case of schizophrenic illness. In fact, recent literature does not support this view. In a careful review, Thornicroft (1990) showed no evidence for a separate diagnosis of cannabis psychosis and concluded that chronic psychosis, apparently as a result of cannabis misuse, is more likely to be due to the onset of schizophreniform disorder or schizophrenia in a vulnerable individual rather than a separate diagnosis of disorder purely induced by cannabis. The view that cannabis psychosis would somehow be less serious than schizophrenia has not been supported by the facts. Cleghorn *et al.* (1991) showed that delusions and hallucinations were more severe in medicated schizophrenia with a history of substance abuse than those with no such history and that, similarly, thought disorder was more severe in substance abusing unmedicated schizophrenics than in those who did not take illicit substances (see Chapter 3).

SCHIZOPHRENIA PRESENTING AS BEHAVIOURAL DISTURBANCE NOT NECESSARILY RECOGNIZED AS ILLNESS

In recent years there has been growing concern about the plight of the mentally abnormal offender (Department of Health and the Home Office 1992). Schizophrenia may be accompanied by severe behavioural disturbance even in its earliest stages (Johnstone *et al.* 1986). A substantial proportion of patients with schizophrenia have had involvement with the police (Mackay & Wright 1984) and, of those, more than 10% may have been convicted of an offence at some time (Johnstone *et al.* 1991). This also applies to those in their first episode of illness (MacMillan & Johnson 1987).

The extent to which such behaviour may occur before the schizophrenic illness is diagnosed was demonstrated by Humphreys *et al.* (1994), who examined the past history and sociodemographic schedules (Jablensky *et al.* 1980) completed in 192 of the 253 cases of first schizophrenic episodes described by Johnstone *et al.* (1986). These schedules refer to the 5 years before admission. Thirty-one patients had had convictions recorded during that time, having committed a total of 55 offences (21 acquisitive, 14 assault, 7 property damage, 3 road traffic, 4 alcohol or drugs, 2 public order, and 4 other). Sixteen people committed offences which were independent of their illness or where the relationship was unclear. Thirteen people, however, committed offences closely associated with psychotic symptoms, some as a direct result of their delusions; at least two more were ill when they were arrested. Examples of the behaviour leading to conviction in these patients were the repeated theft of food by a woman who had believed for years that attempts were being made to poison her and had stolen what she saw as uncontaminated food; also the throwing of a brick through a window by a man in an attempt to prove he was not in the IRA. At the time of conviction, these patients were not known to be experiencing a psychosis and the first time that they were known to have revealed their delusional beliefs to medical staff was at the time of initial admission to hospital, which, in some cases, was some years later. It appears that the disturbed behaviour leading to conviction was one of the presenting features of their schizophrenia which was not diagnosed at the time.

Movement disorders

Movement disorders are not generally included in classifications of psychiatric illness but they are very common in association with psychiatric conditions. They may present in ways which give rise to diagnostic doubt and therefore to management which is not always appropriate.

Whether or not abnormalities of movement are a feature of untreated schizophrenia (Owens *et al.* 1982) has been the subject of some debate, but there is no doubt that the anti-psychotic agents most frequently used in schizophrenia are associated with abnormalities of movement.

Acute disorders include acute dystonias, akathisia and drug-induced pseudo-Parkinsonism. Chronic movement disorders include tardive dyskinesia and tardive dystonia. These disorders may present in various ways which allow them to be misdiagnosed as psychiatric disorders.

ACUTE DYSTONIA

This condition usually appears within a few days of starting anti-psychotic drugs. The movements are uncoordinated and may involve the body, the head and neck and the limbs. Retrocollis, torticollis, opisthotonos and oculogyric crises all occur. Characteristically, these are repeated spasms of the muscles which are distressing and painful. The onset of the symptoms can be very abrupt and they may be conceivably mistaken for epilepsy or meningitis unless a history of anti-psychotic ingestion is obtained. Alternatively, the symptoms may be misdiagnosed as being hysterical. These disorders are common. Addonizio and Alexopoulos (1988) have suggested a prevalence of 23% overall in neuroleptic-treated patients with a figure of 31% in young patients (with a mean age of 26 years). It may seem improbable to psychiatrists that these acute dystonias can be regarded as hysterical but it is worth bearing in mind that surveys have shown that 40% of patients with the generality of dystonia (and it does of course also occur in people who have not had anti-psychotic drugs) are given a diagnosis of conversion hysteria at some point (Fahn 1983). Intramuscular anticholinergic drugs produce a rapid therapeutic response.

AKATHISIA

In 90% of cases, akathisia occurs within 3 months of starting anti-psychotics. It presents as motor hyperactivity with restlessness, shifting posture and an inability to stay still for more than a few moments. Patients complain of a subjective sense of discomfort and associated feelings of tension. Resemblance to agitation may lead to a mistaken diagnosis of agitated depression.

DRUG-INDUCED PSEUDO-PARKINSONISM/AKINESIA

Akinesia develops within days of the first administration of anti-psychotic drugs and is very common although often unrecognized. The patient's spontaneous movements, especially arm swing, are reduced, and there is a lack of facial expression as well as a marked reduction in volitional behaviour. The resemblance between this state and both depression and the schizophrenic defect state has been well described (Rifkin *et al.* 1975) and it is readily misdiagnosed.

TARDIVE DYSTONIA

Tardive dystonia has only been given much consideration in recent years (Burke *et al.* 1982). The majority of tardive dystonias occur in the head and neck but it may be axial, including the so-called Pisa syndrome (Ekbom *et al.* 1972; Gerlach 1979), and can involve the laryngeal muscles causing dysphonia and dysphagia. The altered speech may be regarded as a feature of the patient's mental state rather than the result of neurological abnormality (Owens 1990).

Psychiatric symptoms may be a feature of a number of conditions where the principal problem is a movement disorder. These include Parkinson's disease and its variants, Huntingdon's chorea and Gilles de la Tourette's syndrome.

More topically, the new variant of Creutzfeldt–Jacob disease (CJD) described in the media before it has reached the medical press has been said by those involved in the CJD surveillance programme to be associated with anxiety and depression at its onset in at least some cases (Will *et al.* 1996). Depression is reported to occur in 30–60% of cases of Parkinson's disease (Mindham 1970). Various psychiatric symptoms, including irritability and emotional lability, may be presenting features of Huntington's chorea, and paranoid delusions have been reported in as many as 33% of cases (Bolt 1970).

Gilles de la Tourette's syndrome

Gilles de la Tourette described this syndrome in 1885 and many cases have been reported since. Operational criteria (Shapiro *et al.* 1978) are used for making the diagnosis. The main clinical features include multiple tics (sudden brief movements) beginning in the early teens, or before, with coprolalia and echolalia, and stereotyped movements.

Many cases of Tourette's syndrome have been claimed to have obsessional features (Shapiro & Shapiro 1992) and it unclear what the significance of this relationship is. In its complete form, Tourette's syndrome is not difficult to diagnose, but the full picture is not always present and such cases may be considered to have behavioural disturbances or myoclonic epilepsy.

The treatment of Tourette's syndrome has traditionally been with a combination of behavioural techniques, such as massed practice for tics (Clark 1966) and low-dose haloperidol (Milman 1960). In cases with associated obsessionality, preliminary studies suggest that use of the serotonin re-uptake inhibitor fluoxetine can be helpful (Eapen *et al.* 1996).

'Functional' presentation of 'organic' disease

The classifications of psychiatric illness in current use have their roots in the 19th century. At that time, diseases came to be defined in terms of symptom clusters, lesions and natural history (Berrios 1987). Psychoses were divided into the exogenous and endogenous, these terms being introduced into medicine by the neurologist Mobius in 1893.

The exogenous–endogenous dichotomy lacked clear definition even at this time, and there are semantic uncertainties surrounding the use of such terms (Lewis 1971).

Bonhoeffer (in translation in Hirsch & Shepherd 1974), who described the essential similarity of psychoses relating to diverse organic causes, appreciated the difficulties associated with this dichotomy and wrote, 'We cannot be absolutely certain what is endogenous in the final analysis ... in fact we shall hardly ever be able to deal with pure types of exogenous and endogenous aetiology'. The problems of the alternative terminology of 'organic versus functional' (which is used to convey similar meaning) were appreciated at an early stage by Mendel (1907) who, in referring to functional psychoses, stated:

> On the other hand there is great difference of opinion amongst authors as to how to divide these mental diseases in which no anatomical findings have hitherto been met and which do not belong under any of the forms named. They are designated as functional psychoses, by which it is not said that anatomical changes do not exist but only that we have so far been unable to identify them.

In spite of these difficulties, the idea that on one hand there are psychoses related to identifiable disease of the brain or other parts of the body, and on the other hand psychotic illnesses in which the symptoms and the natural history are in general different from those of the former and in which demonstrable lesions are not usually found, is fundamental to modern classifications such as DSM-IV or ICD-10. There have, however, been reports of apparently typical 'functional' psychotic pictures of both a schizophrenic (Davison & Bagley 1969) and an affective (Krauthammer & Klerman 1978) nature being associated with organic brain disease. Psychiatric illness, particularly schizophrenia, is associated with an increased risk of death (Baldwin 1979; Herrman *et al.* 1983). At least some of this increased mortality results from an enhanced risk of trauma and poisoning which, like the greater liability to infections formerly found in sufferers from schizophrenia (Baldwin 1979), is clearly secondary to the mental disorder. It is the case, however, that not all of the organic disease described by Davison and Bagley (1969) and Krauthammer and Klerman (1978) as occurring in association with schizophrenia or affective psychosis, or with phenomenologically indistinguishable conditions, could be considered to result from any of the social or environmental disadvantages suffered by the mentally ill.

Four possible explanations of the relationship between psychosis and organic disease of the central nervous system (CNS) were suggested by Slater *et al.* (1963):

1   the association is fortuitous;
2   the CNS disorder precipitates 'true schizophrenia';
3   the CNS disorder 'causes' the psychosis;
4   cases occur according to each of these hypotheses.

It has been established that in various organic disorders of the CNS, the association with psychosis phenomenologically indistinguishable from schizophrenia exceeds chance expectation (Davison & Bagley 1969; Davison 1983) and it was concluded by Davison and Bagley (1969) that in the majority of instances the third of these explanations is correct. It is clear that some cases must occur in accordance with the first possibility, and the second may be relevant in those with a family history of schizophrenia.

In a study of first episodes of schizophrenia (Johnstone *et al.* 1986), 462 potential cases were referred. Two hundred and nine of them did not fulfil the study criteria and in 15 of these, this was because of the presence of organic disease of definite or possible aetiological significance. All of these patients had been considered by the referring psychiatrist to be probable cases of first-episode schizophrenia. The organic diagnoses in the 15 patients were syphilis (three cases), alcohol excess (three cases), sarcoidosis (two cases), drug abuse (two cases), and carcinoma of the lung, autoimmune multisystem disease, epilepsy resulting from cerebral cysticercosis, chronic thyroid disease with acute thyrotoxicosis, and head injury with hemiparesis (one case each). It is evident that while in two of the alcohol-related cases and the case of head injury the patients' disturbed behaviour and/or dramatic presentation delayed the full assessment, that would have revealed the organic nature of the disorder. Many of the cases are indeed phenomenologically indistinguishable from schizophrenia.

A further study from the same research group (Johnstone *et al.* 1988) studied 360 consecutive admissions with definite or possible psychosis shortly after they came into hospital. Twenty-three of them were later found to have an organic disorder of definite or possible aetiological significance for their psychosis. The study compared the phenomenology of these patients with that of 92 matched controls drawn from the parent sample who conformed to DSM-III criteria for schizophrenia, mania, or depression. Few significant differences were found and there was considerable overlap between the phenomenology of the different diagnostic groups. The organic conditions in this study are shown in Table 14.2. In these patients the organic condition quickly came to light, but this not the case in the first study, where patients continued to present a picture apparently typical of 'functional' psychosis for weeks or months. A similar situation has been well described in the literature, particularly in respect of syphilis and cerebral tumours, by Davison (1983). In retrospect and on a purely anecdotal basis, the clinicians who saw the patients described by Johnstone *et al.* (1987) considered that

Table 14.2 Organic conditions with significance for psychosis found by Johnstone *et al.* (1988).

Disorder	No. of cases
Amphetamine abuse	2
Alcohol abuse/withdrawal	2
Amphetamines, heroin and cannabis abuse	5
Barbiturates and diazepam abuse/withdrawal	1
Barbiturates/diazepam/alcohol abuse/withdrawal	1
Ephedrine-containing cold cure abuse	1
Hypothyroidism	1
Thyrotoxicosis	1
Syphilis	1
Cerebrovascular accident	1
Frontal astrocytoma	1
Pituitary tumour	1
Ulcerative colitis on steroids	1
Systemic lupus erythematosus	1
Carcinoma of the lung	1
B_{12} deficiency (previous gastric surgery)	1
Uncontrolled insulin-dependent diabetes mellitus	1

they differed from the generality of patients in terms of their minimal response to anti-psychotic treatment.

As far as affective illness is concerned, the most important underlying organic conditions which can mimic the picture of either depression or of mania are endocrine. Thyroid disease is commonly associated with affective illness. It is reported that 10% of severe cases of hypothyroidism suffer a psychotic illness (Whybrow & Hurwitz 1976). This may be paranoid or schizophreniform in nature, but most commonly the picture is of severe depression. Emotional lability, anxiety, poor concentration and restlessness are, of course, features of the generality of cases of hyperthyroidism but major depression, hypomania or paranoid psychoses are seen in about 10% of the more severe cases (Bursten 1961).

Adrenocortical disease is strongly associated with psychiatric symptomatology. About one third to one half of all patients with Cushing's syndrome show some psychiatric disturbance. Ross *et al.* (1966) reviewed 601 cases in 11 published series and noted a 42% incidence of psychological difficulty.

Depression was evident in 39% of a personal series of 36 cases described by Mattingly (1968). Disorder sufficient to be termed psychotic occurs in 5–20% of cases (Ferrier 1987). Affective psychoses are the most common. The prevalence of psychosis is much greater in pituitary-dependent (adrenocorticotrophic hormone (ACTH)-driven) Cushing's disease compared with that found with other pituitary tumours, adrenal tumours or ectopic ACTH-producing neoplasms (Cohen 1980; Kelly *et al.* 1983). Patients treated with pharmacological doses of glucocorticoids frequently exhibit mood changes and the prevalence of psychosis is substantial.

Schizophreniform psychoses occur (see above) and hypomania is said to be more likely than depressive illness (Ferrier 1987).

Lastly, in considering organic disorders which may mimic the typical presentations of 'functional' psychiatric illness, two relatively new disorders should be included. It has become clear that infection with human immunodeficiency virus (HIV) may be associated with a range of psychiatric problems (Catalan 1990). Both psychological reactions (adjustment reactions, neurotic disorders, depressive disorder) and organic brain syndromes (acute and chronic) can occur. A neuropathological picture of encephalitis occurs in AIDS cases and the term 'AIDS dementia complex' has been introduced to describe a chronic syndrome, characterized in the early stages by cognitive and behavioural changes, which tend to progress to global intellectual impairment with major neurological signs (Rosenblum *et al.* 1988). Neurological and neuropsychiatric manifestations may be amongst the presenting features of AIDS, sometimes developing in the absence of other signs of the disease. Psychotic illness, typically resembling mania or schizophrenia, may occur in patients with HIV infection. Symptoms and signs of an organic brain syndrome are not always found, so that the aetiology of the disorder can at times remain unclear. While these disorders could be manifestations of an organic brain process (secondary to HIV infection or its treatment, or to drug misuse), the possibility of a chance association remains (Vogel-Schibilia *et al.* 1988).

This chapter was written in Edinburgh, the site of the UK Creutzfeldt–Jacob Surveillance Project, in the month in which the possibility that a new form of CJD affecting young people and possibly associated with ingestion of beef infected with bovine spongiform encephalopathy (BSE), has been raised, causing widespread concern (Will *et al.* 1996). This issue was discussed in the public domain before it was reported in the scientific literature, but it appears that the early manifestations of this very serious and ultimately fatal organic brain disease are anxiety and depression (Will *et al.* 1996). At present there is no means of knowing whether this disorder will remain very rare or whether the recently reported cases are the first of many. If the latter possibility comes to pass, the question of depressive features in young adults being an atypical presentation of dementia may become a matter which has to be considered in the practice of many psychiatrists. The report of a case of presumed Pick's disease in a 28-year-old woman (Mowadat *et al.* 1993) considered in turn to have a neurotic reaction to pregnancy, a depressive psychosis and schizophreniform illness before the organic nature of her disorder became evident, highlights the difficulties of diagnosing dementing illness in very atypical circumstances.

Conclusions

The practical importance of atypical illnesses lies in the fact that the diagnostic confusion with which they are associated may give rise to inappropriate management. As far as functional disorders with atypical presentations are concerned, this may mean that a patient does not receive readily available treatment which could alleviate his or her condition and that an inaccurate and possibly unduly pessimistic prognosis is given. Particular examples of this would be depressive pseudodementia, where the treatable nature of the disorder is not recognized, or elevated mood or psychosis presenting as behavioural disturbance, which is not recognized as illness at all. Such presentations may result in essentially medical issues being inappropriately handled in the judicial system.

The presentation of 'organic' disorders in a way that is suggestive of a functional condition may result in a patient being deprived of readily available and effective treatment, for example replacement treatment for thyroid insufficiency, but even where no treatment other than palliation is possible (e.g. some malignant tumours), delay in diagnosis of the underlying physical condition can be very distressing for patients, and perhaps especially so for their relatives. The nature of the difficulties concerning appropriate diagnosis of atypical presentations means that it is not possible to give more than crude estimates of their frequency, and certainly some of the situations described do not occur often but some do, and better recognition of, for example, mental illnesses in people with learning disability, and of the problems associated with movement disorder occurring in relation to psychiatric disorder, could provide valuable reductions in morbidity.

Apart from these practical matters, atypical presentations highlight some theoretical issues. The very fact that disorders that are assumed to have different aetiologies, and considered to have different courses and outcomes, may at times seem indistinguishable reminds us of our limited level of our understanding of so many aspects of psychiatric disorder. On the other hand, the evidence provided by atypical presentations has the potential to increase our understanding. The association of adrenocortical disease with affective disorder, and the occurrence of schizophrenia-like psychoses in organic disease affecting the temporal lobes of the brain, are well-known examples of this, but the recognition of the need to include atypical presentations, perhaps those with an essentially behavioural picture, in linkage studies may advance the progress of psychiatric genetics. The importance of the recognition of atypical illnesses is clear, and it is probably worth emphasizing that this rests essentially upon clinical skill. These are usually situations where no battery of tests is a match for competent clinical assessment and a willingness to think again.

References

Addonizio, G. & Alexopoulos, G.S. (1988) Drug-induced dystonia in young and elderly patients. *American Journal of Psychiatry* **145**, 869–871.

American Psychiatric Association (1980) *Diagnostic and Statistical Manual of Mental Disorders*, 3rd edn (DSM-III). American Psychiatric Association, Washington, D.C.

American Psychiatric Association (1994) *Diagnostic and Statistical Manual of Mental Disorders*, 4th edn (DSM-IV). American Psychiatric Association, Washington, D.C.

Asnis, G.M., McGinn, L.K. & Sanderson, W.C. (1995) Atypical depression: Clinical aspects and noradrenergic function. *American Journal of Psychiatry* **152**, 31–36.

Baldwin, J.A. (1979) Schizophrenia presenting and physical disease. *Psychological Medicine* **9**, 611–618.

Berman, I., Kalinowski, A., Berman, S.M. *et al.* (1995) Obsessive and compulsive symptoms in chronic schizophrenia. *Comprehensive Psychiatry* **36**, 6–10.

Berrios, G.E. (1987) Historical aspects of psychoses: 19th century issues. *British Medical Bulletin* **43**, 484–498.

Bolt, J.M.W. (1970) Huntingdon's chorea in the West of Scotland. *British Journal of Psychiatry* **116**, 259–270.

Burke, R.E., Fahn, S., Jankovic, J. *et al.* (1982) Tardive dystonia, late onset and persistent dystonia caused by antipsychotic drugs. *Neurology* **32**, 1335–1346.

Bursten, B. (1961) Psychosis associated with Thyrotoxicosis. *Archives of General Psychiatry* **4**, 267–273.

Catalan, J. (1990) HIV and AIDS related psychiatric disorder: what can the psychiatrist do? In: *Difficulties and Dilemmas in the Management of Psychiatric Patients* (eds Hawton & Cowan) pp. 205–217. Oxford University Press, Oxford.

Clark, D.F. (1966) Behaviour therapy of Gilles de la Tourette's syndrome. *British Journal of Psychiatry* **112**, 771–778.

Cleghorn, J.M., Kaplan, R.D., Szechtman, B. *et al.* (1991) Substance abuse and schizophrenia: Effect on symptoms but not on neurocognitive function. *Journal of Clinical Psychiatry* **52**, 26–30.

Cohen, S.I. (1980) Cushings syndrome: A psychiatric study of 29 patients. *British Journal of Psychiatry* **136**, 317–321.

Connell, P.H. (1958) *Amphetamine Psychosis*. Maudsley Monograph No. 5. Chapman & Hall, London.

Cooper, J.E., Kendell, R.E., Gurland, B.J. *et al.* (1972) *Psychiatric Diagnosis in New York and London*. Maudsley Monograph No. 20. Oxford University Press, London.

Davison, K. (1983) Schizophrenia-like psychoses associated with organic disorders of the nervous system: A review of the literature. In: *Current Problems in Neuropsychiatry* (ed. R.N. Herrington), pp. 113–184. Headley Bros, Ashford, Kent.

Davison, K. & Bagley, C.R. (1969) Schizophrenia-like psychoses associated with organic disorders of the nervous system: A review of the literature. In: *Current Problems in Neuropsychiatry* (ed. R.N. Herrington). Headley Bros, Ashford, Kent.

Department of Health and the Home Office (1992) *Review of Health and Social Services for Mentally Disordered Offenders and Others Requiring Similar Services: Final Summary Report.* HMSO, London.

Dowley, T. (1982) *Schumann: His Life and Times.* Hippocrene Books, New York.

Eapen, V., Trimble, M.R. & Robertson, M.M. (1996) The use of Fluoxetine in Gilles de la Tourette syndrome and obsessive compulsive behaviours: Preliminary clinical experience. *Progress in Neuro-Psychopharmacology and Biological Psychiatry* **20**, 737–743.

Ekbom, K., Lindholm, H. & Ljungberg, L. (1972) New dystonic syndrome associate with Butyrophenome therapy. *Journal of Neurology* **202**, 94–103.

Fahn, S. (1983) High dosage anticholinergic therapy in dystonia. *Neurology* **33**, 1255–1261.

Feinmann, C., Harris, M. & Cawley, R. (1984) Psychogenic facial pain; presentation and treatment. *British Medical Journal* 288, 436–438.

Ferrier, I.N. (1987) Endocrinology and psychosis. *British Medical Bulletin* 43, 672–688.

Folstein, M.F. & Rabins, P.V. (1991) Replacing pseudodementia. *Neuropsychiatry, Neuropsychology and Behavioral Neurology* 4, 36–40.

Freeman, H.L. (1994) Historical and nosological aspects of dysthymia. *Acta Psychiatrica Scandinavica* 89 (Suppl. 383), 7–11.

Freeman, T.W., Clothier, J.L., Pazzaglia, P. *et al.* (1992) A double-blind comparison of valproate and lithium in the treatment of acute mania. *American Journal of Psychiatry* 149, 108–111.

Frith, C.D. (1983) Effects of ECT and depression on various aspects of memory. *British Journal of Psychiatry* 142, 610–617.

Gerlach, J. (1979) *Tardive Dyskinesia*. Laegeforeningens Forlag, Copenhagen.

Goodwin, G.M. (1994a) Lithium revisited: A reply. *British Journal of Psychiatry* 167, 573–574.

Goodwin, G.M. (1994b) Recurrence of mania after lithium withdrawal. *British Journal of Psychiatry* 164, 149–152.

Herrman, H.E., Baldwin, J.A. & Christie, D. (1983) A record linkage study of mortality and general hospital discharge in patients diagnosed as schizophrenic. *Psychological Medicine* 13, 581–593.

Himmelhoch, J.M., Mulla, D. & Neil, J.F. (1976) Incidence and significance of mixed affective states in a bipolar population. *Archives of General Psychiatry* 33, 1062–1066.

Hirsch, S. & Shepherd, M. (eds) (1974) *Themes and Variations in European Psychiatry*. Wright, Bristol.

Hoch, P. & Polatin, P. (1949) Pseudoneurotic forms of schizophrenia. *Psychiatric Quarterly* 23, 248–256.

Humphreys, M., Johnstone, E.C. & MacMillan, M. (1994) Offending among first episode schizophrenics. *Journal of Forensic Psychiatry* 5, 51–61.

Imade, A.G.T. & Ebie, J.C. (1991) A retrospective study of symptom patterns of cannabis induced psychosis. *Acta Psychiatrica Scandinavica* 83, 134–136.

Jablensky, A., Schwartz, R. & Tomov, T. (1980) WHO collaborative study on impairments and disabilities associated with schizophrenic disorders: a preliminary communication — Objectives and methods. *Acta Psychiatrica Scandinavica* 65 (Suppl. 285), 152–163.

Jamison, K. (1993) *Touched with Fire: Manic Depressive Illness and the Artistic Temperament*. Free Press, New York.

Jelliffe, S.E. (1931) Some historical phases of the manic-depressive synthesis. *Association for Research in Nervous and Mental Disease* 11, 3–47.

Johnstone, E.C., Cooling, N.J. & Frith, C.D. (1988) Phenomenology of organic and functional psychoses and the overlap between them. *British Journal of Psychiatry* 153, 770–776.

Johnstone, E.C., MacMillan, J.F. & Crow, T.J. (1987) The occurrence of organic disease of possible aetiological significance in a population of 268 cases of first episode schizophrenia. *Psychological Medicine* 17, 371–379.

Johnstone, E.C., Leary, J., Frith, C.D. & Owens, D.G.C. (1991) Disabilities and circumstances of schizophrenic patients: A follow-up study. Police contact No. 7. *British Journal of Psychiatry* **159** (Suppl. 13), 37–39.

Johnstone, E.C., Crow, T.J., Macmillan, J.F. *et al.* (1986) The Northwick Park study of first episodes of schizophrenia. 1. Presentation of the illness and problems related to admission. *British Journal of Psychiatry* **148**, 115–120.

Johnstone, E.C., Frith, C.D., Crow, T.J. *et al.* (1992) The Northwick Park 'functional' psychosis study: Diagnosis and outcome. *Psychological Medicine* **22**, 331–346.

Kelly, W.F., Checkley, S.A., Bender, D.A. *et al.* (1983) Cushing's syndrome and depression: A prospective study of 26 patients. *British Journal of Psychiatry* **142**, 16–19.

Kraepelin, E. (1919/1971) *Dementia Praecox* (ed. G.M. Robertson, trans. R.M. Barclay). Kruger, New York.

Krauthammer, C. & Klerman, G.L. (1978) Secondary mania. *Archives of General Psychiatry* **35**, 1333–1339.

Lascelles, R.G. (1966) Atypical facial pain and depression. *British Journal of Psychiatry* **112**, 651–659.

Lesse, S. (1993) The masked depression syndrome. *American Jorunal of Psychotherapy* **37**, 456–475.

Lewis, A. (1971) Endogenous and exogenous: A useful dichotomy? *Psychological Medicine* **1**, 191–196.

Lewis, N. & Pietrowski, Z. (1954) Clinical diagnosis of manic-depressive psychosis. In: *Depression* (eds P.M. Hoch & J. Zubin). Greene and Stratton, New York.

Mackay, R. & Wright, R. (1984) Schizophrenia and anti-social (criminal) behaviour: Some responses from sufferers and relatives. *Medicine, Science and the Law* **24**, 192–198.

MacMillan, J.F. & Johnson, A.L. (1987) Contact with the police in early schizophrenia: Its nature, frequency and relevance to outcome and treatment. *Medicine, Science and the Law* **27**, 191–200.

Magni, G.J.N. (1991) The use of antidepressants in the treatment of chronic pain: A review of the current evidence. *Drugs* **42**, 730–748.

Mattingly, D. (1968) Disorders of the adrenal cortex and pituitary gland. In: *Recent Advances in Medicine*, 15th edn (eds D.N. Baron, N. Campsten & A.M. Dawson), pp. 125–169. Churchill, London.

Mendel, E. (1907) *Textbook of Psychiatry* (trans. W.C. Krauss). F.A. Davis, Philadelphia, Penn.

Milman, D.H. (1960) Multiple tics. *American Journal of Psychiatry* **116**, 935–936.

Mindham, R.H. (1970) Psychiatric symptoms in Parkinsonism. *Journal of Neurology, Neurosurgery and Psychiatry* **33**, 188–191.

Mobius, P.J. (1893) *Abriss der Lehre der Nervenkrankheiten.* Abel, Leipzig.

Moncrieff, J. (1994) Lithium revisited: A re-examination of the placebo-controlled trials of lithium prophylaxis in manic-depressive disorder. *British Journal of Psychiatry* **167**, 569–574.

Monfort, J.C. (1995) The difficult elderly patient: Curable hostile depression or personality disorder? *International Psychogeriatrics* **7**, 95–111.

Mowadat, H.R., Kerr, E.E. & St Clair, D. (1993) Sporadic Pick's disease in a 28 year old woman. *British Journal of Psychiatry* **162**, 259–262.

Ogilvie, A., Battersby, S., Bubb, V.J. *et al.* (1996) Polymorphism in serotonin transporter gene associated with susceptibility to major depression. *Lancet* **347**, 731–733.

Owens, D.G. (1990) Dystonia: A potential psychiatric pitfall. *British Journal of Psychiatry* **156**, 620–634.

Owens, D.G., Johnstone, E.C. & Frith, C.D. (1982) Spontaneous involuntary disorders of movement. *Archives of General Psychiatry* **39**, 452–461.

Paykel, E.S. & Norton, K.R.W. (1982) Diagnoses not to be missed: Masked depression. *British Journal of Hospital Medicine* **28**, 151–157.

Post, F. (1996) Verbal creativity, depression and alcoholism: An investigation of one hundred American and British writers. *British Journal of Psychiatry* **168**, 545–555.

Rifkin, A., Quitkin, F. & Klein, D. (1975) Akinesia: A poorly recognised drug-induced extrapyramidal behavioural disorder. *Archives of General Psychiatry* **32**, 672–674.

Rosenblum, M.L., Levy, R.M. & Bredesen, D.E. (eds) (1988) *AIDS and the Nervous System*. Raven Press, New York.

Ross, E.J., Marshall-Jones, P. & Friedman, M. (1966) Cushings syndrome: Diagnostic criteria. *Quarterly Journal of Medicine* **35**, 149–192.

Sachdev, P.S., Smith, J.S., Angus-Lepan, H. & Rodriguez, P. (1990) Pseudodementia twelve years on. *Journal of Neurology, Neurosurgery and Psychiatry* **53** (3), 254–259.

Schou, M. (1979) Artistic productivity and lithium prophylaxis in manic-depressive illness. *British Journal of Psychiatry* **135**, 97–103.

Shapiro, A.K. & Shapiro, E.S. (1992) Evaluation of the reported association of obsessive-compulsive symptoms or disorder with Tourette's syndrome or disorder. *Comprehensive Psychiatry* **33**, 152–165.

Shapiro, A.K., Shapiro, E.S., Bruun, R.D. *et al.* (1978) *Gilles de la Tourette Syndrome*, pp. 581–587. Raven Press, New York.

Sheldrick, C., Jablensky, A., Sartorius, N. & Shepherd, M. (1977) Schizophrenia succeeded by affective illness: Catamnestic study and statistical enquiry. *Psychological Medicine* **7**, 619–624.

Sims, A. (1995) *Symptoms in the Mind: An Introduction to Descriptive Psychopathology*, 2nd edn. Bailliere Tindall.

Siris, S.G., Adan, F., Cohen, M. *et al.* (1988) Postpsychotic depression and negative symptoms: An investigation of syndromal overlap. *American Journal of Psychiatry* **145**, 1532–1537.

Slater, E., Beard, A.W. & Glitheroe, E. (1963) The schizophrenia-like psychoses of epilepsy. *British Journal of Psychiatry* **109**, 95–150.

Sovner, R. & Hurley, A.D. (1983) Do the mentally retarded suffer from affective illness? *Archives of General Psychiatry* **40**, 61–67.

Sturmey, P., Reed, J. & Corbett, J. (1991) Psychometric assessment of psychiatric disorders in people with learning difficulties (mental handicap): A review of measures. *Psychological Medicine* **21**, 143–155.

Thornicroft, G. (1990) Cannabis and psychosis: Is there epidemiological evidence for an association? *British Journal of Psychiatry* **157**, 25–33.

Turner, T.H. (1989) Schizophrenia and mental handicap: An historical review, with implications for further research. *Psychological Medicine* **19**, 301–314.

Tyrer, P., Seivewright, N., Ferguson, B. *et al.* (1993) The Nottingham study of neurotic disorder: Effect of personality status on response to drug treatment, cognitive therapy and self-help over two years. *British Journal of Psychiatry* **162**, 219–226.

Tyrer, S.P. & Brittlebank, A.D. (1993) Misdiagnosis of bipolar affective disorder as personality disorder. *Canadian Journal of Psychiatry* **38**, 587–589.

Vogel-Schibilia, S.E., Mulsant, B.H. & Keshavan, M.S. (1988) HIV infection presenting as psychosis: A critique. *Acta Psychiatrica Scandinavica* **78**, 652–656.

West, E.D. & Dally, P.J. (1959) Effects of Iproniazid in depressive syndromes. *British Medical Journal* **1**, 1491–1499.

Whybrow, P.C. & Hurwitz, T. (1976) Psychological disturbances associated with endocrine disease and hormone therapy. In: *Hormones, Behaviour and Psychopathology* (ed. E.J. Sachar), pp. 125–143. Raven Press, New York.

Will, R.G., Ironside, J.W., Zeidler, M. *et al.* (1996) A new variant of Creutzfeld–Jakob disease in the U.K. *Lancet* **347**, 921–925.

World Health Organization (1973) *Report of the International Pilot Study of Schizophrenia*, Vol. 1. World Health Organization, Geneva.

World Health Organization (1992) *The ICD-10 Classification of Mental and Behavioural Disorders. Clinical Descriptions and Diagnostic Guidelines*. World Health Organization, Geneva.

CHAPTER 15

Culture-Bound Syndromes

DINESH BHUGRA AND K.S. JACOB

Introduction

Culture-bound syndromes (CBS) have attracted attention in medical as well as social sciences because they are rare and exotic. Murphy (1976) proposed that as CBS cause comparatively little damage to humanity, they therefore cast light on important but little understood aspects of human functioning. They need to be understood and categorized in the specific context of comparative psychiatry along with the interface between anthropology and psychiatry.

One of the major problems with the clinical concept of CBS has been in their definition. Considered to be rare, they are not necessarily rarer than anorexia nervosa or even schizophrenia. When considered exotic (because of their rarity) observers have not taken into account cultural contexts. In addition, because these often have a component of chaotic and unpredictable behaviour, their sufferers have been seen as savages and uncivilized. Another major problem with the concept has been their contextualization within Western diagnostic systems, which means that they have not been accepted as a part of mainstream psychiatry but as the exotic syndrome to be studied in parallel with the culture but without allowing the culture to define the levels of distress. As a result, there have been a series of syndromes classified as CBS that have led to the assumptions that there are no obvious links to be found between the cultural beliefs, the environmental stressors, and the symptomatology.

As Hughes and Wintrob (1995) suggest, in order to understand the clinical significance of CBS an enlarged conceptual frame of reference is essential. Since these syndromes cross the range of clinical diagnoses, they do provide the options of looking at alternative methods of assessing and allowing the clinician to attempt to understand alternatives of folk models of healing and caring. In addition, by giving some indications of normality versus pathology, these syndromes allow the societies and cultures to understand idioms of distress and pathways into care along with the social definitions of illness and illness behaviours. However, clinician's and researcher's confusion has led to these being seen as instances of deviance (Hughes 1985a). As Hughes (1985a) goes on to highlight, controversy over whether such episodes or patterns of behaviour are simply culturally based and different and yet normal ways of acting, or as examples of authentic disease and disorder, is ongoing, and the anthropologist is often on one side of this argument and the psychiatrist on the other.

In this chapter we aim to illustrate some of these arguments. Our purpose is not to describe every known CBS but to point out that clinical approaches both from the emic and the etic points are valid if the clinicians are aware of the shortcomings of each approach.

Origin

Culture-bound syndromes have traditionally been considered as variants of the classic disorders described in Europe. Kraepelin (in Hirsch & Shepherd 1974), after studying mental illness in Malaysia, concluded that the similarities of the disorders far outweighed the deviant features. He described *amok* as a variant of epilepsy or catatonia. This theme was incorporated in textbooks of comparative psychiatry, which suggested that reactions seen in non-Western cultures were not new diagnostic entities and were in fact similar to disorders already described in the West (Kiev 1972). Exotic conditions were grouped together based on this focus.

Yap (1962) suggested that the variety of terms used at the time be replaced by 'atypical culture-bound, psychogenic psychoses'. Subsequently, Yap (1969) shortened the phrase to 'culture-bound syndromes'. This phrase has gradually become commonly accepted despite controversy about its implications especially with regard to the restrictiveness of the suffix '-bound'. This term is used in this chapter as it identifies the phenomena under scrutiny.

Conflicting definitions

The underlying problem of reaching clinical diagnosis with the individual CBS is in reality no different from reaching any other clinical diagnosis, especially if clinical definitions and criteria are taken into account along with appropriate cultural limitations of psychopathology. As alluded to earlier, the distinction between locally defined and outside-analyst defined ideas of psychopathology remains an important step in reaching any kind of diagnosis.

These syndromes had been called the 'psychogenic psychoses' (Faergeman 1963), the 'ethnic psychosis' and 'ethnic neurosis' (Devereux 1956), and 'hysterical psychoses' (Langners 1967; Yap 1969). Although Yap (1974) did attempt a complex designation containing several conceptual elements of the atypical culture-bound reactive syndromes in contrast with Arieti and Meth's (1959) 'rare, unclassifiable, collective and exotic syndromes', the myriad of titles given suggest that from the very beginning of the nosology of these syndromes there has been an understandable element of confusion and misunderstanding. The use of the suffix '-bound' to illustrate the boundedness of these syndromes to individual culture is fraught with difficulties. As Hughes (1985a) observes, labels of 'atypical psychoses' and 'exotic syndromes' imply deviance from a standard diagnostic base and this (ab)normality illustrates the problem; the exoticness means 'foreign', exciting, different or deviant — thereby strengthening the notion of the 'other' in the pattern of diagnosis. This has also meant that not only the observed (individual demonstrating behaviour, which may be odd) deviant other, he or she is also the exciting, exotic other, therefore he or she is in double jeopardy. The problems with psychiatric diagnosis generally are beyond the scope of this chapter. These arguments are well known and interested readers are referred to Clare (1979); suffice it to say that the patterns of psychiatric diagnosis are not only ethno- or Euro-centric but also androcentric and anthropocentric.

The rarity (or so-called perceived rarity) of these syndromes, which contributes to their exotic nature, also lands the unwary in trouble in definition. Hughes (1985a) cautions that the rarity of these syndromes be seen in the context of their epidemiological data which, except in the case of one or two CBS, are rare indeed, thereby 'confusing' the rarity of the condition. The specificity of these syndromes to certain cultures is also loaded with problems in that they occur only in certain cultures and in their specific diaspora. However, this is not always the case and whether the term 'culture-reactive' is more appropriate is arguable. Fabrega (1982) suggests that these syndromes have the properties of abrupt onset, relatively short duration and absence of formal thought disturbance. Yap (1969) considered these conditions as variants of disorders described by Western psychiatry. He also reiterated that many labels included under CBS do not denote specific syndromes but refer to generic mental disorders, healing rituals, or supernatural notions of causation (Yap 1974).

Ritenbaugh (1982) suggested the inclusion of notions of aetiology and treatment rather than clinical presentations *per se*, and proposed 'meaning centered definitions'. On the other hand, Prince and Tcheng-Laroche (1987) preferred the exclusion of beliefs related to the causation of these disorders, while Simons (1987) argued for a restriction of the term to 'psychiatric disorders'.

There have been numerous diagnostic systems developed in Western society. Some of these have been clinical, for example, *International Classification of Diseases* (ICD-10; World Health Organization (WHO) 1992) and *Diagnostic and Statistical Manual* (DSM-IV; American Psychiatric Association (APA) 1994) and others have been research orientated, for example, Spitzer *et al.* (1978). As Hughes (1985a) argues, the formulation of American diagnostic systems (e.g. DSM-III and -IV) is explicitly committed to taking a theoretical neutral position with regard to aetiology as well as an explicitly descriptive approach with respect to symptoms, and such an approach is less likely to confound reliability, at least in the initial stages of inquiry. Multiaxial diagnostic systems allow the clinicians to create a diagnostic profile. Hughes (1985a) posits that such systems have the flexibility of fitting various CBS in without loss of local cultural meaning.

Hughes and Wintrob (1995) propose that using DSM-IV or ICD-10 does allow practitioners to take cultural factors into account in diagnostic assessments. This is a relatively new phenomenon and allows the clinician to get away from the traditional stereotypes of CBS as exotic or rare. There is no doubt that a single system cannot take into account all the various ramifications of CBS, thereby making their existence either questionable, on the one hand, or confirmed, on the other.

Sorting the CBS in itself is an ethnocentric phenomenon. Whereas shoplifting, eating disorders, obesity (Ritenbaugh 1982), and petism (Simons 1985c) have been put forward as Western CBS, certainly in the Western psychiatric literature such examples have not been discussed very much as culture-bound or even culture-reactive. Although it can be argued that each CBS can be fully explained by the system of meanings prevalent in the locale where the syndrome is prevalent, such meanings are then often ignored by the clinicians and the researchers alike. Kleinman (1980) has argued that in every instance of sickness, the illness behaviour, as distinct from the disease process, is always culturally determined, and this distinction is important. A major value of such a distinction is the recognition of the interactions of biopsychosocial factors in the genesis of distress. Simons (1985c) emphasized that, although any given CBS is profoundly shaped by the social and cultural realities of the society in which it is found, no amount of description of that shaping disproves the relevance of biology in the shaping of the same syndrome. The question Simons (1985c) asks is, which aspects of any given CBS are shaped in which manner, by what aspects of the material and social environment, and which aspects are shaped by what aspects of the subject's biology? These are important questions.

DSM-IV defines CBS as recurrent, locality-specific patterns of aberrant behaviour and troubling experience which are indigenously considered as illnesses and are restricted to specific areas or cultures. It includes conditions with folk-diagnostic labels with culture-specific meanings. However, it fails to acknowledge the heterogeneity of the disorders included under this label (which include clinical syndromes, aetiologic explanations, folk labels for specific behaviour and idioms of distress).

Levine and Gaw (1995) have recently proposed specific criteria for CBS: (i) the disorder must be a discrete, well-defined syndrome; (ii) it must be recognized as a specific illness in the culture with which it is primarily associated; (iii) the disorder must be expected, recognized and to some degree sanctioned as a response to certain precipitants in a particular culture; and (iv) a higher incidence or prevalence of the disorder exists in societies in which the disorder is culturally recognized, compared with other societies.

The use of the term 'CBS', without an operational definition, has resulted in the non-uniform usage of the term and controversies. Consensus has yet to be arrived at on the essence of these disorders that is widely acceptable across theoretical perspectives.

Explaining the controversies

The basis of classification of mental disorders forms the background for much of the controversies related to CBS. Western psychiatry has given primacy to naturalistic notions of illness. Consequently, the focus has been on the clinical presentation. Symptoms and behaviour have been employed to define clinical syndromes. On the other hand, non-Western societies tend to concentrate on personalistic explanations for illness. As a result, many of the disorders are classified based on notions regarding aetiology, idioms of distress, and other cultural attributions, with a much lesser emphasis on the clinical syndrome.

The difference between the naturalistic explanations and personalistic notions of illness has been the central reason for the controversies related to CBS. While the Western syndrome approach is supposedly atheoretical on possible aetiology of these disorders, many non-Western folk categories are based on presumed aetiology. Both approaches stem from different cultural traditions and compromise is difficult. The major classifications of mental disorders have adopted the clinical syndrome as the basis for classification. Consequently, incorporating presumed aetiology as the basis for including CBS in international classifications is difficult. DSM-IV has included a glossary of CBS but only as an appendix highlighting the problem.

Many attempts at looking for common features across disorders and cultures have been made employing syndromes. Many descriptions of CBS have focused on notions about aetiology and illness attributions rather than the clinical phenomena resulting in problems in comparison. Despite this limitation, the use of clinical syndromes as the basis of classification has resulted in the documentation of similarities and differences between many traditional CBS and Western categories. Consequently, the CBS have been considered as variants of existing Western conditions. However, when importance is given to aetiological and treatment, notions which distinguish them force them to be grouped separately.

Similarly, organizing principles of various disciplines differ. While psychiatry has accepted the primacy of the clinical syndrome in classification, anthropology focuses on cultural issues, including personalistic explanations offered for different CBS. The diametrically opposite nature of their respective positions has resulted in difficulties and the consequent lack of consensus. While many psychiatrists view CBS as culture bound, anthropological perspectives would consider them bound by constructs. The documentation of broad similarities across CBS which exist in apparently different cultures contradicts the basic assumption of cultural specificity. However, an emphasis on detail and on the culture context would argue otherwise.

The lack of consensus on the definition of CBS has resulted in a lack of answers to many important questions related to CBS, including prevalence risk factors, treatment and outcome. However, considering the widely different perspectives on the subject it would require enormous effort to reach a consensus definition.

The impact of biological factors on the 'causation' of CBS is illustrated by the debate on *latah* (for definition, see below). Simons (1985b) argues that *latah* is a variant within the startle matching taxon—the latter includes syndromes from all over the world which are characterized by a variety of odd behaviours locally considered amusing. He argues that matching the words or actions of others is one such frequent and prominent behaviour, hence 'startle matching'. Simons (1985b) proposes that what *latah* looks like and what *latahs* do is dictated by the specific aspects of pan-mammalian neurophysiology. *Latah*, as seen in Malaysia, can be considered a local cultural elaboration of that physiology and therefore *latah* ought to be seen as culture-specific elaboration of the potential of the startle reflex. Kenny (1985) criticized this approach by arguing that *latah* should be best considered in terms of local meanings within their societies of origin. He argues that if one can demonstrate the symbolic meaning of *latah*, the allegation that physiological factors are important in its shaping is logically unnecessary and therefore misguided. Simons (1985a) reports that syndromes essentially like *latah* have been reported from Burma (where it is called *yaun*), Thailand (*bahschi*), and the Philippines (*mali-mali* or *silok*) (Yap 1969). It has been reported from Siberia (*myriachit, ikote, amurakh*) (Czaplicka 1914), Lapland ('Lapp panic'; Collinder 1949) and among the Ainu in Japan (*imu*; Nakagawa 1973). Comparing these descriptions to those of American hyperstartlers who are startled easily and frequently and describe broadly similar patterns of behaviour suggests that there may well be an underlying neurophysiological mechanism said to be located in the limbic system. However, three different types of *latah* also suggest that there may well be a continuum of responses. Simons (1985c) has put forward startle as an emergency override system response which is activated automatically when a sudden unexpected environmental event requires immediate first priority attention which is thus the whole-body equivalent of the single segment spinal reflex. There have been some suggestions that these responses are linked with marginal social status and *latah* also has asymmetric sex distribution—both points take the argument away from the biological aspects and universality of hyperstartle response. Kenny's (1985) critique of Simons' proposal mentioned earlier is based upon his observation that the condition has a profound internal relation to Malayo-Indonesian culture and on the observation that psychiatric and anthropological interpretation of *latah* and kindred states here have been superficial. Kenny argues that *latah* conveys the marginal status and the distress of the individual to the observer and the society and allows this in a number of ways which are not pathologizing. Hilarity, disorder, marginality, supernaturalism, transition and loss of self itself are all intricately linked within the cultural matrix of the *latah* pattern. This loss of self in itself raises some interesting questions. Is it the real self? Is it the real loss? Is it a symbolic communicating pattern? Is it an ambiguous boundary condition with the framework of ritual or within the related framework of an individual life?

As noted earlier this 'disorder' can be perceived as pathological and it can also be put to uses where pathology has no part at all. The social demonstration is more likely to occur in states with culturally ascribed attitudes. Kenny (1985) argues forcefully that this performance of the disorder is to do with culture-specific exploitation of a meaning potential implicit in a limited human repertoire of concept pertaining to order, disorder and self-identity. Each of the individual components of *latah* has to be understood in the cultural and social context before any claims could be made to comprehend the whole. Kenny (1985) also dismisses the psychoanalytic explanation of *latah* on broadly similar grounds. Simons (1985d) replied to Kenny by putting forward the explanations of the basis of what he called 'ethological' framework, which means that symbolic significance does not by itself preclude biological significance. The paradigm of marginality is not reflected by Simons but put in the context of psychological as well as physiological and social and cultural factors. The debate between these two authors reflects the dichotomy between psychiatry and anthropology and it is worth restating.

Skultans (1993) too highlights the distinction between anthropology and psychiatry in their respective approaches to clinical and cultural relationships. She argues that at the theoretical level two positions represent a continuum—the relativist and the universalist positions. Whereas the psychiatrists cluster near the universalist pole, the anthropologists gather near the relativist pole. The use of familiarity with a culture as a starting point before the translation of such culture's activities starts to take place is recommended. Fabrega (1989) revives the notion of cultural relativism and argues that this process refers of the differences in beliefs, feelings, behaviours, traditions, local practices, and technological arrangements that are found among diverse peoples of the world. Such differences are related because they are linked with differences in culture. The distinction between etic and emic observation, investigation and appropriate diagnosis remain the key features of such an approach. The differences between universalist and relativist approaches are clearly important because if psychiatry is to succeed a holistic biopsychosocial model of diagnosis is essential. The differences between relativist and universalist approaches highlight clinical dilemmas if psychopathology and its understanding is to be committed to exegetical analysis.

The initial application of cultural relativism to clinical psychiatry emerged from the perceptions and definitions of normal and abnormal behaviours. Culture and personality theorists used these ideas to emphasize the following logically derived categories, as highlighted by Fabrega (1989):

1   behaviour that was definitely considered abnormal in our society but might be considered normal in others;
2   behaviour that was considered normal in our society but might be considered abnormal in others;
3   behaviour that might be considered normal in all societies;
4   behaviour that might be considered abnormal in all societies; and
5   abnormal behaviour or normal behaviour, considered as such that would be seen in one or some but not in all societies.

Thus, it would make sense that while universalist approaches in psychiatry play down the uniqueness of CBS, cultural relativism is able to signify an important factor of the existence of these syndromes. The debate on *latah*, for example, between Simons (1985a) and Kenny (1985) has to be seen in this context. Hughes (1989) cautions that the pervasive role of 'culture' in the dynamics of human behaviour (including psychiatric disorder) remains to be fully operationalized and incorporated into the diagnostic repertoire of the practitioner. He suggests that the emphasis should be on relative culturalism rather than cultural relativism. Westermeyer (1985) emphasizes that clinicians might observe more psychopathology than in fact exists, viewing a patient's culture-bound belief as delusion, whereas at the other end of the spectrum, the clinician might fail to perceive the patient's psychopathology through the layers of culture-bound expression—thereby making knowledge of cultural mores and norms almost mandatory (see Chapter 8).

Pfeiffer (1982) suggests that four varying dimensions of culture-specific areas—stress, shaping of conduct, interpretations and interventions—have to be borne in mind while ascertaining any cultural influences on pathogenesis and pathoplasty of illness. All four dimensions deserve to be understood in relation to all CBS.

Culture itself can induce stress on individuals by family and societal structure. The development of culturally approved patterns of exceptional behaviour and promotion and suppression of certain other kinds of behaviours means that the normality and abnormality by behaviour — including development of disease into illness—are very much dictated by the culture.

Culture-bound syndromes therefore court controversy at several levels. Using a prism of culture, individual and the social as well as cultural factors are to be taken into account, but the physiological and neurobiological factors too remain important. Hughes (1985a) took on the task of producing a glossary for CBS, this being an initial attempt to systemize and bring some cross-referenced order to the names used for various conventional CBS. As he goes on to emphasize, the systematization of the names for these syndromes is only the first step towards ordering the content and integrating the concept of CBS into other conceptual schema. Whether these are seen as sub-classified variants within folk psychiatric disorders or fully fledged diagnostic concepts remains a matter for debate.

A further complicating factor associated with CBS needs to be highlighted here. The clinical management of CBS depends upon the behaviour, how it is labelled, and who is seen as the most appropriate individual to deal with it. The healers or shamans may follow an approach in reaching diagnosis and making management plans, thereby perhaps destigmatizing the behaviour but also allowing the sufferers or their carers to seek help. It is possible that these healers deal with the illnesses and problems of their patients at a symptomatic phenomenological level and necessarily at a psychodynamic level.

Some commonly described culture-bound syndromes

Hughes (1985a) listed 163 CBS (not including synonyms) in his glossary. We do not aim to describe all these syndromes but will focus on following six which highlight some of the controversies and some of the management difficulties. Table 15.1 lists some of the common CBS with their variants and places of description. We will describe *koro*, *latah*, *dhat*, *amok*, *nervios*, and *susto*.

KORO

Definition

Koro or *shook-yang* is said to occur predominantly in men of Chinese origin living in southern China or the countries of southeast Asia. The origin of the work *koro* may be related to the Javanese word for 'tortoise' (Yap 1965). *Shook-yang* means 'shrinking penis' and was described by Pao in 1834 (Ngui 1969).

Symptoms

The set of symptoms are related to a primary feeling that the man's penis is retracting into the body with a fear of impending death. This is often accompanied by feelings of intense panic which have physiological symptoms of palpitations, sweating, feeling faint, breathlessness, visual blurring, pain and

Table 15.1 Some culture-bound syndromes.

Syndrome	Region/culture	Presentation	Variants described
Amok	Malaysia	Homicidal frenzy preceded by brooding and followed by amnesia	*Cathard* (Polynesia), *pseudonite* (Sahara), *mal de pelea* (Puerto Rico), *whitko* (Cree Indians), *imu* (Japan), *myriachit* (Siberia)
Latah	Malaysia	Hypersensitivity to sudden fright with echopraxia, echolalia, command obedience, trance-like behaviour	*Amurakh, irkunni, ikota, olan, menkeiti, bahschi, imu, mali-mali, silok*
Pibloktoq	Inuit	Extreme excitement followed by apparent seizures and transient coma	*?Amok*
Shin-byung	Korea	Anxiety and somatic complaints followed by dissociation attributed to ancestral spirits	
Ataque de nervios	Latin America	Symptoms of anxiety and aggressive behaviour followed by convulsive movements and amnesia	Puerto Rican syndrome
Dhat	India	Extreme anxiety and hypochondriasis associated with discharge of semen	*Jiryan* (India), *sukra prametra* (Sri Lanka), *shen-K'uei* (China)
Koro	Asia	Extreme anxiety due to belief that penis will retract into body	*Shuk yang, shook yong, suo yang* (China), *jinjinia* (Assam), *roo-joo* (Thailand)
Kayak angst	Inuit	Extreme anxiety of drowning while at sea	*Nangiapok*
Brain fag	West Africa	Fatigue due to stress of school	*Ori ode* (Nigeria)
Shenjing shuairuo	China	Physical and mental exhaustion, difficulty in concentration, memory loss, dizziness	Neurasthenia

Continued

Table 15.1 *Continued.*

Syndrome	Region/culture	Presentation	Variants described
Anorexia nervosa	Western cultures	Obsessive preoccupation with weight loss, distortion of body image	
Chronic fatigue syndrome	Western culture	Extreme fatigue associated with somatic symptoms and psychological complaints	
Susto	Latin America	Physical and emotional symptoms due to fear that the soul will leave the body	*Espanto, pasmo, tripa ida, perdida del alma, chibih*

feelings of impending doom. These physiological and psychological reactions lead the individual to develop some preventing strategies, for example attaching weights to the penis to stop it from retracting. The strength of the belief will dictate elements of actions necessary. Men present with shrinking penises and women with retracting breasts. Men largely overwhelm the number.

Epidemiological data

Epidemics of *koro* were described in the late 1800s. Poor education and social and geographical isolation have been linked with epidemics. However, for reasons related to the perception of Western psychiatrists, these epidemics were often regarded as a novelty rather than an event to be taken seriously and studied further.

One of the first clinicians to study *koro*, Yap (1965), described 19 cases and argued that *koro* ought to be seen as a depersonalization syndrome whose form and content are determined by social and cultural factors. In 1967, there was an outbreak of *koro* in Singapore lasting a period of 10 days and 469 cases were recorded (Mun 1968; Ngui 1969). The onset of the epidemic was related to newspaper stories about various chemicals present in the bodies of animals which would also affect human beings. This led to a panic of *koro* after a group of individuals consumed the heart of a pig which had received inoculation against swine fever. Rumours spread that the affected meat led to penile retraction. Within 5 days the numbers of people presenting with symptoms of *koro* increased dramatically. Of these, 95% were men and 5%, women. Women presented with complaints of shrinking breasts. The vast majority were Chinese and the rest Malaysian or Indian. Only three cases were educated through secondary school. The predominant symptoms were fear (90%), belief about shrinking of the genitals (74%), and retraction of the penis (61%), and principal remedies were manual restraint by the afflicted individuals (72%) and placebo (74%).

The North Bengal *koro* epidemic occurred in 1982. A total of 405 cases (357 male, 48 female) were identified over a $2^1/2$-year period, although a total of 82% of cases were seen in 1 month, by Chowdhury *et al.* (1988), who divided the whole outbreak into three epidemic types—sudden onset, explosive; explosive with identifiable prodromal phase; and rebound outbreak.

Dutta (1983) describes an epidemic in northeast India known colloquially as *jinjini bemari*, indicating a disease characterized by a tingling sensation and the patient going on to develop other symptoms. This was precipitated by a rumour that a lethal disease had struck the people bringing instant death or making the person impotent. The epidemic disappeared after mass media education campaigns. The Singapore epidemic (Ngui 1969) was directly related to an outbreak of swine fever. Although six cases below the age of 6 were reported, the youngest was 7 months old—without doubt, victims of parental anxiety. The majority (79%) of cases were aged between 16 and 40 years. More than three quarters (76.8%) were single. Only two cases were related to direct sexual activity and a quarter had the attack during micturition. Tseng *et al.* (1988) surveyed 232 cases, although more than 2000 persons were said to be the victims of the 1984–85 epidemic. An incidence of 3.2/1000 was reported, although in some areas rates of 63.4/1000 were observed. Of these 232 cases, 195 (84%) were men and the rest, women. More than half (53%) of the men were aged between 15 and 24 and almost one third (31%) were aged between 10 and 14. Two thirds had primary school education. Most attacks started at night and most individuals had seen others have the attack and were themselves involved in the rescue. Onset of chills was followed by feeling of shrinking of penis and then anxiety, palpitations, shouting, sweating, etc. followed. Substances full of *yang* qualities were fed to the individuals and family and relatives were involved in physically pulling the penis out.

Suwanlert and Coates (1979) interviewed 350 people out of a total of 2000 who had developed *koro* in an epidemic in 1976 in Thailand. Of these, 338 were men and the vast majority were between the ages of 11 and 20.

Prodromal phase lasted 20 minutes and included vertigo, genital pain, numbness and diarrhoea, followed by the penile shrinking phase where genital numbness, feeling of penis shrinking, and nipple pain accompained by panic reaction were reported. A majority (70%) sought treatment from folk healers and only 25% by Western facilities. Only 6% gave a psychological reason as the reason for their disturbance and 94% felt they had been poisoned.

Ilechukwu (1992), reporting on a *koro*-like epidemic from Nigeria, suggested that the epidemic had been precipitated by impending political changes. But, the fear of loss of sexual organs remained a paramount one.

Local explanations

Yap (1965) suggested that as traditional beliefs about sexuality are based on the theory of an equilibrium between *yin* and *yang*—the female and male principles—and these are said to be affected by environment, different kinds of food, and the sexual act itself. The vulnerability to sexual imbalance has a crucial role in day-to-day functioning of individuals. The worry and guilt over sexual activity with the precipitation of *koro* is not unknown. Yap (1965) believed that *koro* belief is not only pathoplastic but actually pathogenic—a view also put forward by Gwee (1963, 1968) and Rin (1963). They argue that conflicts portrayed by the patients are sexual or sex-related and deal with masturbation, nocturnal emission (see also *dhat*, below) and promiscuity. The underlying theme of preserving *yang* is important. The traditional medicine also recognizes a neurasthenic state (*sun-k'uai*) associated with sexual excess and the symptoms of this condition were thought to be giddiness and debility (both physical and mental), as well as aching in the loins and excessive shivering at the end of micturition (Yap 1965). Fears of semen loss are well known in other cultures; however, without the *koro* and related beliefs, only a small proportion of persons so troubled will present to the physicians. Despite having emigrated from China, the population of the Chinese diaspora are still influenced by the Chinese traditional medical system. Although occasional cases have been described among other cultures, the Chinese remain the predominant group to be affected. Tseng *et al.* (1988) argue that Rin had overgeneralized its occurrence. It has been argued that often the cause is seen as unfriendly ghosts who do not have penises and are therefore after the individual. It would appear that one village would be affected for several days and the people would be involved in the effort of rescuing the victims and in chasing away the evil. Once a new case is reported from the neighbouring village, the ghost is said to have moved on and the panic starts to subside. Sociocultural explanations put forward by Suwanlert and Coates (1979) suggest the possibility of 'attacking' a vulnerable community through economic effects.

The spread of *koro* from the Chinese community to the northeastern parts of India is related to a metamorphosis of the syndrome and is likely to be caused by experiencing a threat to their socio-economic, ethnic, cultural and biological survival (Jilek & Jilek-Aall 1985). Prince (1992) proposes that Sino-Japanese folklore, with its emphasis on fox maidens and ghosts, suggests that these *koro* syndromes can be generated within cultures that harbour a wide variety of world views. The most parsimonious explanation for these wide-ranging disorders is that there is a pan-human male dread of castration and sexual impotence and danger of the ubiquitous fantasy of the destructive female.

Chowdhury (1989a) developed a graphomotor projective test — the draw-a-penis test — which elicits the penis image of the patient, both of a normal penis and his perception of his own penis. It also elicits the nature of perceptual processes concerning the penile state change. From the original sample of 405 cases, the author selected 77 cases to participate in this test. From this test, the author went on to conclude that *koro* patients perceived a shorter penis, whether it was their own or that of a normal individual. This perception was reported both for flaccid and erect states. Chowdhury (1989b) then went on to look at the perceptions of these individuals regarding various parts of the penis, for example the root, the shaft and the gland, and concluded that even in the follow-up this perception of small penis remained. However, this cannot and should not be attributed to *koro* because the dysmorphophobic perception in the pre-*koro* state is not known. Rin (1965) has related these epidemics to oral personality. However, these explanations are put forward in the Western psychiatric context without any clear reference to the cultural explanations. Although Yap (1974) had suggested that *koro* might occur in patriarchal societies with institutionalized polygamy and cultural emphasis on male potency, it is difficult to believe that Oedipal and castration anxieties are universal and will occur in every culture and, much less, have the same effect.

Differential diagnosis

Bernstein and Gaw (1990) suggest that a subset of genital retraction disorder be considered where underlying urological and organic brain disorders must be ruled out. Secondly, the clinician should rule out the possibility of a somatoform disorder and, thirdly, the cultural sanctioning of the belief should be identified and sociocultural dimensions added to the diagnosis. However, in view of the short and often self-limiting epidemics with a clear precipitating event the diagnosis can be straightforward.

From a diagnostic viewpoint, *koro* has been considered as a form of anxiety, a variant of obsessive-compulsive illness, an imaginary organic illness based on folk belief, acute castration anxiety, and a psychotic delusional state (Gwee 1963, 1968; Rin 1963; Yap 1965; Rubin 1982). All these need to be recognized or excluded. *Koro*, as Rubin (1982) suggests, fulfils the criteria of a syndrome complex and should be seen as a collection of symptoms stemming from diverse aetiologies.

Management

General principles of managements of CBS are outlined below. Management of *koro* specifically includes managing overt anxiety with moderate doses of anxiolytics and supportive psychotherapy. The range of therapies has included using benzodiazepines, antidepressants and psychotherapies. Cognitive behavioural therapy may have a more appropriate and prominent part to play when compared with psychoanalytic therapies.

In the Singapore epidemic, 81% had only one attack, 8% had two, and 11% had more than two attacks among the males. Three quarters had been treated with supportive psychotherapy. Tan (1981) recommends an intravenous injection of calcium gluconate, when faced with a case of *koro* in the emergency room situation. This gives an immediate sensation of warmth running through the whole body, and is an effective form of acute management. Having thus reduced the anxiety and the panic, the patient can then be sedated for the night and his conflicts can be dealt with on a psychotherapeutic basis the following morning.

LATAH

Definition

Latah, already alluded to earlier, remains one of the classic examples of CBS sparking off a debate between the universalist and the relativist ends of the spectrum. A dissociative state, provoked usually in the form of a shout, a loud noise or a prod in the ribs associated with altered consciousness, coprolalia, echolalia, echopraxia and, in more severe cases, 'command automatism'. Yap (1952) described the condition ocurring in middle-aged women of the Malay or other indigenous races in southeast Asia. However, a number of cases have been described among males as well. It was first described in the 19th century.

Clinical features

Friedmann (1982) suggests that a number of afflictions that seem to be similar to *latah* have been reported from several nations. Although supposedly rare, its distribution is very wide. Friedmann (1982) goes on to summarize the symptoms of *latah* and the *latah*-like syndromes as follows:

1   usually sudden onset after an acute fright;
2   variability of symptoms depending on the culture and the individual;
3   features of echopraxia, echolalia, coprolalia;
4   episodic nature;
5   episodes may be triggered off by tickling or startling the victim;
6   episodes accepted by the culture as state rather than disease and may be entertaining;
7   poorly educated and low social class individuals;
8   may be linked up with violence and may have a variable course.

Epidemiological studies

Chiu *et al.* (1972) studied over 12 000 Malaysians—half of Malay origin and half of Iban origin. Among these, they found 50 cases who fit the criteria for *latah*. Among the 50, seven had a firm clinical diagnosis of neurosis, schizophrenia, or adjustment reaction. However, 14 had a mixed range of diagnoses. All were women and several sexual conflicts appeared to have a role in many of these cases. Depression was the prevailing affect. Its distribution is said to be quite widespread around the world (Murphy 1976).

Simons (1985a) collected information on a number of individuals presenting with *latah*-type phenomena and reported that suddenness of the stimulus in the perceptual field triggers a startle response. Ingestion of caffeine and certain other stimulants of the central nervous system can increase arousal, monitoring, and ease of startle elicitation along with the strength of startle response. Simons (1985a) described three types of *latah*: immediate response, attention capture and the role *latah*. It is the role *latah*,

Simons argues, who go on to respond to social factors. Two further points, of *latah* as having marginal social status and as having asymmetric sex distribution, are worth making.

Local explanations

This condition is locally often seen as an eccentricity which may well have some social value. Subjects of *latah* are often in great demand at social occasions such as marriages, and will provide comic relief by uttering obscenities when provoked by the members of the wedding party or others. Yap (1952) suggests that the coprolalia allows a publicly sanctioned expression of sexual utterances providing light relief.

Friedmann (1982) suggests that *latah* may well represent a final common pathway for a wide spectrum of disorders and, as much of it is not classifiable in Western psychiatric terms, it needs to be seen in cultural context. Although there was increased incidence of *latah* after colonization, gradually this appears to be going down as cultural norms are beginning to change.

Murphy (1976) posited that final feature of *latah* was related to the frankly sexual dream that often precipitated it. Underlying hyperstartle response to ticklish responses may well perpetuate this phenomenon. As noted earlier, Simons (1985a) highlighted the differences between three types of *latah* and suggested that purely cultural explanations of *latah* do not take into account universality of these symptoms and its occasional appearance in persons in societies without a cultural tradition to account for *latah* behaviour. Kenny (1985) counters this by suggesting that the condition has a profound internal relation to Malayo-Indonesian culture and is clearly related to local witchcraft beliefs, midwifery, shamanism, folk art and fundamental ideas pertaining to the gaining of religious insight and power through loss of self.

Although similar conditions have been described in other countries, the basic tenet needs to remain as specific to cultural institutions. The symbolism of the body has a key role in these actions.

Psychiatric explanations

Putting aside Simons' (1985a) views on the aetiology and universality of *latah*, it is worth looking at the psychoanalytic explanations. Murphy (1976) lists these as follows:

1   repressed wishes;
2   stimulus generalization where non-sexual stimuli are being misinter-
preted as sexual;
3   masochistic tendency;
4   dissociative child-rearing practices;
5   rewarding of hypersuggestibility in adults;
6   suppression of lengthier dissociations;
7   inflexibility of impulse control.

The first three are said by Murphy to be the equivalent of producing neurosis in Western adults or some sexual perversion, but the *latah* subject does not demonstrate any clear continuous conflict. It is possible that milder *latah* cases have a weaker id–ego relationship, thereby differentiating them from those who are more seriously affected and go into a *latah* state several times a day. Simons (1987) points out that Malayan dictionaries define *latah* as neurological disease and a disorder of attention.

Management

Management of *latah* will include excluding hysterical dissociation and treating the individual with appropriate sedative medication along with supportive psychotherapy. Rarely, family work may be indicated.

DHAT

A few of the CBS defined in psychiatry have sexual contents and anxiety-related semen loss is well described.

Definition

The Indian *dhat* syndrome has been described as a cultural neurosis of the Orient (Malhotra & Wig 1975). The *dhat* syndrome constitutes a clinical entity where nocturnal emissions are said to relate to severe anxiety, somatic symptoms with elements of hypochondriasis, and sexual impotence. The patient blames nocturnal emissions for feelings of weakness and tiredness, and remains tense and preoccupied and roams from physician to physician requesting help in stopping the night emissions or seeking a cure for the imaginary loss of semen with urine. Similar observations have been reported from Sri Lanka (Kodagoda 1978; Kulanayagam 1979).

Clinical features

Vague physical symptoms are very common. Often tiredness, headache, vague aches and pains, lethargy, weakness, and a general sense of ill-health present as a syndrome and only on close questioning are the causative factors discovered. There may be additional psychological symptoms of anxiety, poor concentration and poor memory, and specific sexual symptoms of erectile difficulties and premature ejaculation.

Epidemiological studies

There have not been any epidemiological studies, though clinic populations have been reported on. Singh (1985) studied 50 consecutive males with potency disorders and reported that 40% complained of semen in urine. Akhtar (1988) states that a majority of those affected live in villages and belong to families with very conservative attitudes to sex and may have low educational status.

Local explanations

In Ayurvedic explanations, formation of semen can be affected by any number of factors including diet and seasons, and impotence could result from infections, poor diet, changing seasons, etc. Semen is vital for life. Ayurvedic texts suggest that food and its juices after digestion produce blood, which goes on to produce flesh, which goes on to produce fat, which leads to production of bone, which produces marrow, which then leads on to production of semen. Thus, in an exponential manner, 40 drops of one product produce one drop, thereby confirming the importance of semen (see Bhugra & Buchanan 1989; Bhugra 1992). This model also fits in with the traditional Hindu way of thinking that suggests that the first 25 years (a quarter of one's lifespan) should be spent as a celibate individual, thereby making the loss of semen even more threatening. Digestive causes are also said to contribute to this state.

Using a case vignette of nocturnal emission, when Malhotra and Wig (1975) interviewed 110 respondents across all socio-economic strata, they reported that across all social classes semen loss was seen as harmful, whereas its preservation was linked with longevity and supernatural powers, and deemed to be a guarantee of good health. Foods perceived to be hot were seen as possible contributors to *dhat* and therefore ought to be avoided, whereas foods with cooling effects were seen as essential, especially among the lower socio-economic class. Medical intervention was recommended by respondents from social classes III and IV, and marriage was a recommended treatment.

Ayurvedic physicians in India and Sri Lanka promote and perpetuate these beliefs through advertising in the popular media and roadside hoardings, and there is an element of gradation in the contents of medication dependent upon the individual's ability to pay (Bhugra & de Silva 1993). These physicians will carry out tests using alum to 'clear' the urine and prove the existence of *dhat* (see Bottéro 1991).

Psychiatric explanations

Bottéro (1991) reported that between 15% and 20% of those consulting an Ayurvedic physician are likely to have anxiety related to semen loss syndrome. Paris (1992) suggests that the urine often seen as opaque is attributed to the presence of semen (but it is more opaque with a vegetarian diet and fluctuations in this may well provide a basis for symptom formation). Carstairs (1957) speculated that if *dhat* is more common in North India it may be a reflection of the family structure. Although these symptoms are reported from other parts of the world as well (Dewaraja & Sesaki 1991), lack of sexual experience has a role in the aetiology. A more systematic study of this phenomenon was reported by de Silva and Dissanayake (1989), who assessed 38 males attending a sexual dysfunction clinic in Sri Lanka. Of these 38, 15 were independently given a clinical diagnosis of hypochondriasis and 21 were diagnosed as suffering from anxiety state. These authors saw this as a variant of the Indian *dhat* syndrome and called it loss of semen syndrome. In the 50 cases studied by Singh (1985), nearly three quarters had symptoms of headache, fatigue and weakness. Depression and anxiety were also common. However, it was difficult to ascertain which appeared first — depression or semen-loss anxiety.

Management

Management must include specific treatment for the underlying condition as well as education and reassurance. The traditional views of abstinence may well contribute to the confusion and perplexity in the minds of young adults who may have to get married at an early age and have to procreate, thereby adding to feelings of conflict, anxiety, tension, guilt, shame and sexual problems. Rather than challenge the individual's views, Agarwal (1970) proposed reassurance along the lines of 'Maybe energy *is* lost in emissions but the body has got a self-regulatory mechanism which recoups this loss quickly.' The need for education and dealing with superstition is paramount in this group and, combined with specific behavioural and cognitive tasks along with multivitamins, may enable the patient to develop confidence in ongoing therapy. Themes of parental dominance and neurotic fears of damaging male genitalia during intercourse often surface and could be tackled using analytic methods (Gupta *et al.* 1989). The traditional healers will use their skills to reassure them and avoid causing further anxiety, for they are well aware that suggestibility of such patients can be due to weakening of their mental faculties induced by sperm deficiency. Bhatia and Malik (1991) reported best responses from antidepressant and anxiolytic groups. They suggest that improvement with antidepressants may be due to treating underlying mood disorder. However, giving placebo with consent is likely to worsen the underlying anxiety and if given without consent is unethical.

AMOK

Amok is a Malaysian term used to describe a syndrome which has often elements of dissociation in it. A variety of syndromes have been described as being *amok*-like from a wide number of countries and cultures around the world (Levine & Gaw 1995).

Definition

The term '*amok*' refers to a violent or furious assault of homicidal intensity and is associated with the indigenous people of the Malay archipelago (Carr & Tan 1976). Such a furious and violent assault is often found in farmers or mountain dwellers, unrelated to suicide, drugs or alcohol but related to physical stress in the form of fright, anger, grief, or nervous depression. However, recent reports have suggested a lack of agreement on the causation (see below). Although *amok* is described in DSM-IV as representing a dissociative state, the predominant and most dramatic aspect of the syndrome is mass assault, which would warrant placing it in the impulse control disorders category. In some of the varieties described from around

318 | *Chapter 15*

the world, dissociation remains the main feature, but there is no mass assault.

Epidemiological data

Earlier reports of this condition, dating from the middle of the late 19th century to the middle of the 20th century, were from a literary point of view. One of the earliest descriptions dated to 1786 when *amok* was reported in a Javanese prisoner in South Africa (Bradlow 1991). Her account is based on the report of a British officer, although it had been described in the Indian islands before. Predisposing emotions noted were the spirit of revenge, with an impatience of restraint. Murphy (1973) suggested that a history of *amok* went through three phases over a 400-year period. Between the 16th and 18th centuries, the individual was seen as initiating his actions consciously and deliberately and avoided attacking people known to him. In the first half of the 19th century, the attacker's eyes were closed, friends could be victims, and mass killings occurred, with subsequent amnesia. In the latter half of the 19th century, *amok* became associated with psychosis and the true incidence of *amok* declined.

Carr and Tan (1976) studied 21 *amok* subjects found among 134 patients of the male security ward of a hospital in West Malaysia. This description had been used by the local police. The act was seen as unconscious, indiscriminate and without purpose.

Local explanations

As outlined, the historical concepts and local explanations have changed over the past three centuries, although, as Carr and Tan (1976) highlight, the Malay view of *amok* was that mental illness was very threatening and was feared by society. The phenomenon is believed to have had its origins in the cultural training for warfare which the early Javanese and Malays adopted from the Hindu states of India. Carr (1985) suggests that *en masse* attacks by warriors brandishing a dagger and screaming 'Amok! Amok!' were popular tactics among Malay warriors. They were intended to terrify the enemy. It was a highly regarded and culturally reinforced tactic.

Malay cultural features allowed individuals to carry weapons and, by supporting *amok* as a behavioural alternative, have supported violent outbursts. Within Malay society, where balance and distribution of power are informal and social rather than written and legal, *amok* may have functioned over the centuries as a means for limiting the power of hereditary rulers, since arbitrary dictums might elicit *amok* violence (Gullick 1958). Decrease in *amok* violence after colonization has been related to a stable socio-economic, political, and cultural climate and taking away the cultural sanctions by punishing the perpetrators by long stays in prisons.

Psychiatric explanations

Of the 10 cases who were seen as true *amok* subjects by Carr and Tan (1976), a majority (seven) were showing inappropriate behaviour, manifesting delusions and/or hallucinations at the time of admission.

Westermeyer (1985) studied 18 subjects in Laos, all aged between 17 and 35, and none of the individuals had suffered from psychosis, convulsion, mental retardation, or incapacitating physical disability. This is in contrast to Van Loon (1927), who suggested that cerebral malaria was a cause, and Burton-Bradley (1968), who stated that all his cases were of transient psychosis. Carr and Tan (1976) identified attacks precipitated by vertigo (fever) and visions (influences). Physical stress may well have precipitated it in some cases.

Certain authors have suggested the role of alcohol (see Westermeyer 1982) and psychodynamic theorists have suggested projection—blaming of others for one's own difficulties — and extraordinary sensitivity and over-investment in control and decorum such that failure of these rigid and overdetermined defences results in a total abandonment of restraint.

Loss of social standing has been put forward as a possible precipitating event along with stresses of migration, loss of significant other, and lack of social support all contribute to the pattern of *amok* (for details, see Westermeyer 1982, 1985). There may be associated suicidal thoughts.

Management

The behaviour may well hide underlying psychiatric pathology such as paranoid states or schizophrenia which would need to be treated in its own right. Psychological and physical investigations may well give a clue to risk factors, and preventive actions may be more relevant. Once the attacks have already happened, the legal system of the country will have to decide on the subsequent referral of such patients if they are deemed to be psychiatrically ill.

This syndrome is seen in the Latin American population and has also been called the Puerto Rican syndrome.

Definition

Symptoms include shaking, palpitations, flushing and numbness, often accompanied by shouting or striking out, and followed by falling convulsive body movements or amnesia. An attack can resemble panic disorder followed by amnesia. DSM-IV differentiates between *ataques* and panic disorder on the basis that the former has a precipitating event and frequent absence of the hallmark symptoms of acute fear or apprehension.

Epidemiological data

Often seen in people of the Spanish-speaking Caribbean, it has since been reported in the Spanish diaspora. Its coexistence with a number of psychiatric disorders make its phenomenology and epidemiological data difficult to obtain.

Rothenberg (1964) characterized *ataque* as a sudden onset of violence, uncommunicativeness, and hyperkinesia and swearing and striking out at others are common. There may be 'suicidal fits' which may have two phases — firstly, the patient flees from a stressful scene and, secondly, the patient impulsively attempts suicide (Trautman 1961). Oquendo *et al.* (1992) suggest that these descriptions have three common denominators — suddenness of onset, the disruption in ability to communicate, and the action-orientated result.

It usually begins at a funeral, at the scene of an accident, or at a family fight, where strong emotional expression is culturally sanctioned. Guarnaccia *et al.* (1989) and Grace (1959) describe how the individual falls to floor and either convulses or acts as if dead. Another prominent feature is the effect of *ataque* on the social support network — it mobilizes an individual's family and friends, all of whom come together and attempt to alleviate the stress as best they can.

Local explanations

Ataque is an expression of anger and grief resulting from the disruption of family systems, the process of migration, and concerns about family members in the country of origin (Guarnaccia *et al.* 1989). Some form of *ataque* may be expected of a good woman at the death of a close relative or when witnessing violence within the family (Garrison 1977). A suicidal fit may stop a relationship from ending and, among women, the *ataque* represents a condoned, perhaps even expected, pattern of behaviour in response to stress (Oquendo *et al.* 1992). The family in turn may facilitate a reconciliation. The fit causes a major upheaval in the family, eliciting strong guilt feelings and a show of attention and affection toward the patient.

Among the Hispanic group, culturally sanctioned beliefs such as *espiritisimo* (Bird & Canino 1981) or *santeria* (Sandoval 1977) may influence both the experiences and interpretations of hallucinatory perceptions. Thus, cultural and spiritual beliefs appear to have an important role in the formation and the interpretation of perceptual experiences.

Psychiatric explanations

Oquendo *et al.* (1992) suggest a number of essential features along with a series of associated features as important for diagnosis.

Some cases may meet the diagnosis of adjustment reaction or brief reactive psychosis, whereas others may need to de differentiated from conversion or dissociative reactions. Drug-induced states need to be differentiated. Borderline personality disorders and factitious disorders need to be excluded.

Family disturbances along with life events may be clear precipitants of this condition.

Management

In some cases, following the rallying of the family, the symptoms may well disappear, whereas others may need family work. Taking complaints seriously but within the context of the culture is a major step forward for the clinician. As Oquendo *et al.* (1992) propose, the use of diagnostic criteria would facilitate understanding of the symptoms and a reliable recognition would have important therapeutic implications.

SUSTO

The word 'susto' means 'fright' or some loss and represents a disorder among Latinos in the US, Mexico and Central and South America. The main worry is related to fear.

Definition

Susto is attributed to a 'frightening event that causes the soul to leave the body and results in unhappiness and sickness' (DSM-IV, p. 848) or social withdrawal. It is believed that sudden fright will cause the soul to leave the body, thereby making the body vulnerable to a variety of symptoms. Such feelings may last for years after the initial fright. Such a fright may result from an animal, accident, violent events, or being left in an unfamiliar place. The core symptoms include lack of appetite (or excess appetite), too much (or too little) sleep, feeling low, poor motivation, and low self-worth, and somatic symptoms of muscle aches, pains, headache, stomach ache and diarrhoea may occur. Diagnosis may be confirmed by family or friends and especially by a traditional healer in order to identify the cause of the fright.

Epidemiological data

Rubel *et al.* (1984) studied a sample of 38 Chinantec, 26 Zapotec and 36 Mestizo individuals. All individuals had presented with illness and had sought medical assistance. One half of the sample attributed their illness to *susto*. A clear correlation between social stress and the reported experience of the illness was observed (see below).

The indication in general in their findings was that organic disease can be implicated in the *susto* illness—although the type and the exact relationship are not clear in the study.

Folk explanations

In both Latino and American Indian explanatory terms, the separation of the human spiritual components from its body is understood to result from a frightening experience. Spanish people will use the word *susto* to describe a folk illness caused by fright (Rubel *et al.* 1985).

The folk interpretation of this condition, especially if it is seen as a health problem, is that there is a distinction between spiritual and organic components and that the former can be detached from the latter. Rubel *et al.* (1985) suggest that two conditions can lead to the detachment, one relating to unsettling experiences which disturb the normally existing equilibrium assumed to exist within a healthy organism, and the second resulting from the spirit beings or forces associated with features of the natural environment which may well seize and control the detached spirit. The spiritual element may be a unitary indivisible substance or a conglomerate of units with hierarchial functions. Various synonyms are used to describe the same basic experience which Simons and Hughes (1985) place under the fright illness taxon.

Psychiatric explanations

In the study mentioned earlier, Rubel *et al.* (1985) suggested that in their sample social inadequacy was an important feature. Rubel (1964) had integrated the interplay between one's social role performance, biological state of health, and personality system. Recognizing factors in the social system was seen as essential for understanding this disorder. Their findings did not find any equation with anaemia, cancer, rheumatism or any other disease, but 80% of their patient sample had infection with onchocerciasis. Mortality rates on follow-up were found to be high. However, more emotional difficulties were diagnosed in those suffering from the disorder than in controls. Hypoglycaemia has been put forward as a cause, with a proposal that *susto* should be seen as a syndrome of physically recognizable diseases (Bolton 1981).

Management

Susto needs to be differentiated from malingering and from underlying physical illness. If an underlying physical condition is discovered, it would need to be treated. A patient of *susto* can be managed with tranquilizers and supportive and family work. Holloway (1994) proposes that, under conditions of worsening health and the pressure to continue treatment, the 'best' solution for the victim appears to be 'to pull the victims out of the medical system', to desocialize him or her from semi-institutionalization, and to use social and informal structures for support to encourage the patient to start building his or her self-esteem, personal integrity and sense of control of his or her own life.

Overview

A brief introduction and description of six CBS suggests that CBS cannot be slotted into neat pigeonholes of anthropological or medical categories. It must be emphasized that although Tan (1981) equated CBS with psychiatric

Table 15.2 Culture-bound syndromes and their equivalents (Tan 1981).

CBS	Psychiatric diagnosis
Koro	Acute anxiety state
Spermatorrhoea syndrome	Hypochondriacal neurosis with sexual symptomatology
Spirit possession	Mostly psychotic states
Amok	Schizophrenia

diagnosis, it is not always possible to find conceptual equivalence (Table 15.2).

Hughes and Wintrob (1995) propose that widespread throughout the world are five basic categories of events or situations that, in folk aetiology, are believed to be responsible for illness: sorcery, breach of taboo, intrusion of a disease-producing object, intrusion of a disease-causing spirit, and loss of soul (Clements 1932). The discussion about cultural matrix of psychiatry, mental illness and its management is beyond the scope of this chapter. However, the role of CBS in Western psychiatric systems is beginning to be established with the introduction of the concept in DSM-IV categories.

Levine and Gaw (1995) divide the CBS into those which appear to be 'true syndromes' and those which are not, with the subclassification of the former categories as follows.

1 Dissociative phenomena
    (a) *Amok*
    (b) *Latah*
    (c) *Pibloktoq*
    (d) *Grisi sikris*
2 Anxiety state
    (a) *Ataque de nervios*
    (b) *Dhat*
    (c) *Koro*
    (d) *Kayak angst*
3 Affective/somatoform disorder
    (a) Brain fag
    (b) Anorexia nervosa
    (c) Chronic fatigue

4   Psychotic states
   (a) *Bouffée délirante*
   (b) *Qi-gong*
5   Illness of attribution
   (a) Induced by anger
   (b) Induced by fright
   (c) Induced by witchcraft
   (d) Induced by the 'evil eye'
   (e) Induced by perceived organic cause
   (f) Induced by possession
6   Idioms of distress

We propose that three basic categories of psychiatric classification can contribute to the classification of CBS that are likely to appear. These are shown in Fig. 15.1.

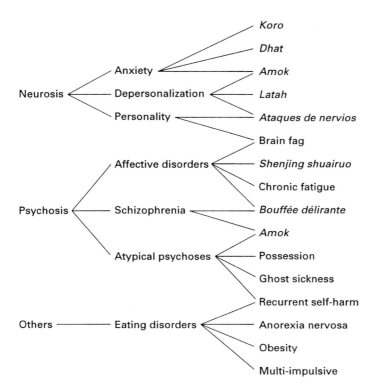

Fig. 15.1 Interaction between psychiatric diagnosis and culture-bound syndromes.

The understanding of CBS has been explained by Hahn (1985) as one of three alternative understandings. One is whether by being culture bound, these syndromes are excluded in other cultures. The second way of understanding maintains that all human events have cultural and natural and cognitive and psychodynamic aspects, although some may be more profoundly shaped than others. The third way asserts that all human conditions are equally natural and cultural and social, cognitive, psychosocial and psychodynamic, etc.

Jilek and Jilek-Aall (1985) argue that it is fallacious to classify human behaviour as either culture specific or universal. They go on to suggest that in order to understand CBS the clinicians and researchers alike have to look beyond individual psychodynamics and culture-specific traits, and it is useful to understand geopolitical, socio-economic and ideological circumstances of an ethnic group. It is important that the observer does not see and view CBS as an esoteric, exotic or cultural oddity but as a condition which needs to be understood in the context of a much broader canvas. Karp (1985) proposed that the term 'CBS' be dropped altogether but the disorder should be studied and understood in the context of the local meaning. Swartz (1985) proposed that CBS be seen as a constellation of symptoms which has been categorized as a dysfunction or disease and characterized by one or more of the following.

- It cannot be understood apart from its cultural and subcultural context.
- Its aetiology summarizes and symbolizes core meanings and behavioural norms of that culture.
- Its diagnosis relies on culture-specific technology as well as ideology.
- Its successful treatment is accomplished only by participation in that culture.

Corollaries of this observation are as follows.

- Symptoms may be recognized and simultaneously organized elsewhere but are not categorized as the same dysfunction or disease.
- Treatment judged as successful in one cultural context may not be understood as successful from another perspective.
- The fact that biomedicine does not include culture in its basic explanatory model leads to:
    (a) a failure to recognize CBS within Western cultures and within the biomedical system;
    (b) a redefinition of syndromes from other cultures into biomedical

terms so that potentially important cultural patterns (may) become irrelevant to diagnosis or treatment.

We firmly believe that the whole concept of CBS needs to be questioned and abandoned. As we noted from the six CBS we described, there is a lot of overlap in clinical features and diagnostic overlap. Having CBS as a separate taxonomic and nosological entity allows the traditions of exotic/esoteric/amusing/challenging 'savages' or 'the colonized' continue to highlight the supremacy of Western diagnostic systems without adding anything to our understanding. Instead, we should have cultural factors (at a broader level) in the aetiological axes of all psychiatric diagnoses and at global level inclusion of geopolitical and socio-economic factors. Getting away from a simplistic single diagnostic entity through to the multiaxial diagnostic systems and adding social and cultural factors that matter will enable the researcher and the clinician alike to understand the role of culture. It will also encourage treatment and management plans which are culturally appropriate and culturally sensitive. In addition, the role of culture in genesis, perpetuation and management will become useful. This will bring the folk and the scientific explanations of illnesses and illness behaviour closer together, thereby making psychiatry a clinical discipline better equipped to deal with patients and their carers in an appropriate and acceptable manner.

General principles of management

The importance of cultural issues in the management of individuals with psychiatric disorders is being increasingly acknowledged in literature (DSM-IV; Mezzich *et al.* 1996). The need for a cultural formulation which systematically reviews, from a cultural perspective, the individual's background, the explanations for the illness, psychosocial factors, and the patient–therapist relationship are highlighted. These formulations emphasize the role of cultural factors and their influence on diagnosis and management. The general principles in the management of these disorders are briefly mentioned.

A feature common to all mental disorders is the heterogeneity within categories. Individuals within the same diagnostic label seem to differ with regard to their response to treatment, course and outcome. In addition, the absence of category-specific treatment implies that most therapies are essentially symptomatic. Despite the lack of systematic investigations of CBS and their management, it would be prudent to assume that these disorders would behave similarly. This would suggest the need to use an eclectic approach to the managemnt of CBS which may have to be based on pragmatic considerations rather than on any theoretical constructs. Care would have to be tailored to meet individual needs.

The diagnosis would involve different approaches. Attempts will have to be made to identify the clinical syndrome. The explanatory models of the illness and the cultural context would have to be elicited. While psychiatrists are familiar with the recognition of the clinical syndromes, eliciting the explanatory models of the illness from the patient and relatives would require an understanding of the local culture. The approach suggested by Kleinman (1980) is very useful. Simple questions regarding the name of the illness, the nature of the problem, its cause, consequences, and its treatment usually elicit the emic explanations for the illness. This facilitates the use of cultural models in addition to those employed traditionally by psychiatrists (e.g. biomedical, cognitive, social, psychological, etc.). Adding cultural models to the existing eclectic practice increases the therapeutic armamentarium.

Pharmacological agents can also be employed. Anti-psychotic medication and anxiolytics can be used if the clinical presentation is one of psychotic proportions or if the individual presents with extreme anxiety. Antidepressant medication may prove useful in those individuals with persistent major depressive features. Such medication is helpful in reducing distress and in facilitating psychological treatment.

The first step in psychological intervention is the establishment of a relationship with the patient. This would require a knowledge of the local culture and an empathic understanding of the issues involved. The elicitation of the patient's explanatory model of the illness and his or her expectation of treatment would give insights into the emic understanding of the problem. These explanations would have to be employed in therapy. The gap between reality and patients' expectations will have to be assessed. Large gaps suggest greater need for psychological assistance. The process would involve abreaction, support, reassurance, and the provision of alternative culturally acceptable explanations for the illness, and other principles of brief psychotherapies are useful. While the individuals with milder forms of these disorders respond rapidly, the help of local experts may be necessary for the more resistant conditions.

Conclusions

A culture-bound syndrome is an expression of complex processes. Undoubtedly, when fully developed, the response of the culture or the society has to be seen in the context of the individual's biopsychosocial circumstances. The universal spread of technical civilization and of the scientific medicine pertaining to it has caused the disappearance of well-defined syndromes previously thought to be specific to a certain culture (Pfeiffer 1982). This process of globalization often indicates that individual cultural forms are ignored, to be blindly replaced by totally inappropriate methods of intervention.

Culture-bound syndromes have been useful in highlighting the role of culture in defining illness behaviour and pathways into care. Idioms of distress have been identified and clearly defined categories have emerged over the past two centuries. However, their subdivisions and classifications have added little except to exoticize the conditions, their sufferers, their carers, and sometimes society at large. It becomes clear that anthropologists and clinicians have looked at these categories from opposite ends of the spectrum, following relativist or universalist positions in which the individuality of the patient has often been lost. The diagnostic categories often have an overlapping area which cannot be defined very clearly. The psychiatric diagnostic categories have not been much help in creating clear nosological entities. Abandoning such fruitless pursuits of exotic disease hunting is the best way forward, and combining the role of specific culture in the diagnostic axes will allow this role to be recognized and used in an appropriate style to encourage understanding of the folk models of illness.

References

Agarwal, A. (1970) Treatment of impotence. *Indian Journal of Psychiatry* 2, 88–96.

Akhtar, S. (1988) Four culture-bound psychiatric syndromes in India. *International Journal of Social Psychiatry* 34, 70–74.

American Psychiatric Association (1994) *Diagnostic and Statistical Manual of Mental Disorders*, 4th edn (DSM-IV). American Psychiatric Association, Washington, D.C.

Arieti, S. & Meth, J. (1959) Rare, unclassifiable, collective and exotic syndromes. In: *American Handbook of Psychiatry* (ed. S. Arieti). Basic, New York.

Bernstein, R. & Gaw, A. (1990) Proposed classification for the DSM-IV. *American Journal of Psychiatry* 147, 1670–1674.

Bhatia, M. & Malik, S. (1991) Dhat syndrome. *British Journal of Psychiatry* 159, 691–695.

Bhugra, D. (1992) Psychiatry in ancient Indian texts. *History of Psychiatry* 3, 167–186.

Bhugra, D. & Buchanan, A. (1989) Impotence in ancient Indian texts. *Sexual and Marital Therapy* 7, 87–92.

Bhugra, D. & de Silva, P. (1993) Sexual dysfunction across cultures. *International Review of Psychiatry* 5, 243–252.

Bird, H. & Canino, F. (1981) The sociopsychiatry of Espiritisimo. *Journal of the American Academy of Child Psychiatry* 20, 725–740.

Bolton, R. (1981) Susto, hostility and hypoglycaemia. *Ethnology* 20, 201–276.

Bottéro, A. (1991) Consumption by semen loss in India and elsewhere. *Culture, Medicine and Psychiatry* 15, 303–320.

Bradlow, E. (1991) Mental illness or a form of resistance? The case of Spera Brotto. *Transcultural Psychiatric Research Review* 28, 219–229.

Burton-Bradley, B.G. (1968) The Amok syndrome in Papua New Guinea. *Medical Journal of Australia* i, 252–256.

Carr, J.E. (1985) Ethno-behaviourism and the culture-bound syndrome: The case of amok. In: *The Culture-bound Syndromes: Folk Illnesses of Psychiatric and Anthropological Interest* (eds R.C. Simons & C.C. Hughes), pp. 199–224. Reidel, Dordrecht.

Carr, J. & Tan, E. (1976) In search of the true amok: Amok as viewed within the Malay culture. *American Journal of Psychiatry* 133, 1295–1299.

Carstairs, G. (1957) *The Twice-born*. Haworth Press, New York.

Chiu, T., Tong, T.E. & Schmidt, K. (1972) A clinical survey of latah in Sarawak, Malaysia. *Psychological Medicine* 2, 155–165.

Chowdhury, A., Pal, P., Chatterjee, A., Roy, M. & Das Choudhury, P.O.B. (1988) Analysis of North Bengal koro epidemic with 3-years follow-up. *Indian Journal of Psychiatry* 30, 69–72.

Chowdhury, A.N. (1989a) Penile perception of koro patients. *Acta Psychiatrica Scandinavica* 80, 183–190.

Chowdhury, A.N. (1989b) Dysmorphic penis image perception: The root of koro vulnerability. *Acta Psychiatrica Scandinavica* 80, 518–520.

Clare, A. (1979) *Psychiatry in Dissent*. Tavistock, London.

Clements, F.E. (1932) Primitive concepts of disease. In: *Publications in American Archaeology and Ethnology*, Vol. 32, pp. 185–252. University of California Press, Berkeley, Calif.

Collinder, B. (1949) *The Lapps*. Greenwood Press, New York.

Czaplicka, M.A. (1914) *Aboriginal Siberia*. Clarendon, Oxford.

De Silva, P. & Dissanayake, S. (1989) The loss of semen syndrome in Sri Lanka. *Sexual and Marital Therapy* 4, 195–204.

Devereux, G. (1956) Normal and abnormal. In: *Some Uses of Anthropology* (eds J.B. Casagrande & T. Gladwin). Anthropological Society of Washington, Washington, D.C.

Dewaraja, R. & Sesaki, Y. (1991) Semen loss syndrome: A comparison between Sri Lanka and Japan. *American Journal of Psychotherapy* 45, 14–20.

Dutta, D. (1983) Koro epidemic in Assam. *British Journal of Psychiatry* 143, 309–310.

Fabrega, H. (1982) Culture and psychiatric illness. In: *Cultural Conceptions of Mental Health and Therapy* (eds A.J. Marsella & G.M. White). Reidel, Dordrecht.

Fabrega, H. (1989) Cultural relativism and psychiatric illness. *Journal of Nervous and Mental Disease* 177, 415–425.

Faergeman, P. (1963) *Psychogenic Psychoses*. Butterworth, London.

Friedmann, C.T.H. (1982) The so-called hystero-psychoses: Latah, windigo and pibloktoq. In: *Extraordinary Disorders of Human Behaviour* (eds C.T.H. Friedmann & R.A. Faguet), pp. 215–228. Plenum, New York.

Garrison, V. (1977) The Puerto-Rican syndrome in psychiatry and espiritisimo. In: *Case Studies in Spirit Possession* (eds V. Crapanzano & V. Garrison). Wiley, New York.

Grace, W.J. (1959) Ataque. *N.Y. Medicine* 15, 12–13.

Guarnaccia, P.J., Delacancela, V. & Carillo, E. (1989) The multiple meanings of ataque de nervios in the Latino community. *Medical Anthropology* 2, 47–62.

Gullick, J.M. (1958) Indigenous political systems in Western Malaysia. *LSE Monographs on Social Anthropology*, No. 17.

Gupta, P., Bannerjee, G. & Nandi, D.N. (1989) Modified Masters and Johnson technique in the treatment of sexual inadequacy in males. *Indian Journal of Psychiatry* 31, 63–69.

Gwee, A.L. (1963) Koro: A cultural disease. *Singapore Medical Journal* 4, 119–122.

Gwee, A.L. (1968) Koro: Its origin and nature as a disease. *Singapore Medical Journal* 9, 3–5.

Hahn, R.A. (1985) Culture-bound syndromes unbound. *Social Science and Medicine* 21, 165–171.

Hirsch, S.R. & Shepherd, M. (eds) (1974) *Themes and Variations in European Psychiatry*. Wright, Bristol.

Holloway, G. (1994) Susto and the career path of the victim of an individual accident: A sociological case study. *Social Science and Medicine* 38, 989–997.

Hughes, C.C. (1985a) Glossary of 'culture-bound' or folk psychiatric syndromes. In: *The Culture-bound Syndromes: Folk Illnesses of Psychiatric and Anthropological Interest* (eds R.C. Simons & C.C. Hughes), pp. 469–505. Reidel, Dordrecht.

Hughes, C.C. (1985b) Culture bound or construct bound. In: *The Culture-bound Syndromes: Folk Illnesses of Psychiatric and Anthropological Interest* (eds R.C. Simons & C.C. Hughes), pp. 3–24. Reidel, Dordrecht.

Hughes, C.C. (1989) Commentary on Fabrega and cultural relativism. *Journal of Nervous and Mental Disease* 177, 426–430.

Hughes, C. & Wintrob, R.M. (1995) Culture-bound syndromes and the cultural context of clinical psychiatry. In: *Review of Psychiatry*, Vol. 14 (eds J.M. Oldham & M. Riba), pp. 565–597. American Psychiatric Association, Washington, D.C.

Ilechukwu, S. (1992) Magical penis loss in Nigeria: Report of a recent epidemic of a korolike syndrome. *Transcultural Psychiatric Research Review* 29, 91–108.

Jilek, W. & Jilek-Aall, L. (1985) The metamorphosis of culture-bound syndromes. *Social Science and Medicine* 21, 205–210.

Karp, I. (1985) Deconstructing culture-bound syndromes. *Social Science and Medicine* 21, 221–228.

Kenny, M. (1985) Paradox lost: The latah problem revisited. In: *The Culture-bound Syndromes: Folk Illnesses of Psychiatric and Anthropological Interest* (eds R.C. Simons & C.C. Hughes), pp. 63–76. Reidel, Dordrecht.

Kiev, A. (1972) *Transcultural Psychiatry*. Penguin, Harmondsworth.

Kleinman, A. (1980) *Illness and Disease in the Context of Culture*. University of California Press, Berkeley, Calif.

Kodagoda, N. (1978) Some psychosexual problems of Asian adolescents. *Journal of Biosocial Sciences* (Suppl. 5), 227–233.

Kulanayagam, R. (1979) Semen-losing syndrome. *Journal of the Psychiatric Association of Thailand* 24, 152–158.

Langners, L.L. (1967) Hysterical psychosis: The cross-cultural evidence. *American Journal of Psychiatry* 124, 143–152.

Levine, R. & Gaw, A. (1995) Culture-bound syndromes. *Psychiatric Clinics of North America* 18, 523–536.

Malhotra, H.L. & Wig, N.N. (1975) Dhat syndrome: A culture-bound sex neurosis of the Orient. *Archives of Sexual Behaviour* 4, 519–528.

Mezzich, J.E., Kleinman, A., Fabrega, H. & Parron, D. (1996) *Culture and Psychiatric Diagnosis*. American Psychiatric Association Press, Washington, D.C.

Mun, C. (1968) Epidemic Koro in Singapore. *British Medical Journal* 1, 640–641.

Murphy, H.B.M. (1973) History and the evolution of syndromes: The striking case of latah and amok. In: *Psychopathology* (eds M. Hammer, K. Salzinger & S. Sutton). John Wiley, New York.

Murphy, H.B.M. (1976) Notes for a theory of latah. In: *Culture-bound Syndromes* (ed. W. Lebra), pp. 3–21. University of Hawaii Press, Honolulu.

Nakagawa, H. (1973) Imu of the Ainu. Cited in: *The Culture-bound Syndromes: Folk Illnesses of Psychiatric and Anthropological Interest* (eds R.C. Simons & C.C. Hughes), p. 62. Reidel, Dordrecht.

Ngui, P.W. (1969) Koro epidemic in Singapore. *Australia and New Zealand Journal of Psychiatry* 3, 263–266.

Oquendo, M., Horwath, E. & Martinez, A. (1992) Ataque de nervios: Proposed diagnostic criteria for a culture-specific syndrome. *Culture, Medicine and Psychiatry* 16, 367–376.

Paris, J. (1992) Dhat: The semen-loss anxiety syndrome. *Transcultural Psychiatric Research Review* 29, 109–118.

Pfeiffer, W.M. (1982) Culture-bound syndrome. In: *Culture and Psychopathology* (ed. I. Al-Issa), pp. 201–218. University Park Press, Baltimore, Md.

Prince, R. (1992) Koro and the fox-spirit on Hainan island (China). *Transcultural Psychiatric Research Review* 29, 119–132.

Prince, R. & Tcheng-Laroche, F. (1987) Culture-bound syndromes and international disease classification. *Culture, Medicine and Psychiatry* 11, 3–19.

Rin, H. (1963) Koro: A consideration on Chinese concept of illness and case illustrations. *Transcultural Psychiatric Research Review* 15, 23–30.

Rin, H. (1965) A study of the aetiology of koro in respect to the Chinese concept of illness. *International Journal of Social Psychiatry* 11, 7–13.

Ritenbaugh, C. (1982) Obesity as a culture bound syndrome. *Culture, Medicine and Psychiatry* 6, 347–361.

Rothenburg, A. (1964) Puerto Rico and aggression. *American Journal of Psychiatry* 120, 962–970.

Rubel, A. (1964) The epidemiology of a folk illness: Susto in Hispanic America. *Ethnology* 3, 268–283.

Rubel, A., O'Neill, C. & Collado, R. (1984) *Susto: A Folk Illness.* University of California Press, Berkeley, Calif.

Rubel, A., O'Neill, C. & Collado, R. (1985) The folk illness called susto. In: *The Culture-bound Syndromes: Folk Illnesses of Psychiatric and Anthropological Interest* (eds R.C. Simons & C.C. Hughes), pp. 333–350. Reidel, Dordrecht.

Rubin, R.T. (1982) Koro (shook yang): A culture-bound psychogenic syndrome. In: *Extraordinary Disorders of Human Behaviour* (eds C.T. Friedmann & R. Faguet), pp. 155–172. Plenum, New York.

Sandoval, M. (1977) Afro-cuban concepts of disease and its treatment in Miami. *Journal of Operational Psychiatry* 8, 52–63.

Simons, R.C. (1985a) The resolution of the latah paradox. In: *The Culture-bound Syndromes: Folk Illnesses of Psychiatric and Anthropological Interest* (eds R.C. Simons & C.C. Hughes), pp. 43–62. Reidel, Dordrecht.

Simons, R.C. (1985b) The startle matching taxon. Introduction in: *The Culture-bound Syndromes: Folk Illnesses of Psychiatric and Anthropological Interest* (eds R.C. Simons & C.C. Hughes), pp. 41–42. Reidel, Dordrecht.

Simons, R.C. (1985c) Sorting the culture-bound syndromes. In: *The Culture-bound Syndromes: Folk Illnesses of Psychiatric and Anthropological Interest* (eds R.C. Simons & C.C. Hughes), pp. 25–38. Reidel, Dordrecht.

Simons, R.C. (1985d) Latah II: Problems with a purely symbolic interpretation. In: *The Culture-bound Syndromes: Folk Illnesses of Psychiatric and Anthropological Interest* (eds R.C. Simons & C.C. Hughes), pp. 77–89. Reidel, Dordrecht.

Simons, R.C. (1987) A feasible and timely enterprise: Commentary on 'Culture-bound syndromes and international disease classification' by Raymond Prince and Françoise Tcheng-Laroche. *Culture, Medicine and Psychiatry* 11, 21–28.

Simons, R.C. & Hughes, C.C. (eds) (1985) *The Culture-bound Syndromes: Folk Illnesses of Psychiatric and Anthropological Interest.* Reidel, Dordrecht.

Singh, K. (1985) Dhat syndrome revisited. *Indian Journal of Psychiatry* 27, 119–122.

Skultans, V. (1993) The case of cross-cultural psychiatry: Squaring the circle? *International Review of Psychiatry* 5, 125–128.

Spitzer, R., Endicott, J. & Robins, E. (1978) Research diagnostic criteria: Rationale and reliability. *Archives of General Psychiatry* 35, 773–782.

Suwanlert, S. & Coates, D. (1979) Epidemic koro in Thailand: Clinical and social aspects. *Transcultural Psychiatric Research Review* 16, 61–64.

Swartz, L. (1985) Anorexia nervosa as a culture-bound syndrome. *Social Science and Medicine* 20, 725–730.

Tan, E.S. (1981) Culture-bound syndrome among overseas Chinese. In: *Normal and Abnormal Behaviour in Chinese Culture* (eds A. Kleinman & Y. Lin), pp. 371–386. Reidel, Dordrecht.

Trautman, E.C. (1961) The suicidal fit. *Archives of General Psychiatry* 5, 98–105.

Tseng, W.S., Kan-Ming, M., Hsu, J. *et al.* (1988) A socio-cultural study of koro epidemics in Guangdong, China. *American Journal of Psychiatry* 145, 1538–1543.

Van Loon, F.H.G. (1927) Amok and latah. *Journal of Abnormal and Social Psychology* 21, 434–444.

Westermeyer, J. (1982) Amok. In: *Extraordinary Disorders of Human Behaviour* (eds C.T. Friedmann & R.A. Faguet), pp. 173–190. Plenum, New York.

Westermeyer, J. (1985) Sudden mass assault with grenade: An epidemic amok form from Laos. In: *The Culture-bound Syndromes: Folk Illnesses of Psychiatric and Anthropological Interest* (eds R.C. Simons & C.C. Hughes), pp. 225–235. Reidel, Dordrecht.

World Health Organization (1992) *The ICD-10 Classification of Mental and Behavioural Disorders. Clinical Descriptions and Diagnostic Guidelines.* World Health Organization, Geneva.

Yap, P.M. (1951) Mental diseases peculiar to certain cultures: A survey of comparative psychiatry. *Journal of the Mental Sciences* 97, 515–564.

Yap, P.M. (1952) The latah reaction: Its psychodynamics and nosological position. *Journal of the Mental Sciences* 98, 515–564.

Yap, P.M. (1962) Words and things in comparative psychiatry, with special reference to exotic psychoses. *Acta Psychiatrica* 38, 157–182.

Yap, P.M. (1965) Koro: A culture-bound depersonalisation syndrome. *British Journal of Psychiatry* 111, 46–50.

Yap, P.M. (1969) The culture-bound syndromes. In: *Mental Health Research in Asia and the Pacific* (eds W. Caudill & T.Y. Lin), pp. 33–53. East–West Center Press, Honolulu, Hawaii.

Yap, P.M. (1974) Nosological aspects of the culture-bound syndromes. In: *Comparative Psychiatry: A Theoretical Framework* (eds M.P. Lau & A.B. Stokes), pp. 84–110. University of Toronto Press, Toronto.

CHAPTER 16

Conclusions

DINESH BHUGRA AND
ALISTAIR MUNRO

Introduction

The aim of the clinical diagnosis cannot be underestimated. Irrespective of the problems of using labels of diagnosis, it is essential that the clinician and the patient know what condition is being dealt with and the exact process involved in it. On the other hand, the researcher needs to know for the purposes of epidemiological enquiry as well as service planning. In the introductory chapter of this volume, we alluded to the problems and paradigms in reaching a diagnosis. This may include problems where the therapist–patient interaction across a divide is dictated by the respective power held by each participant and difficulties with the definitions of 'normal' and 'abnormal' across different cultures and societies.

The development of newer diagnostic systems such as DSM-IV (American Psychiatric Association (APA) 1994) and ICD-10 (World Health Organization (WHO) 1992) means that various cultural components are being taken into account. However, even though the diagnostic processes have been homogenized to some degree, it appears that there remain several significant areas of contention. We have made an attempt to cover some of these in this volume and they are to be seen as mere illustrations for some of the issues rather than a comprehensive overview on how to do it. The success of this project depends upon individual clinicians being aware of some of the problems in diagnosis, areas of diagnosis which are under-recognized and also undertreated. The reason for these processes remain in flux. The purpose of such a volume is to make clinicians aware of some of the underlying processes.

The past

The clinical diagnosis emerges from the stage at which a patient with a disorder presents to the clinician. This means that often clinical descriptions were just that—a detailed description of a general set of symptoms as evinced by the classical paper by Shepherd (1961) on morbid jealousy. Thus, the diagnosis was sometimes made by ignoring the underlying cause and sometimes by incorporating both aetiology and the cause of the illness. This stage in the history of psychiatry is not dissimilar to that period of history of medicine where underlying structural pathological changes were not known and the clinician simply made that diagnosis in syndromes. Advances in pathological techniques meant that structural dysfunction was identified which could be linked with impaired functioning and production of distress. Scadding (1967) argues that the diagnosis may not deal with actual process of disease but focus on a collection of a set of symptoms.

As noted earlier, if these biopsychosocial models of aetiology of mental disorder are to be followed, the aetiological as well as management factors in all three areas must be taken into account. Premorbid personality, past experiences, biological factors and social factors like unemployment, housing, social support, will all dictate the time and the method of presentation. The shift from the syndromes to more focused aetiological factors has been a gradual one simply because of the development of aetiological theories such as psychoanalytic models and behavioural models. With multiaxial approaches taking these factors into account it is obviously of essence that a simple medical approach to diagnosis is not followed.

The present

With the development of scanning and imaging techniques, it has become apparent that the underlying biological and biochemical changes are being identified more readily and the management of certain conditions has become more sophisticated and focused. With increasing knowledge of the function of neurotransmitters, newer drugs are beginning to be developed which target neurotransmitters selectively thereby reducing side-effects. The appearance of DSM-III (APA 1980) has been likened to the arrival of a breath of fresh air because of its focus on operational definition, multiaxial format and innovative regrouping of categories (Wig 1994).

The clinical problems which have sometimes defeated diagnosticians and researchers alike have been conditions such as acute psychosis, reactive psychosis, psychogenic psychoses, or personality disorders and have to be studied in the specific social and cultural contexts of this existence. In recent years, only the concept of explanatory models has been advocated and developed further. Fabrega (1994) proposes that the existing tenets regarding mineral classification of psychiatric diagnosis suggest that all persons do not have enormous variations in the light of genetic structures, cultural characteristics and historical circumstances and secondly, that all persons are vulnerable to developing a finite common set of behavioural manifestations of disorders that are in the process of being identified by the clinical branch of psychiatry. The demonstration of difficulties in using DSM-IV and ICD-10 have been illustrated in some of the preceding chapters. The argument and debate between the relativists and universalists is beyond the scope of this discussion (see Skultans 1993 for a brief overview).

The future

Atypical conditions or under-recognized clinical conditions need to be seen in the specific context of culture and society at a macro-level and individual patients and their clinicians at a micro-level. Fabrega (1994) suggested that the previous correctionist agenda, anchored in an awareness that the psychiatric disorders were rooted in the social problems and also impacted on them, had several problems—the foremost being the growth of the scientific appreciation of psychiatric disorders was delayed. The interactions between biology, psychology and social factors and behaviours remains in itself a culture-bound syndrome.

CLINICAL

A major step forward in improving the diagnostic method and not losing the purpose of diagnosis has to be an awareness of description of what Fabrega (1994) has called human behavioural breakdown (HBB), which includes virtually all psychiatric categories in its rubric. The sense of the universalist approach to psychiatry needs to be abandoned with a clear mandate for a more focused and individualist approach and clearly defined guidelines which allow both the clinician and the patient to come to some degree of agreement and lead on from the therapeutic encounter. The conditions which have been highlighted in this volume are from a Western perspective as is most of psychiatry and the rarity and the atypicality of this conditions should be seen in that particular context. These conditions are for the clinician's consciousness so that they are recognized and dealt with and the patient does not suffer unnecessarily.

RESEARCH

Wig (1996) has recently argued that a lot of 'minor' emotional disturbances such as jealousy should be taken out of psychiatric nosology, failing which he urges that other emotional conditions such as anger and tearfulness be included in the psychiatric diagnostic categories. In a way, the researchers have the luxury of being very selective in their case recruitment and are more likely to use operational criteria in the process. Under the circumstances, clinical approaches often do not yield the same results as the research approaches do. Perhaps one way forward would be to have both narrow and broad criteria for inclusion in the research trials thereby making the generalizability and applicability easier.

References

American Psychiatric Association (1980) *Diagnostic and Statistical Manual of Mental Disorders*, 3rd edn (DSM-III). American Psychiatric Association, Washington, D.C.

American Psychiatric Association (1994) *Diagnostic and Statistical Manual of Mental Disorders*, 4th edn (DSM-IV). American Psychiatric Association, Washington, D.C.

Fabrega, H. (1994) Epilogue: A universal approach to psychiatric diagnosis. In: *Psychiatric Diagnosis: A World Perspective* (eds J.E. Mezzich, Y. Honda & M.C. Kastrup), pp. 317–329. Springer-Verlag, New York.

Scadding, J. (1967) Diagnosis: The clinican and the computer. *Lancet* ii, 877–882.

Shepherd, M. (1961) Morbid jealousy: Some clinical and social aspects of a psychiatric symptom. *Journal of Mental Sciences* 107, 607–653.

Skultans, V. (1993) The case of cross-cultural psychiatry: Squaring the circle? *International Review of Psychiatry* 5, 125–128.

Wig, N.N. (1994) An overview of cross-cultural and national issues in psychiatric classification. In: *Psychiatric Diagnosis: A World Perspective* (eds J.E. Mezzich, Y. Honda & M.C. Kastrup), pp. 3–10. Springer-Verlag, New York.

Wig, N.N. (1996) Psychiatry East and West. Paper presented at Regional Meeting of the Royal College of Psychiatrists, Nov. 28–Dec. 1, Hyderabad.

World Health Organization (1992) *The ICD-10 Classification of Mental and Behavioural Disorders. Clinical Descriptions and Diagnostic Guidelines*. World Health Organization, Geneva.

World Health Organization (1993) *The ICD-10 Classification of Mental and Behavioural Disorders. Diagnostic Criteria for Research*. World Health Organization, Geneva.

Index